Burkhart's View of the Shoulder

A COWBOY'S GUIDE TO ADVANCED
SHOULDER ARTHROSCOPY

Burkhart's View of the Shoulder

A COWBOY'S GUIDE TO ADVANCED SHOULDER ARTHROSCOPY

STEPHEN S. BURKHART, MD

The San Antonio Orthopaedic Group
San Antonio, Texas

IAN K. Y. LO, MD, FRCSC

Department of Surgery
University of Calgary
Calgary, Alberta

PAUL C. BRADY, MD

Orthopaedic Surgeon
Tennessee Orthopaedic Clinics
Knoxville, Tennessee

Illustrated by Nancy D. Place, MS, AMI

. Lippincott Williams & Wilkins
a Wolters Kluwer business
Philadelphia · Baltimore · New York · London
Buenos Aires · Hong Kong · Sydney · Tokyo

Acquisitions Editor: Robert Hurley
Managing Editor: Jenny Kim
Production Manager: Dave Murphy
Senior Manufacturing Manager: Benjamin Rivera
Marketing Manager: Sharon Zinner
Design Coordinator: Holly McLaughlin
Compositor: TechBooks
Printer: C&C

Library of Congress Cataloging-in-Publication Data
Burkhart, Stephen S., 1949–
    Burkhart's view of the shoulder : a cowboy's guide to advanced shoulder arthroscopy / Stephen S. Burkhart, Ian K. Y. Lo, Paul C. Brady ; illustrated by Nancy D. Place.
        p. ; cm.
    Includes bibliographical references and index.
    ISBN 0-7817-8000-4 (alk. paper)
    1. Shoulder joint—Endoscopic surgery.   2. Arthroscopy.   I. Lo, Ian K. Y.
    II. Brady, Paul C.   III. Title.   IV. Title: View of the shoulder.
    [DNLM: 1. Shoulder—surgery.   2. Arthroscopy—methods.
    WE 810 B959b 2006]
    RD557.5.B87 2006
    617.5′720597—dc22

                                                                              2005036674

Care has been taken to confirm the accuracy of the information presented and to describe generally accepted practices. However, the authors, editors, and publisher are not responsible for errors or omissions or for any consequences from application of the information in this book and make no warranty, expressed or implied, with respect to the currency, completeness, or accuracy of the contents of the publication. Application of this information in a particular situation remains the professional responsibility of the practitioner.

The authors, editors, and publisher have exerted every effort to ensure that drug selection and dosage set forth in this text are in accordance with current recommendations and practice at the time of publication. However, in view of ongoing research, changes in government regulations, and the constant flow of information relating to drug therapy and drug reactions, the reader is urged to check the package insert for each drug for any change in indications and dosage and for added warnings and precautions. This is particularly important when the recommended agent is a new or infrequently employed drug.

Some drugs and medical devices presented in this publication have Food and Drug Administration (FDA) clearance for limited use in restricted research settings. It is the responsibility of the health care provider to ascertain the FDA status of each drug or device planned for use in their clinical practice.

To purchase additional copies of this book, call our customer service department at (800) 638-3030 or fax orders to (301) 223-2320. International customers should call (301) 223-2300.

Visit Lippincott Williams & Wilkins on the Internet: at LWW.com. Lippincott Williams & Wilkins customer service representatives are available from 8:30 am to 6 pm, EST.

10 9 8 7 6 5

To Nora. Thanks for sharing the trail with me. Vaya con Dios.

S.S.B.

To my mentors of science, Graham King, Sandy Kirkley, and Cy Frank; to my mentors of shoulder surgery, Bob Litchfield, Bob Hollinshead, and Evan Flatow; to Dr. Burkhart, who taught me so much about shoulders and even more about life; and to my wonderful wife Elaine and our precious daughters, Katelyn, Madison, and Isabella, the loves of my life.

I.K.Y.L

For all her love and support I thank my wife Jennifer—you're the greatest. To my wonderful children (Meredith, Davis, Garrett, and baby on the way) who had to give up much "Daddy Time" for this endeavor—I say, "You rock, dudes." Thanks mostly to the master healer ... my Lord Jesus ... for giving me the privilege of helping the hurting and letting me learn from the best—Drs. David Martin, Gary Poehling, and of course Stephen S. Burkhart.

P.C.B.

Acknowledgments

The authors wish to thank Nancy Place for her magnificent artwork, her photoediting, and her total dedication to a project that consumed far too many of her weekends; Gina Ruelas for her tireless efforts in compiling, transcribing, and proofreading the manuscript; Bob Merrill for his technical video support; Jenny Kim for her work as managing editor; Mark Flanders for his work as video editor; and finally, Bob Hurley and Eileen Wolfberg at Lippincott Williams & Wilkins for believing in the cowboy code and for recognizing that sometimes the book that will make the most difference is the book that is the most different.

Stephen S. Burkhart, MD
Ian K. Lo, MD
Paul C. Brady, MD

Contents

Preface ix
Foreword xv, xvii
  James C. Esch and Stephen J. Snyder
Messages from the Fellows xix

PART I. THE BASIS OF COWBOYIN'
There Ain't a Horse That Can't Be Rode, There Ain't a Man That Can't Be Throwed

1 Visualization 3

2 Angle of Approach 7

3 Creating a Stable Construct 33

4 Understanding and Recognizing Pathology 53

5 The Tough Stuff: Massive Contracted Adhesed Rotator Cuff Tears, Subscapularis Tears, and Biceps Pathology 110

6 Exposing the Hidden Arthroscopic Landmarks 147

7 Insurmountable Problems— Bone Deficiency 156

8 Gaining Speed and Tricks of the Trade 169

9 Order of Steps 191

10 Rotator Cuff Tear Patterns: Repairing a Tear the Way It Ought to Be 193

11 Postoperative Rehabilitation 203

PART II. PLAYIN' WITH FIRE
A Cowboy's Guide to Cookin' (Workin' Smooth), Smokin' (Workin' Fast), and Brandin' (Leavin' Your Mark)

12 Operating Room Set-up 215

13 Instability 217
  A. Arthroscopic Bankart Repair 217
  B. Arthroscopic Latarjet Procedure 220
  C. Arthroscopic Treatment of Multidirectional Instability 220

D. Nonengaging Hill-Sachs Lesion 222
E. Open Latarjet Reconstruction 223
F. Posterior Bankart and SLAP Repair 226
G. Repair of a Bony Bankart Lesion 227
H. Repair of Reverse Humeral Avulsion of Glenohumeral Ligament (RHAGL) Lesion 230
I. Repair of Triple Labral Lesion 232
J. Arthroscopic Repair of Humeral Avulsion of Glenohumeral Ligament (HAGL) Lesion 234

14 SLAP Repair 236

15 Subacromial Procedures (Non-cuff) 239
  A. Arthroscopic Acromioplasty 239
  B. Arthroscopic Distal Clavicle Excision 241
  C. Coplaning of Distal Clavicle 242
  D. Os Acromiale Excision 243

16 Stiffness 245
  A. Capsular Release for Adhesive Capsulitis 245
  B. Capsular Release for Postoperative Stiffness after Rotator Cuff Repair 246
  C. Manipulation Under Anesthesia 247

17 Rotator Cuff 249
  A. Completion of a PASTA Lesion to a Full-Thickness Cuff Tear 249
  B. Coracoplasty with Nonretracted Subscapularis Tendon 250
  C. Double-Pulley Technique of Double-Row Repair 251
  D. Double-Row Rotator Cuff Repair 252
  E. L Shaped Tear Assessment 254
  F. Margin Convergence to Bone in a Reverse-L Tear 255
  G. Massive Adhesed Rotator Cuff Tear: Repair by Modified Double Interval Slide 257
  H. PASTA Repair: One Anchor Repair 261
  I. Repair of a Partial (Upper) Subscapularis Tendon Tear 263
  J. Repair of Bursal Sided Rotator Cuff Tear 265
  K. Repair of Complete Subscapularis Tendon Tear 266

L. Repair of Interstitial Rotator Cuff Tear 268

M. Reverse L-Shaped Tear: Evaluation and Repair 269

N. Small Bursal-Surface Crescent Tear with Single Lateral Row Fixation 269

O. The "Bubble" Sign: A Method of Detecting an Interstitial Rotator Cuff Tear 270

P. The "Triple Double" Technique of Rotator Cuff Footprint Reconstruction 271

Q. The Roller-Wringer Phenomenon 274

R. The "Shoestring" Technique of Knotless Lateral Row Fixation 274

S. Tuberoplasty: Arthroscopic Treatment of Greater Tuberosity Malunion 275

T. Margin Convergence to Bone: Double-Row Repair of a Small U-Shaped Tear 277

U. Double Interval Slide Technique 279

V. Routine Margin Convergence Technique 281

W. Double-Row Margin Convergence to Bone 282

X. Two Anchor Transtendon PASTA Repair via the Double-Pulley Technique 284

Y. Anterior Interval Slide in Continuity 286

Z. Anterior Interval Slide 287

18 Biceps 289

A. Arthroscopic-Assisted Biceps Tenodesis for Retracted Biceps Tendon Tear: The Cobra Procedure 289

B. Biceps Tenodesis without Supraspinatus Tendon Tear 291

C. Biceps Tenodesis with Torn Supraspinatus Tendon 293

19 Tricks and Tips 294

A. Arthroscopic Knot-Tying Using the Sixth Finger Knot Pusher 294

B. Anchor Removal from Glenoid Using OATS Harvester 297

C. Anchor Removal from Greater Tuberosity Using OATS Harvester 298

D. Arthroscopic Suprascapular Nerve Release at the Suprascapular Notch 298

E. Compaction Bone Grafting Using OATS Harvester 301

F. Exposing the Scapular Spine 302

G. Salvaging a Loose Anchor by the "Buddy Anchor" Technique 303

H. The "Suture Weave" Technique of Reloading an Anchor 304

I. Pull the Right One: How to Ensure That You Don't Unload a Suture Anchor 305

20. Assorted Conditions 306

A. Calcific Tendinitis 306

B. Minicapsular Plication in the Overhead Athlete 307

C. Stretching and Strengthening Exercises: Patient Education Video 308

21. The Future 309

A. BioForkLok Bankart Repair 309

B. FiberChain Plus Swivel-Lok Double-Row Rotator Cuff Repair 309

Index 311

Preface

I swore I would never write a book on shoulder arthroscopy. For those of you who heard me say this, I imagine that this book must come as a bit of a surprise.

The problem in writing a technical book is that the author must overcome two major obstacles. First of all, he or she must accept the fact that, for a rather extended time period, the book will dominate the author's life. Until the book is finished, the author will not sleep well; the author will seem distant and distracted during dinner conversation; and likely become a bit short-tempered from time to time. Secondly, in the case of a rapidly developing technical discipline such as shoulder arthroscopy, the book must be written over a fairly short time period so that it will not be out of date by the time it is printed. The challenge to the author is to produce a book that is timely yet timeless—an obviously impossible task that creates even further insomnia.

So why bother to write this book? First of all, I knew that I would have tremendous help with this daunting project from my outstanding former fellows, Dr. Ian Lo and Dr. Paul Brady, as well as from my immensely talented medical illustrator, Ms. Nancy Place. Furthermore, I never would have begun the book without Ian Lo's repetitive encouragement to write it, plus his promise to be a coauthor. As it turned out, Paul Brady's abundant skills at video editing were a perfect complement to round out our team. But I'm sure that the greatest incentive of all was the opportunity, finally, to consolidate my rather extensive collection of previously published concepts, ideas, and research in a single place. The way this research came about has a story of its own.

When I was first beginning to consider the possibility of arthroscopic rotator cuff repair, I firmly believed that if it were to be done, its technique would need to have a sound biomechanical basis to become accepted as a reasonable alternative to open repair. My previous training in mechanical engineering was quite useful in providing me the necessary background to devise a series of experiments designed to determine optimized rotator cuff repair constructs. These experiments were set up to identify the weak link in a standard repair, then to test new constructs and methods that would shift the weak link to a different component of the construct. I would then test new constructs to optimize the weak link, so that the weak link shifted to another component of the repair. This sequence of experimentation would continue until finally the weak link was shifted to the weakest biologic substrate (i.e., tendon). Obviously, the biologic tissue had an intrinsic mechanical strength over which I

had no control, so once we had isolated it as the weak link, we had optimized our repair construct.

After I had identified the optimized constructs, I set out to devise instrumentation to assemble these constructs arthroscopically, a task that is much like building a ship in a bottle. I began with very simple devices which we gradually expanded and refined, so that now we have a wide array of instrumentation and implants that assure a secure arthroscopic repair every time.

Obviously, I could never have done this work alone. Dr. Kiriacos (Kerry) Athanasiou was an invaluable and inspired collaborator on the basic research. As for the instrumentation, I was privileged to work with Don Grafton and his engineering team in developing most of the instruments and implants used in the surgical procedures described in this book. Reinhold Schmieding, president of Arthrex, gave me great support and assistance in the development of these procedure-specific devices.

Fortunately, I was not facing the open shoulder establishment alone. Two of the greatest visionaries in shoulder arthroscopy, Dr. Steve Snyder and Dr. Jim Esch, also became my best friends during the early years of shoulder arthroscopy. Over the years, we have come to be called "The Three Amigos," and the name has stuck. The value of having loyal friends united in a common cause cannot be overstated. Revolutions are never won by an individual.

One aspect of my work that deserves special mention as a true group effort is that of the disabled throwing shoulder. Dr. Craig Morgan, Dr. Ben Kibler, and I pooled our ideas and taught each other a great deal in the process. To a washed-up baseball player such as myself, this project was a lot of fun.

Another combined effort was my collaboration with Dr. Joe DeBeer of Cape Town, South Africa, on the consequences of bone loss in patients with anterior shoulder instability. It is a tribute to the state of our current communications systems that two researchers from opposite sides of the globe could combine and analyze their data to reach conclusions with important implications for patients and surgeons around the world.

Now, I'm sure you are wondering why we chose to call this book a "cowboy's guide" to shoulder arthroscopy. I'll confess that this was entirely my idea. I've often been called a cowboy, and I take that as a compliment. Where I grew up, in central Texas, there were two ways to do things: the easy way and the cowboy way. I was fortunate to grow up with role models who always tried to do the right thing, and who passed on pithy pearls of cowboy wisdom in their everyday speech. For example, it doesn't take a genius to figure out what the cowboy means when he says, "Never drink downstream from the herd." But it takes a genius to put it so succinctly.

The cowboy spirit has pervaded the personalities of those most responsible for the development of shoulder arthroscopy. It seems only fitting that each chapter should begin with a nugget of cowboy wisdom, paraphrased to the best of my memory from my childhood mentors.

So, here it is. We have tried to write a book that is different from all the rest—a book with a consolidated section on the principles that underlie successful operative shoulder arthroscopy, followed by an extensive section devoted to details, tricks, and technical tips on the latest arthroscopic techniques. Specifically, we tried to emphasize the surgical pearls (tricks and tips) that are most useful to surgeons, yet are rarely found in books.

This book serves to further a mission to which I have felt called from the very beginning. That mission has been to do all that I can to facilitate the development and teaching of shoulder arthroscopy so that it becomes the "new gold standard" for shoulder surgery around the world. In my opinion, that has already happened; however, because of the marked resistance of certain open shoulder surgeons to operative arthroscopy, I think that "piling on" is justified. I hope this text, with its liberal use of digital video, will accelerate the dissemination of the art, the science, and the technique of shoulder arthroscopy.

Finally, I have felt some urgency to finish this book. Over the past year, after treatment for recurrent prostate cancer, I have been acutely aware of my own mortality and of the precious frailty of life. I believe that God wants all of us to pass on any of our ideas that have merit and that have the potential to help our fellow man. I would like this book to serve as a tribute to the preservation of worthwhile ideas.

Philosophically, the ascendancy of shoulder arthroscopy is the only acceptable outcome. It is a significant medical advancement, and it is gratifying to be a part of that advancement. Two years ago, I tried to crystallize my thoughts on arthroscopy and arthroscopic surgeons for my Presidential Address to the Arthroscopy Association of North America. My sentiments have not changed. We're still a bunch of cowboys.

PRESIDENTIAL ADDRESS

Stephen S. Burkhart, MD
Presented at the 22nd Annual Meeting of the Arthroscopy Association of North America; Phoenix, Arizona; April 26, 2003.

The Arthroscopic Surgeon: Cowboy and Scientist

Ladies and gentlemen, members and guests: My heroes have always been cowboys. Growing up in a small Texas town, it's hard to imagine that they could have been anything else. To me, Roy Rogers was not an actor on the small screen. He was real; and he was exactly the type of man I wanted to be.

Now more than ever, people feel the need to know their history, to know where they came from. But they also need to know their mythology, to know who they are trying to be. Our history tells us who we are, and our myths tell us who we hope to be.

The West, with a capital W, became the mythical landscape of America's home-grown hero, the cowboy. This hero, of course, was not the real cowboy, but the mythical cowboy, the one that talked slow, rode fast, shot straight, and called every woman "Ma'am." This cowboy was generally dependable, but he could be brash and impetuous, and he was easily offended. And once he set out to do something, he was tenacious. Relentless. He simply would not give up.

When I attended my first meeting of the Arthroscopy Association of North America (AANA) in the early 1980s, I had a sensation that I had never experienced during all my years of medical training, a sensation that I had stumbled into the camp of a major group of cowboys. And that's a compliment.

This group of cowboys, assembled at the infancy of arthroscopic surgery, presented papers on arthroscopic ligament reconstruction of the knee in broad daylight, and discussed them in an open forum as if these procedures were okay to perform. And it didn't stop with the knee. These renegades had the audacity to discuss arthroscopic procedures of the shoulder and to predict that such procedures would someday become the standard of care for the shoulder. And they were so sure of themselves that they didn't care what any of the open surgery experts of the day thought.

I was so impressed by my first encounter with the Arthroscopy Association of North America that I immediately applied for membership. Unfortunately, the membership committee was less impressed by me than I was by the Association, and they deferred my application, advising me to reapply in a year. I was crushed. But like the rodeo bronc-riders I admired, I got back on that bucking horse and tried again, and the second time I was successful. Ironically, I am the first president of the Arthroscopy Association of North America who was not accepted to membership on his first application.

What does that mean? That I'm stubborn, tenacious, and bull-headed? That I'm an over-achiever? That I can't take a hint? Maybe it means a little bit of all those things. But maybe it means I'm a cowboy. After that first rejection, I could have ridden into the sunset and found another professional organization to which I could devote my time and energy. That would have been the easy way, but it wouldn't have been the cowboy way.

As a Texan, I have observed the cowboy way all my life. The hallmarks of the cowboy are tenacity and self-reliance.

These qualities are also the hallmarks of the surgeon. But as arthroscopic surgeons, we must recognize that the cowboy way did not survive, and we must discover how to avoid that same fate.

The great flaw of the cowboy was his lack of adaptability. Once the open range was fenced, he was reduced to a caretaker of cattle—cattle that were taken to market by railroads rather than by cattle drives. As time went on and the focus of transportation changed from the horse to the automobile, the cowboy became irrelevant. But his values never became irrelevant. Now, more than ever, we should be able to appreciate that "doing the right thing" will never be out of date.

As arthroscopic surgeons, we have had to be very adaptable, and that is where we have surpassed the cowboy. To accomplish this, we have had to take on the characteristics of an entirely different and ultimately adaptable type of human—the scientist.

Arthroscopy has become increasingly dependent upon technology, and we, as arthroscopists, have had to embrace technology. But that embrace has had to be selective, and we have been forced to scientifically choose the best technology for our purposes—technology not only for treating our patients but also for teaching the next generation of surgeons. In short, the arthroscopic surgeon has had to become a blend of cowboy and scientist, an "adaptable cowboy."

The history of surgery is a fascinating story of adaptation. Before the development of inhalation anesthesia, a surgeon's speed was the measure of his skill (1). Robert Liston, professor of surgery at University College of London in the 1830s and 1840s, was widely regarded as the world's best surgeon due to his speed in the operating room, where his practice consisted primarily of amputations. He routinely performed major amputations in less than 3 minutes. As a result, he attracted visiting surgeons from throughout Europe and the United States (2–4).

In his quest for speed, Liston sometimes amputated more than he intended. In one case, he performed an accidental orchiectomy along with amputation of the patient's leg. At times, he would injure observers who stood too close to the operating table. One of his leg amputations resulted in the demise of three people: a visiting surgeon died from a slash wound, the patient died of sepsis several days later, and Liston's assistant died from an overwhelming infection after he lost several of his fingers in the operation. But the speed that made Liston famous lost its significance when ether anesthesia became commonplace during his own career. Even so, he refused to use ether, publicly proclaiming that it offered no advantage to a surgeon who was fast. His failure to embrace this new technology assured his rapid retreat into obscurity. Liston did not adapt.

As a shoulder surgeon and a Texan, I'm proud to relate that the first surgical procedure in North America was a combined shoulder and chest surgery performed in Texas in 1535 by Cabeza de Vaca (5). The Spanish explorer had been shipwrecked off Galveston Island in 1528. He subsequently developed a reputation among the Indians as a healer, treating the sick and injured with herbs and poultices. He had been wandering across Texas for 7 years when the Jumano Indians brought to him a young brave who had been hit in his right shoulder by an arrow, and the arrowhead had lodged in the chest, superficial to the ribs.

"The point was aslant and troublesome to take out," Cabeza de Vaca later wrote. "I continued to cut, and putting in the point of the knife, at last with great difficulty I drew the head forth. With the bone of a deer, and by virtue of my calling, I made two stitches that threw the blood over me, and with hair from a skin I stanched the flow." The wound healed and the Indian recovered. After he finally made it back to Spain, Cabeza de Vaca wrote, "In consequence of this operation, they had many of their dances and festivities. This cure gave us control throughout the country." Cabeza de Vaca was adaptable—and very lucky.

Surgery on the Texas frontier progressed largely due to the efforts of Dr. Ferdinand Herff and Dr. George Cupples (5), the first surgeons in Texas. These men had very busy practices in San Antonio by the 1850s. They understood the importance of clean water in surgery, and actually boiled the water that was to be used for the operation, unlike many of their contemporaries. Furthermore, they used ether anesthesia, but they were acutely aware of its high flammability. For that reason, they performed most of their surgery outdoors under bright sunlight to avoid the fire danger posed by an indoor lantern. Naturally, they tried to operate on days when there was not much wind. These surgeons had results that were far better than those of their peers. In 1886, Dr. Cupples reported to the Texas State Medical Association's Committee on Surgery that his mortality rate for major surgery was only 16%; for minor surgery it was only 8%. Only 1 out of 12 people who had *minor* surgery died. Dr. Herff and Dr. Cupples were adaptable. And they were masters of spin.

As surgeons, it is imperative that we embrace new technology, but we must do so with a discerning eye. The technology must be scientifically proven. Too often, patients demand "the next best thing," and that creates an environment more conducive to marketing than to science.

At the beginning of the Great Depression, Dr. John Brinkley of Del Rio, Texas, was determined to give the people what they wanted. In 1931, when other Americans were standing in bread lines, Dr. Brinkley bought air time from a super-powered radio station across the Rio Grande in Ciudad Acuña, Mexico. For $750, he offered to restore a man's sexual energy by implanting goat testicles beneath the skin of his abdomen. There were many goats in the Del Rio area, and many gullible men listening to the radio. Before he died in 1942, Dr. Brinkley claimed that he had implanted 16,000 sets of goat testicles (5). Dr. John Brinkley had been guilty of what we must always strive to avoid: embracing a procedure or a technology for purely personal gain, regardless of its impact on patients. I should point out that Dr. Brinkley, although he lived and worked in South Texas, was not a cowboy. A cowboy does not compromise his ideals; he always does the right thing, regardless of personal consequences.

Dr. Red Duke, this year's Presidential Guest Speaker, has been a friend for a long time. We've gone on a yearly deer hunt on the Mexican border, along with other friends, for the past 20 years. This hunt is truly like an old-time Texas deer hunt, complete with tall tales and lively dinner conversation at the camp house. About 10 years ago, the conversation turned to occupational hazards of being a surgeon. Naturally, protection against HIV exposure was mentioned, and one doctor at the table expressed his concern about the fact that HIV infection was uniformly fatal, unlike any of the other occupational risks to which we were exposed. Red Duke, who has been a trauma surgeon his entire career, spoke up about the impossibility of avoiding contact with blood in his profession. Then, with his trademark cowboy drawl, he said, "The way I look at it, if you're livin', you're dyin'." The table became quiet. We all knew what he meant. He wasn't minimizing the danger of HIV infection. He was just putting things into perspective. A doctor, like a cowboy, does what is right, even if it has deadly consequences. And a doctor faces up to reality; he knows that death waits around the corner for all of us, sooner or later. Dr. Red Duke is a cowboy.

Let's leave the cowboy for now and move on to the scientist. The word science comes from the Latin word *scientia*, which means knowledge (6). Science differs from other types of knowledge in that scientific progress depends on new ideas expanding or replacing old ones. In contrast, great works of art produced today do not replace the masterpieces of the past. But with science, new discoveries expand the knowledge base on which technology, or applied science, can develop.

The science of medicine is unique in that it sometimes gets confused with the art of medicine. The art of medicine is a subtle blend of opinion and technique, and it is more easily manipulated by strong personalities into dogma than is the science of medicine. Manipulators of the art of medicine have done more to stifle the science of medicine than any government regulations. Their dogma, exempt from the rules of the scientific method, has done immeasurable harm by autocratically denying to the human race the benefits of the natural rate of scientific advancement. Often, this dogma is concealed within the legalistic language of standards of care or accepted medical practice. But it is there, and it is destructive to medical progress, and it has been destructive to the advancement of arthroscopic surgery. This is not the fault of the art of medicine, but the result of the devious manipulation of the art of medicine for personal gain.

At this point, you may be wondering if I am suggesting that all standards of medical practice be suspended; that the tablets of the medical rulemakers be broken. And the answer, of course, is no. All aspects of a civilized society must have rules. I am simply suggesting that medical advancement would be much more rapid and more meaningful if science were allowed to take precedence over dogma. Which is precisely why I treasure my relationship with the Arthroscopy Association of North America.

At its inception, this organization was criticized for being based on a specific technology—arthroscopy—which would some day become obsolete. Nothing could have been further from the truth. This organization was based on the hypothesis that minimally invasive surgery was better for patients than equivalent procedures done by open techniques. That hypothesis was submitted to scientific examination, and was freely discussed and debated at our meetings and in our journal. The organization, the science, and the technology have developed in accordance with the scientific validity of that hypothesis and its corollary hypotheses. To me, the Arthroscopy Association of North America has been the ultimate success story of the application of the scientific method to medicine. And the key to this success has been the principle of allowing science to dominate over dogma.

The history of scientific advancement is fascinating. The pioneering scientist must be, in large measure, a cowboy. Until a scientist's theories are confirmed by others, he must stand alone, much like the cowboy, with only his convictions to shield him from the criticism of his peers. Most of us would never consider Albert Einstein a cowboy, but an excerpt from the esteemed journal *Science*, in 1929, underscores the isolation that a scientific pioneer must be willing to face. "Albert Einstein announced January 20, 1929, that he has found a key to the formulation of a unified gravitational field theory—a group of equations applicable not only to gravitation but also to electromagnetics and subatomic phenomena. His six pages of equations, however, are unprovable, incomprehensible, ignore quantum mechanics, and are incorrect" (7). Einstein stood by his hypotheses and was vindicated when his equations were proved correct by the experiments and observations of his peers. But this did not happen overnight. And until it did, Einstein had to stand alone and exposed, with only his belief in himself and his ideas to comfort him.

Where do ideas come from? How can we explain the creative process? Albert Szent-Gyorgi, the 1937 Nobel Prize winner in medicine, said, "Discovery consists of seeing what everyone else has seen and thinking what no one else has thought" (8). This simple statement explains the spark that separates the creators of knowledge from the collectors of knowledge.

I have been privileged to know a handful of brilliant scientists and researchers in my life, people who have thought what no one else has thought. But I have not always recognized the implications that their work would have on my life and on my career. As a freshman engineering student at Rice University in 1969, I had no clue that

Dr. Robert Curl, the mild-mannered professor who taught my inorganic chemistry class, would win the Nobel Prize in chemistry 22 years later. I had no concept that his discovery of "bucky balls" (carbon-60 fullerenes which are one nanometer, or one billionth of a meter, in diameter, the first of the nanomaterials) would open up a whole new realm of nanotechnology that would have direct application to my future career in arthroscopic surgery.

Nanotechnology deals with "molecular machines," and it is very different from the top-down approach known as miniaturization. Nanotechnology devices are built from the bottom up, one molecule at a time (9). They may be powered by physical energy or by biochemical energy. Rotating molecular shafts with small knobs and dents to encode logic operations can function as molecular computers to regulate the release of arthroscopically implanted substances such as growth factor. Growth factor and other therapeutic compounds can be attached to nanomaterials such as the "bucky balls" that Dr. Curl discovered, so that they can be arthroscopically delivered to aid in biologic repair and regeneration of biologic tissues such as bone and articular cartilage.

In 1969, as I listened to Dr. Curl's chemistry lectures, I didn't dwell on the fact that history runs in both directions and that some things simply haven't happened yet. If I could have read the future, I would have seen 30 years forward, to a time when my good friend Dr. Kiriacos (Kerry) Athanasiou, this year's AANA Scientific Presidential Guest Speaker, would be conducting groundbreaking research on articular cartilage and polymer scaffolds in that very same building on the Rice University campus where Dr. Curl taught my freshman chemistry class. And I would have recognized the importance of that research, which could easily make Dr. Athanasiou a Nobel Prize candidate. Research that could change the way we do orthopaedic surgery. So you see, history runs in both directions, and time weaves it into a complete story.

As my year as President of AANA draws to a close, I am proud of what this organization has been able to accomplish, and I am honored to have been elected to preside over it for the past year. Our mission is education, and we have been able to reach more surgeons with our educational programs than ever before. We had record-breaking attendance this past year at the Fall Course and Specialty Day, and we routinely filled the hands-on cadaver courses at the Orthopaedic Learning Center (OLC) in Chicago. In August, we staged the first live remote interactive surgery transmission from San Antonio to an OLC course, using high-speed phone lines to transmit high-quality digital video images. This technology has created a highly effective teaching tool for us to use in training surgeons both here and abroad. These educational initiatives would not have been possible without the AANA members who have served as instructors, faculty, and committee members, as well as our industry partners.

On a personal level, I have many people to thank for a very successful year: the AANA staff in Chicago (Ed Goss, Holly Albert, Pam Beaumont, Donna Nikkel, and the rest of the staff); our Executive Vice President, Dr. Whit Ewing; the AANA Board of Directors; the AANA committee chairmen and committee members; the *Arthroscopy Journal* staff and editors, led by Editor-in-Chief Dr. Gary Poehling; the Journal Board of Trustees; the Education Committee and its chairman, Dr. Rick Ryu; my Program Chairman Dr. Don Johnson; the audiovisual team that has provided state-of-the-art digital presentations for all our meetings; my secretary Judy Collins; my nurse Mary Hatter; and my partners in The San Antonio Orthopaedic Group, two of whom (Dr. Brad Tolin and Dr. David Gonzalez) are here today.

As for my professional development, I am indebted to my two greatest role models: the late Dr. Mark Coventry of the Mayo Clinic, who demonstrated to me the true meaning of intellectual integrity; and Dr. John Hinchey, my late senior partner, who taught me the sanctity of our profession. I am grateful to Steve Snyder and Jim Esch for being both teachers and my best friends. And I want to thank Dr. Gary Poehling for publishing my early biomechanical concepts when they were considered too "edgy" for traditional orthopaedic journals. As for these biomechanical concepts, I am indebted to Kerry Athanasiou and Don Grafton for their input and contributions to the end result.

Family, of course, is always of paramount importance. My parents, Claude and Gene Burkhart, provided me with a classic small-town upbringing surrounded by real-life characters that were every bit as honest and straightshooting as Roy Rogers. Yet they encouraged me to reach beyond our sheltered environment, to sample the greater world outside of Taylor, Texas, and to believe that I might actually have some impact on that world. I regret that my mother Gene cannot be here today because she would be beaming at me from the audience, but I am happy that my dad Claude Burkhart was able to make the trip.

I am very proud that my son Zack and daughter Sarah are here today. Zack will graduate next month from Notre Dame, summa cum laude, and has been accepted to medical school. He is engaged to Jenny May and they will be married in December. Sarah is a freshman at Rice University, my alma mater, where she is excelling in the mechanical engineering curriculum. It has been a blessing to watch Zack and Sarah develop into such wonderful people. They started out as my biggest responsibility and have become my greatest accomplishment. They have enriched my life, and I am so proud of them.

That brings me to the most important influence in my life, my wife Nora. I'll share a very personal story with you, because it illustrates the great strength and direction that Nora has given me, particularly in the past year and a half.

In 2001, I was scheduled to go to Japan as a guest speaker at the annual meeting of the Japan Shoulder

Society. Nora and I were to leave on September 12, 2001. Needless to say, the events of September 11 caused our trip to be canceled. I found myself at home in San Antonio with a few days off work, so I decided to do something I'd never done before—go to the doctor for a check-up. After a battery of blood tests and routine referrals to specialists for long-overdue tests such as a cardiac evaluation and a stress test, I was feeling confident and quite smug about my apparent good health. The tests were confirming what I had always assumed, that I was healthy and that bad things only happened to other people. After all, I was a doctor, and doctors see themselves as invincible.

I was in California at an arthroscopy meeting when I received the call about my final test, a prostate biopsy. My urologist, not known for his tact, said, "You've got cancer. It's a big one and it may not be curable. I'm sending you to the Mayo Clinic for surgery."

I felt as if I had just been shot. I felt small, helpless, insignificant, and out of control. I spent the first of many sleepless nights.

Two months later, lying in my hospital bed after the surgery, I sustained another direct hit when my surgeon came to my room and explained that he had not been able to get clear margins completely around the tumor. I stared past him in disbelief. At first, I wanted to blame someone. Then, I illogically wanted to run out of the hospital, but with my spinal anesthetic still in effect, I couldn't move my legs. I was terrified. I felt empty and alone. Abandoned. That same day, when Nora was gone from my room, my friend Dr. Shawn O'Driscoll, an orthopaedic surgeon at the Mayo Clinic, dropped by, and I shared the news with him. The first thing he asked was, "Are you equipped spiritually to deal with this?" The question caught me totally off guard. I couldn't answer. I just began to cry.

Then Shawn reached out and held my hand and said, "Let's pray about it." And we did. And for the first time, I felt at peace.

When Nora returned to the room that evening, I told her the story, and I asked her to pray with me. Nora is a person of great faith, and has always prayed for me. She had been praying for me all along but due to my stubbornness and denial she had not been praying with me. But this was the point at which I put everything into God's hands, and we prayed together.

From that moment on, Nora was the rock that I relied on, that pulled me through. She taught me the meaning of faith, and the meaning of life. Without her, I couldn't have made it. But with her as my spiritual guide, I realized that the best thing that ever happened to me was to get cancer, because by facing death through faith I learned to appreciate life.

Nora, I thank you for sharing my life and restoring my faith. And I thank you for being the most entertaining person I have ever known. We have great fun together, and

life with you has been the greatest party I could ever have imagined.

The other positive viewpoint to emerge from my cancer experience was the notion that ideas are a continuum over time, a cement that connects one generation to the next. If our ideas are worthwhile, they can live on through our students long after we're gone. In the early days of arthroscopy, those of us involved in arthroscopic education were often ridiculed by the "experts" of the day. They openly stated that arthroscopy would not catch on, that its results would never be as good as open surgery, and that we were wasting our time. I tried to respectfully disagree with them, but their lack of approval bothered me. Even so, I was gratified by the response of the arthroscopic students that I taught.

Years later, I read the preface to Dr. E. A. Codman's classic book *The Shoulder* (10), and one passage from this great teacher stood out as particularly meaningful to me: *Through much of my life I have suffered somewhat from a sense of isolation, because I have always been thinking, or saying, one thing or another, with which other doctors did not agree. . . . My regrets are for wasting so much time on the opinions of a previous generation and not realizing that it was the approval of my pupils, rather than of my masters, that was desirable.*

Codman was a cowboy (even Bostonians can be cowboys), and Codman was a scientist of the first order. And his ideas set us on a trail of discovery that we hope will never end. As arthroscopic surgeons, we need to recognize our heritage as cowboys and scientists, so that we will always be adaptable cowboys. That will assure the survival of our discipline.

Arthroscopic surgery has come a long way in the past 20 years, but there's still so much to do. Although the history of arthroscopy has been very exciting, the future promises to be nothing short of breathtaking. So, ladies and gentlemen, cowgirls and cowboys, let's take a deep saddle and hold a loose rein, because we've got a long way to go.

Happy Trails

REFERENCES

1. Fenster JM. *Ether Day*. New York: Harper Collins, 2001.
2. Gordon R. *Great Medical Disasters*. New York: Stein and Day, 1983.
3. Thorwald J. *The Century of the Surgeon*. New York: Pantheon Books, 1957.
4. Buckwalter JA. Advancing the science and art of orthopaedics: Lessons from history. *J Bone Joint Surg Am* 2000;82:1782–1803.
5. Cox M. Frontier medicine: Texas doctors overcome disease and despair. *Texas Med* 2003;99:19–26.
6. Mish FC, ed. *The New Merriam-Webster Dictionary*. Springfield, MA: Merriam-Webster, 1989.
7. Trager J. *The People's Chronology*. New York: Henry Holt, 1994.
8. Holliman K. Orthopedic surgeons should become involved in research. *Orthop Today* 2002;22:17–18.
9. Reitman EA. *Molecular Engineering of Nanosystems*. New York: Springer-Verlag, 2001.
10. Codman EA. *The Shoulder*. Boston: Thomas Todd, 1934.

Foreword

This book by Stephen S. Burkhart, Ian K. Lo, and Paul C. Brady is a must read for any surgeon who wishes to be in the forefront of arthroscopic shoulder surgery. Dr. Burkhart brings his unique skills as a mechanical engineer, research scientist, arthroscopic surgeon, and Texas rancher to arthroscopic shoulder surgery. His creative discoveries on the suspension bridge, margin convergence, awning effect, stable force-couples, and loop-knot security have created a paradigm shift in rotator cuff surgery. Arthroscopic repair is now the preferred method of any shoulder surgeon who has taken the time to learn these techniques.

Drs. Burkhart, Lo, and Brady share their technical pearls that make our surgery easier and benefit our patients. The basic techniques of good visualization with appropriate portals using fluid control principles serve the beginning arthroscopic shoulder surgeon and are good reminders for the advanced surgeon. Finally, the chapters on bone loss in our patients with instability are their reminder to take another look at our patients with instability, especially our failures.

All of us are fortunate that Drs. Burkhart, Lo, and Brady have taken their time and effort to put down their ideas in words, drawings, and photographs that will make our surgery easier and benefit our patients. *Burkhart's View of the Shoulder: A Cowboy's Guide to Advanced Shoulder Arthroscopy* belongs next to your bed as you review your shoulder surgery for tomorrow.

James C. Esch, MD
Tri-City Orthopaedics
Oceanside, California

Foreword

It is a pleasure for me to write this foreword for *Burkhart's View of the Shoulder: A Cowboy's Guide to Advanced Shoulder Arthroscopy*, Dr. Stephen S. Burkhart's new book on the treatment of complex rotator cuff tendon pathology using the latest shoulder arthroscopic techniques. I have known Steve as a loyal friend and have respected and learned from him for almost 20 years. This book is yet another example of his dogged devotion to advancing the field of shoulder arthroscopy education for all of us in the field.

Dr. Burkhart is well known as a "thought" leader, an innovator, an exceptional surgeon, a zealous organizer, and a tireless teacher who generously devotes a great deal of time and effort to his favorite area of interest, that of shoulder arthroscopy. His enthusiasm is contagious. I have known him to mesmerize an entire room during a lecture on orthopaedic biomechanics, a generally soporific topic. Steve can skillfully imbue his audience with theories and facts that clarify complex topics such as fluid dynamics or fixation strength of suture anchors in bone. To solidify his lessons, he often uses clever, memorable vignettes that help his audience understand and retain the important points.

Steve draws on many of his talents to disseminate his messages. He sprinkles his lectures with colorful Texas humor, often portraying himself as a simple-thinking, straight-talking cowboy whose goal is to do an honest day's work and keep the bad guys in check. But believe me, Dr.

Burkhart is no simple thinker. His supercomputer genius never rests. His "free" time is consumed with creative writing of scientific works and novels as well as musical lyrics. He has a rare knack for solving difficult surgical problems by either altering and improving an existing technique or inventing new instruments and methods to facilitate the complicated task. It is this creative gift that sets Steve aside from most of us. Although he is gifted, he is humble, self-deprecating, and approachable, traits that make him all the more effective as a paradigm developer and educator.

Steve has been accompanied and supported throughout his professional life by his wife Nora and his children Zack and Sarah. Both children are following in Steve's footsteps. Zack is enrolled in medical school and Sarah is studying biomedical engineering. Nora is not only Steve's wife, but a true complementary partner and lifelong friend. She has traveled the world helping him to stay on course and add important balance to their lives. Recently, the Burkhart family has discovered a special site to spend some much deserved slow-down time. I suspect and hope that Steve will continue to solve problems with shoulder arthroscopy while at work as well as when relaxing with his family and friends at his beautiful "Cloud Nine" Ranch.

Stephen J. Snyder, MD
SCOI Shoulder Clinic
Van Nuys, California

Messages from the Fellows

To be selected from innumerable applicants to be a fellow under Dr. Burkhart is truly a life-changing experience. It is distinct from any other fellowship. It is a true one-on-one apprenticeship to learn from a pioneering master of shoulder arthroscopy. Although the knowledge gained in the theory, rationale, and technical aspects of shoulder disorders and shoulder arthroscopy are unsurpassed, it is the delivery of such information that is completely unique. Dr. Burkhart personifies what it means to be a Texas gentleman. We are eternally grateful to him, his wife Nora, and their wonderful family for providing us fortunate few with an experience like no other. The fellowship year is justifiably one of the greatest years of our lives, and we are honored and humbled to be considered fellows of Dr. Stephen S. Burkhart.

I am proud to have been Dr. Burkhart's first fellow and will forever thank him for taking a chance on me. In my opinion, he defines the term "renaissance man" and if he didn't invent "thinking outside the box," then he certainly fine-tuned it. I am eternally grateful for the experience.

Charles Pearce, MD
Fellow 1997–1998

I honestly didn't see much of the Hollywood-type "cowboy" in Dr. Stephen Burkhart, but I did see that he was, and continues to be, the intellectual "cowboy" of shoulder arthroscopy. Dr. Burkhart is known for taking on a herd of intellectual doubt and controversy regarding various topics in shoulder arthroscopy. With dedication, persistence, and intellect he routinely educates the orthopedic community about various shoulder arthroscopy issues and techniques. This approach leads surgeons to his "ranch of reason," where we can see shoulder-related problems and treatments through his eyes. And with quiet deference, as you would expect of a gentleman and a cowboy, he then lets us come to our own conclusions regarding what he has seen.

Dr. Burkhart often said "I'm no stranger to controversy." It is these simple few words that belie the intellect, passion, and strength of a man who continues to single-handedly reshape the field of shoulder arthroscopy. It is a distinct honor to have worked with such a distinguished cowboy. And I look forward to where he will lead us next.

Steven Danaceau, MD
Fellow 1998–1999

It is an honor to be a part of Steve's view of the shoulder. I owe so much of my success and happiness to him. He is a leader and visionary in many ways and on many levels. People do not care how much you know, until they know how much you care. Thanks for everything, Steve.

Armin M. Tehrany, MD
Fellow 1999–2000

Not a day passes that I don't draw on clinical and surgical lessons learned from my time spent with Dr. Burkhart. He is a complete mentor: an unparalleled teacher, an innovative scientist, a gentleman, and, of course, a cowboy. I will always remain thankful for his guidance and expert instruction, as will my patients.

Peter Parten, MD
Fellow 2000–2001

To say that Dr. Burkhart has been at the frontier of shoulder arthroscopy over the last two decades is an understatement. He has literally defined and continues to redefine the field of arthroscopic shoulder surgery. When I first saw Dr. Burkhart in the operating room, I was in complete awe. Despite my residency training at a respected sport medicine center, I had never seen anyone evaluate or treat a shoulder arthroscopically in a similar fashion. It was a truly awe-inspiring and humbling experience. He remains light-years ahead of the rest of us. It has been an honor and privilege to be a fellow under Dr. Burkhart and hopefully in some small way contribute to his ongoing legacy. I wish to thank Dr. Burkhart, Nora, and their family for providing our family one of the best years of our lives (and a little Texan also).

Ian Lo, MD, FRCSC
Fellow 2001–2002

"How many subscaps have you repaired?" This was one of the first questions Dr. Burkhart asked me during my first case with him as a fellow. As it turned out, this was just the beginning of my arthroscopic shoulder experience, as I was continually introduced to newer and more advanced concepts. I feel fortunate to have been taught and trained by an innovative and progressive thinker that certainly has changed how future orthopaedic surgeons will deal with shoulder pathology. Not only has he been a great teacher, mentor, and example, he has been a genuine friend. As I mentioned to Dr. Burkhart on my last day of fellowship, my advanced shoulder experience in San Antonio was one of the greatest experiences of my life.

David P. Richards, MD, FRCSC
Fellow 2003–2004

Far from my wonderful country of France I took the challenge to visit one of the most famous shoulder arthroscopists of North America. I had the wonderful experience of spending 6 months with a unique surgeon-cowboy. He is not only a wonderful teacher but also a great man and human being who welcomed me as a son in his own family. I want to thank Dr. Burkhart for the wonderful time spent with him in the "West." I am now trying to spread all of the knowledge I learned with him in Grenoble and France.

Johannes Barth, MD
Research Fellow 2003–2004

I came to San Antonio to learn shoulder arthroscopy. Soon I figured out that I wasn't facing just a skilled surgeon but a man with the attitude to live every day and every case as a challenge. To optimize tomorrow what he was doing in that moment. His knowledge, skills, and overall approach to arthroscopy and life were an inspiration to me, and I went home knowing more about the difference between good surgeons and great men. I am honored to have worked with him. Thanks.

Paolo Arrigoni, MD
Research Fellow 2004

In residency I asked Dr Gary Poehling (my chairman) what he would to if he were just finishing his residency. Without hesitation he said, "I'd go work with Steve Burkhart—he's taking our field to the next level." After just a few days with Dr. Burkhart I realized the truth in that statement. Thank you, Dr. Burkhart, for sharing your knowledge and your gift with me.

Paul Brady, MD
Fellow 2004–2005

In 2005 I had an amazing opportunity to visit Dr. Burkhart for 6 months. I traveled from Rio de Janeiro, Brazil, to San Antonio, Texas. I was afraid because I didn't know what was waiting for me, but I knew Dr. Burkhart was a great teacher and doctor.

He has two wonderful attributes: he never loses his posture, and he shares his knowledge with his fellows.

I am very thankful for how you have opened my eyes to arthroscopic shoulder surgery.

Alexandre Alves Campos, MD
Research Fellow 2005

Thank you for taking on what you may now have realized to be one of your life's greatest challenges: teaching me how to approach and treat ailments of the shoulder. I appreciate your patience and generosity in sharing your wisdom. I am inspired by your love for your work and your dedication to helping your patients.

David P. Huberty, MD
Fellow 2005–2006

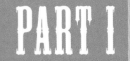

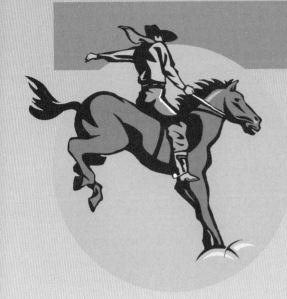

PART I

THE BASIS OF COWBOYIN'

There Ain't a Horse That Can't Be Rode,
There Ain't a Man That Can't Be Throwed

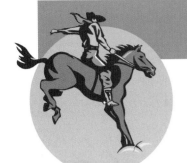

Visualization

COWBOY PRINCIPLE 1

A blind horse can see just as well from either end.

Surgeons on the Texas frontier recognized the need for clear visualization. To achieve that goal in the 1850s, Dr. George Cupples and Dr. Ferdinand Herff of San Antonio operated outdoors in bright sunlight. Not only did this technique afford them superior visualization, but it avoided the fire hazard of an indoor lantern in the presence of flammable ether anesthesia. These cowboy-surgeons not only developed ways to see well, they also displayed a great vision for the future. We would do well to follow their example.

How many times in the past, during open surgery, have you heard the old adage, "exposure is everything" or "you can't fix what you can't see." Complete, unobstructed visualization of the pathology at hand is essential in all types of surgery. This same principle should be religiously adhered to during arthroscopic surgery. Ignoring this principle is the number one reason why many potential arthroscopic surgeons cannot perform certain procedures effectively and efficiently. A major difference between open and arthroscopic surgery is that during arthroscopic surgery considerably more variables need to be considered in obtaining a complete, unobstructed field of view than during open surgery.

Bleeding during any surgery can inhibit visualization. During arthroscopic shoulder surgery, however, even a small capillary vessel can completely "red-out" a field of view. The amount of blood flow into the shoulder joint from this vessel is a balance between the patient's blood pressure, the intra-articular or subacromial pressure, and fluid flow.

To minimize potential bleeding in the shoulder, the first principle is to build a relationship with an understanding and accommodating anesthesiologist. Although this may be difficult in certain health care settings where the anesthesiologist can change on a daily basis, it is important for the anesthesiologist to appreciate the importance of maintaining the patient's blood pressure within a reasonable range. Assuming the presence of no specific medical contraindications, we prefer the systolic blood pressure to be maintained at ≤ 100 mm Hg. To balance the patient's systolic blood pressure, we maintain the arthroscopic pump pressure at 60 mm Hg and infuse normal saline as arthroscopic fluid.

The second principle is to avoid creating bleeding vessels. In the shoulder, although all areas are vascular and potentially sources of bleeding, certain areas are more apt to bleed during dissection, such as the coracoid region, medial subacromial bursa, and the anterior coracoacromial ligament region, because of the acromial branch of the thoracoacromial trunk. In these regions, an electrocautery ablation device such as the OPES wand (Arthrex, Inc.; Naples, FL) is helpful in coagulating bleeding.

When encountering bleeding during arthroscopy, it is necessary to resist the temptation to coagulate every incidence of bleeding in the field. This can be frustrating, time-consuming, and ineffective. When massive bleeding is encountered, particularly when it appears from every possible area in the field of view, the more common culprit is "turbulence" rather than actual uncontrolled bleeding vessels (1). In addition, the reflex solution of elevating the pressure of the irrigation fluid by increasing the arthroscopic pump pressure or elevating the irrigation fluid bags (in a gravity-infusion system) rarely improves visualization because this usually creates more turbulence.

TURBULENCE CONTROL AND THE BERNOULLI EFFECT

The Bernoulli Effect stems from the Bernoulli Principle, which states that a fluid stream creates a force perpendicular to the stream and varies directly with the velocity of the fluid stream (2,3). This effect can be demonstrated in a bathroom shower. When the shower curtain is closed and the shower is turned on, the curtain is pulled toward the streaming jet of water because of the negative pressure gradient created by the Bernoulli Effect (Fig. 1-1). This negative pressure gradient literally pulls or sucks the bathroom curtain toward the stream of water from the shower head.

In the shoulder, this effect is commonly seen in the subacromial space. For example, while performing an arthroscopic rotator cuff repair we are visualizing through the posterior portal. We have an anterior inflow cannulated portal and an uncannulated lateral working portal. In this example, fluid will flow readily out the uncannulated lateral portal because it is constantly pumped under pressure into the subacromial space through the anterior portal. Fluid will exit the lateral portal with considerable velocity because it is moving from the high pressure of the subacromial space to the relatively low ambient barometric pressure outside the body. This creates a situation analogous to the bathroom shower curtain. The fluid that exits the lateral portal is a fast-moving stream (similar to the jet of water from the shower nozzle), which creates a negative pressure gradient that literally sucks blood from the lumens of bleeding vessels (Fig. 1-2). It is not only the absolute volume of blood

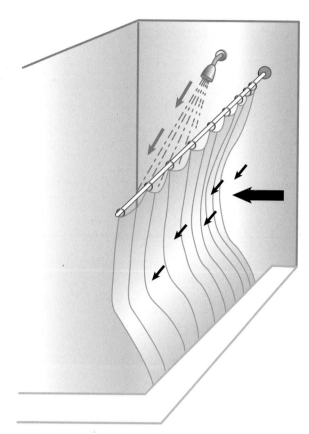

Figure 1-1   A jet of water from a shower nozzle creates a negative pressure gradient perpendicular to the jet (Bernoulli Effect) that pulls the curtain toward the stream of water. (From Burkhart SS, Danaceau SM, Athanasiou KA. Turbulence control as a factor in improving visualization during subacromial shoulder arthroscopy. *Arthroscopy*. 2001;17:209–212, Fig. 1; with permission.)

that obscures visualization, but the rapid mixing of blood with arthroscopy fluid, as the fluids collide at right angles to each other, creating a complex flow field that produces a bloody fluid mixture (Fig. 1-3). Furthermore, the negative

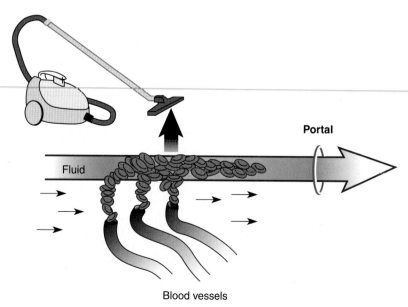

Figure 1-2   The fast-moving arthroscopy fluid that exits the arthroscopic portal that does not contain a cannula creates a negative pressure gradient (suction effect) on the small blood vessels adjacent to the anterior portal. This suction effect is a manifestation of the Bernoulli Principle of fluid mechanics.

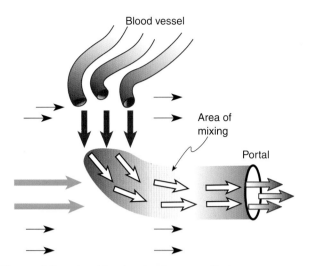

Figure 1-3 When blood and arthroscopy fluid mix as a consequence of flowing together at right angles to each other, the first effect is a blended flow pattern with a bloody opacity because of the mixing effect. (From Burkhart SS, Danaceau SM, Athanasiou KA. Turbulence control as a factor in improving visualization during subacromial shoulder arthroscopy. *Arthroscopy.* 2001;17:209–212, Fig. 4; with permission.)

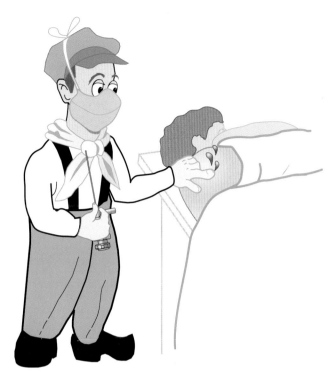

Figure 1-4 A traditional Dutch technique (plugging the hole) is used to control turbulence by eliminating the Bernoulli Effect of fluid streaming out of the portal. (From Burkhart SS, Danaceau SM, Athanasiou KA. Turbulence control as a factor in improving visualization during subacromial shoulder arthroscopy. *Arthroscopy.* 2001;17:209–212, Fig. 5; with permission.)

pressure gradient produced by the arthroscopy fluid on the blood vessels creates turbulence, which rapidly produces an opaque bloody mixture, obscuring visualization and frustrating the arthroscopic surgeon.

How can we prevent this from happening? The answer is simply by controlling turbulence. Similar to the traditional Dutch boy technique, the surgeon or capable assistant can use a finger to completely occlude the portal and prevent the stream of fluid from exiting the portal (Fig. 1-4). Make sure, however, the flow through the portal is completely occluded. Turbulence control will usually yield a

clear field of view in a matter of seconds even if some of the vessels are not coagulated (Fig. 1-5). In contrast, allowing turbulence to continue while coagulating and controlling all bleeding points by electrocautery can be a time-consuming, exhausting, and frustrating experience. During

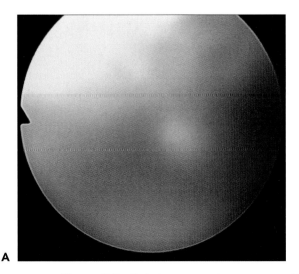

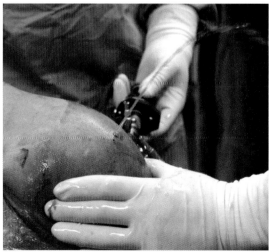

Figure 1-5 Turbulence control as a means of improving visualization. **A:** Blood obscures the anatomic details of this subacromial view. **B:** Turbulence associated with free egress of arthroscopy fluid causes the bloody field.

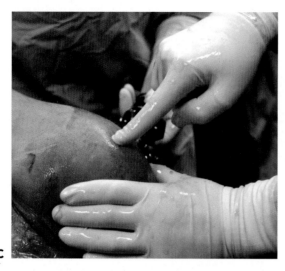
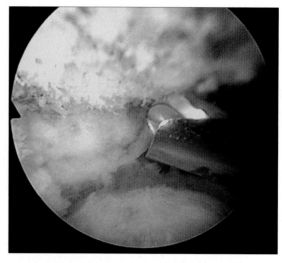

C   **D**

Figure 1-5. *(continued)* **C:** Digital pressure over the noncannulated portal stops the turbulent flow. **D:** The same field as in **(A)** after 10 seconds of digital pressure over the portal. Visualization has been dramatically improved.

arthroscopic rotator cuff repair, we commonly use several noncannulated subacromial portals for repair. This leaves several foci for the Bernoulli Effect, compounding its potential for disrupting visualization. We routinely have an assistant apply digital pressure over all noncannulated portals, occluding the flow at each site. This simple maneuver of turbulence control can dramatically improve visualiza-tion, leaving the surgeon free to proceed with the arthro-scopic procedure.

REFERENCES

1. Burkhart SS, Danaceau SM, Athanasiou KA. Turbulence control as a factor in improving visualization during subacromial shoulder arthroscopy. *Arthroscopy.* 2001;17:209–212.
2. Hall S. *Basic Biomechanics.* St. Louis: Mosby-Year Book; 1991:434–437.
3. Nakayama K, Boucher RF. *Fluid Mechanics.* London: Arnold;1999:56–70.

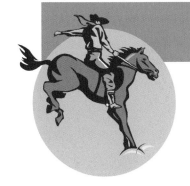

Angle of Approach

Shoot straight or not at all.

Cowboys have always aspired to be straight shooters, both literally and figuratively. They understand that the shortest distance between two points is a straight line, whether they're throwing a rope or driving cattle to market. A cowboy's life can depend on his ability to be a literal straight shooter. Equally important, his reputation rests on his consistency as a figurative straight shooter. After all, the cowboy's word is his bond.

Angle of approach has a direct impact on the ability both to visualize the area of interest and to treat effectively the pathology at hand. To reach all areas of the shoulder, it is essential to become familiar and facile with any combination of arthroscope angles (i.e., 30° and 70° arthroscopes), reconstructive instruments, portals, and their requisite angle of approach to the pathology.

ARTHROSCOPE ANGLES

Angled arthroscope use is the most common method of increasing the field of view available to the arthroscopist. Although a straight 0° arthroscope, at first, may seem the easiest to maneuver within a joint, this straight-ahead view requires a linear, unobstructed pathway toward the area of interest to be effective—a very uncommon scenario in a joint. By rotating the arthroscope and using the angle of the arthroscopic lens to the surgeon's advantage, however, it is possible to obtain exponentially more fields of view without actually changing the position of the arthroscope (Fig. 2-1). Nowhere is this more important than in the shoulder, where looking "around the corner" is a common necessity.

Although we are most familiar with the 30° arthroscope during joint arthroscopy, keep in mind that scopes come with various lens angles, diameters, and lengths. In our surgical cases, we frequently use a 70° arthroscope during shoulder arthroscopy. We find the acute angle of a 70° arthroscope essential, particularly during more advanced arthroscopic procedures such as subscapularis repair, subcoracoid decompression, and double interval slides (Fig. 2-2). The 70° arthroscope, can also be helpful during other standard arthroscopic reconstructions.

For example, when performing a Mumford procedure (i.e., distal clavicle excision), it is essential to ensure adequate decompression and excision superiorly and posteriorly. Failure to excise the distal clavicle completely, particularly the posterosuperior portion of the bone, can lead to ongoing pain, especially with cross-body adduction. Although some authors have proposed indirect methods of decompression (e.g., using a burr or instrument to feel for retained bone), nothing is better than direct visualization. When using a 30° arthroscope, an unobstructed view of the superior and posterior clavicle can be difficult, particularly if the acromioclavicular joint is sloped (Fig. 2-3A). This visualization can be improved by excising some of the medial acromion, but we prefer not to remove additional acromial bone just for the sake of visualization. Use of the 70° arthroscope, with its ability to look straight up into the acromioclavicular joint, is our preferred method for viewing the superior and posterior

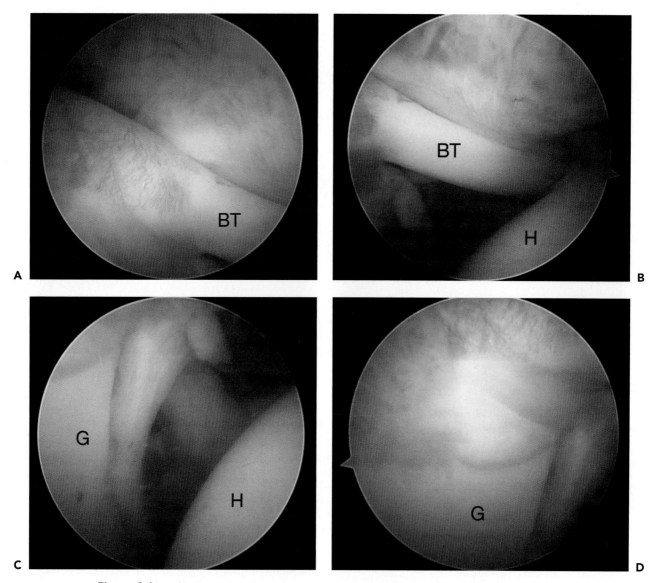

Figure 2-1 Arthroscopic view from a posterior glenohumeral portal of a right shoulder demonstrating an expanded field of view using the 30° arthroscope **(A)** angled superiorly; **(B)** angled laterally; **(C)** angled inferiorly; **(D)** angled medially. BT, biceps tendon; G, glenoid; H, humeral head.

acromioclavicular joint (Fig. 2-3B). Because approximately 30% of acromioclavicular joints are sloped from inferomedial to superolateral, use of the 70° scope will prevent inadvertent "amputation" of the superolateral tip of the distal clavicle. In fact, we use the 70° arthroscope in almost all cases of distal clavicle excision. Although this might be considered overkill, it is useful to perform this exercise routinely to gain familiarity with the 70° arthroscope.

The other common use of the 70° arthroscope is during repair of anterior supraspinatus tears. These tears are often small tears (i.e., ≤1 cm), and it can be difficult (when using a posterior subacromial viewing portal) to visualize the medial aspect of the footprint in this area, even when exter-

nally rotating the arm (Fig. 2-4A). By using the 70° arthroscope, however, the footprint comes into view, allowing easy preparation and fixation of the rotator cuff (Fig. 2-4B).

PORTALS

Accurate portal placement is one of the most important steps to master during shoulder arthroscopy. In fact, we have heard other expert shoulder arthroscopists comment that, when training Fellows, this is the last step they are allowed to perform on their own because improper portal position can frustrate the arthroscopist for the entire duration of the case.

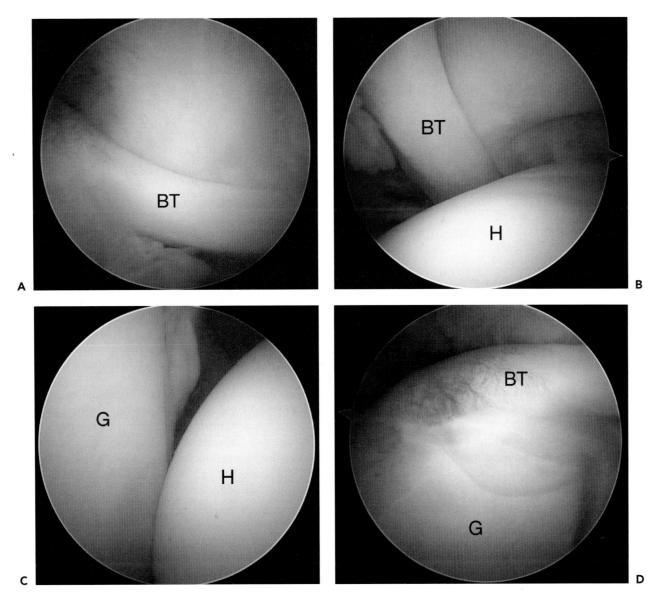

Figure 2-2 Arthroscopic view from a posterior glenohumeral portal of a right shoulder demonstrating an expanded field of view using the 70° arthroscope **(A)** angled superiorly; **(B)** angled laterally; **(C)** angled inferiorly; **(D)** angled medially. Note same position of the arthroscope as in Figure 2-1. BT, biceps tendon; G, glenoid; H, humeral head.

Glenohumeral Arthroscopy Portals

The most commonly used glenohumeral arthroscopy portals are the posterior portal, anterior portal, 5 o'clock portal, anterosuperolateral portal, Port of Wilmington portal, and posterolateral portal (1) (Fig. 2-5). Once the posterior portal is established, we create all the other portals with an outside-in technique, using a spinal needle to determine the proper angle of approach before making the skin puncture. Then, a switching stick is "walked" down beside the needle, and a cannula is placed over the switching stick.

Posterior Portal

Many arthroscopic surgeons create their posterior portal a finger-breadth medial (1–2 cm) and inferior (1–2 cm) to the posterolateral corner of the acromion. We, however, find this location to be too superior and too lateral for two reasons. First of all, if the joint is entered from this location, the scope enters the joint adjacent to the posterosuperior labrum in such close proximity that this structure can be difficult to evaluate. Second, during long or complex cases, subcutaneous swelling can begin to shift the skin incision further superiorly and laterally. If this happens, the surgeon has a continual struggle fighting

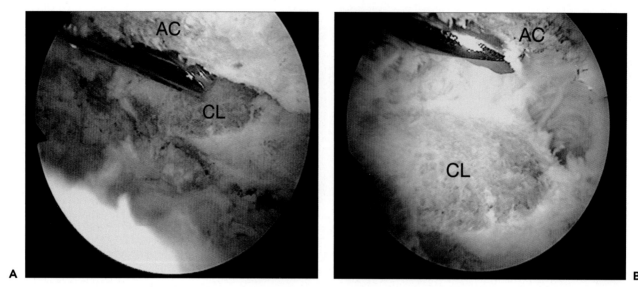

Figure 2-3   Arthroscopic view through a lateral subacromial portal of a left shoulder during arthroscopic distal clavicle excision. **A:** 30° arthroscope; **B:** 70° arthroscope. Note: With the 70° arthroscope, a direct view to the superior and posterior aspect of the acromioclavicular joint is easily obtained. AC, acromion; CL, clavicle.

to get around the "corner" of the acromion, which now partially obstructs the straight-line approach to the pathology. To ensure the proper placement of this portal, we initially palpate for the soft spot or triangle created by glenoid medially, the humeral head laterally, and the rotator cuff superiorly (Fig. 2-6). Because we perform shoulder arthroscopy in the lateral decubitus position,

the glenohumeral joint is essentially parallel to the floor. A skin puncture is made approximately 4 to 5 cm distal to the posterior acromion and the arthroscope sheath with its blunt trocar is directed toward the coracoid. The joint is entered while manual traction is being exerted on the arm. The posterior portal is approximately 3 to 4 cm medial to the posterolateral corner of the acromions, but

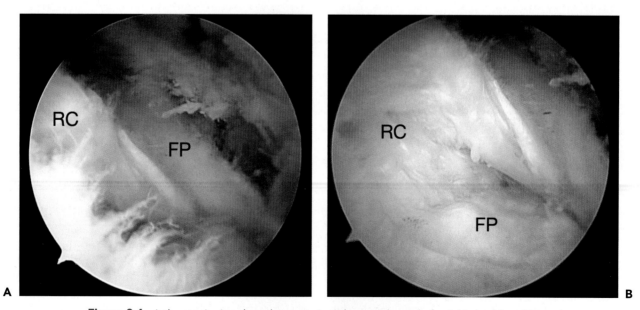

Figure 2-4   Arthroscopic view through a posterior subacromial portal of a right shoulder with an anterior leading edge, partial thickness bursal surface supraspinatus tear. The arm is in maximal external rotation. **A:** 30° arthroscope. Note: It is difficult to completely see the tear, particularly along the medial aspect of the footprint. **B:** 70° arthroscope. Note: The 70° arthroscope provides an expanded view of the rotator cuff tear, including the medial footprint, allowing easy débridement and repair of the rotator cuff. RC, rotator cuff; FP, footprint.

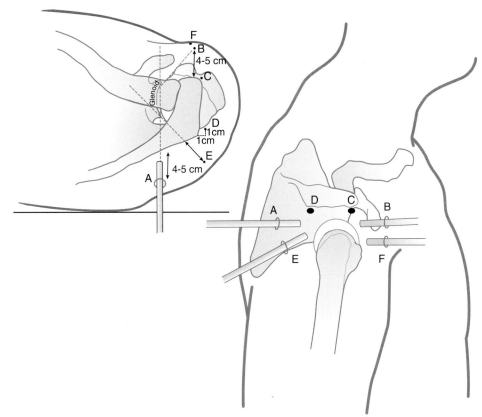

Figure 2-5 Schematic diagram demonstrating the relative positions of the **(A)** posterior portal; **(B)** anterior portal; **(C)** anterosuperolateral portal; **(D)** Port of Wilmington portal; **(E)** posterolateral portal; **(F)** 5 o'clock portal.

this can differ from patient to patient. The exact position of this portal is determined by palpation. The posterior portal entrance is commonly below the equator of the glenoid, in the posteroinferior quadrant of the glenohumeral joint (Fig. 2-7).

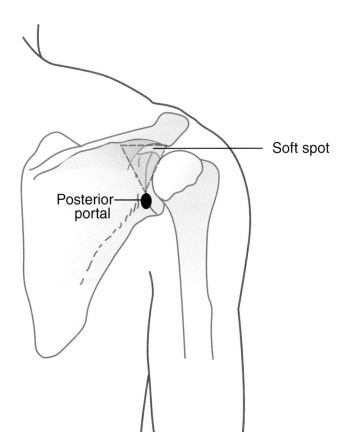

Figure 2-6 Schematic diagram demonstrating the posterior portal position at the lowest point of the soft spot of the shoulder.

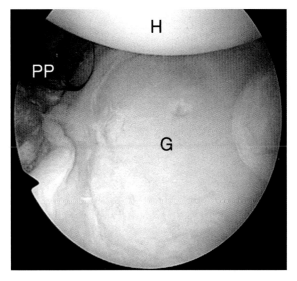

Figure 2-7 Arthroscopic view through an anterosuperolateral glenohumeral portal of a left shoulder, demonstrating the intra-articular position of the posterior portal, which lies in the posteroinferior quadrant. G, glenoid; H, humeral head; PP, posterior portal.

Anterior Portal

While viewing through the posterior portal, a low anterior portal (our standard anterior portal) is usually the second portal created. This portal is established just above the lateral half of the subscapularis tendon, medial to the "sling" of the biceps tendon (Fig. 2-8). This portal allows access to the superior glenoid neck for preparation of the bone bed during a superior labrum anterior and posterior (SLAP) repair and also provides a 30° to 45° angle of approach to the glenoid for anchor placement (in the 3 o'clock and 4 o'clock positions) during Bankart repair. For more inferior anchor placement, we almost always use a 5 o'clock portal.

The 5 O'clock Portal

The 5 o'clock portal is established approximately 1-cm inferior to the low anterior portal through the most lateral part of the subscapularis tendon (Fig. 2-9). This portal is established to allow access for anchor placement at the 5 o'clock position on the glenoid during Bankart repair. Although not always necessary, we use this portal most of the time to get squarely down to the 5 o'clock position without an inferior–oblique angle of approach that can fracture the anterior–inferior glenoid during anchor placement. We use this portal only for suture anchor placement and use the low anterior portal for passage of sutures from the 5 o'clock anchor.

Anterosuperolateral Portal

The anterosuperolateral portal is established approximately 1- to 2-cm lateral to the anterolateral corner of the

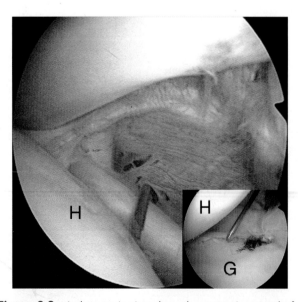

Figure 2-8 Arthroscopic view through a posterior portal of a left shoulder, demonstrating anterior portal placement just superior to the lateral half of the subscapularis tendon and medial to the medial sling of the biceps tendon. Note: The anterior portal allows a 45° angle of approach to the anterior mid-glenoid position for anchor placement (*inset*). H, humeral head; G, glenoid.

acromion. This portal is used for SLAP repair, allowing a 45° angle of approach to the corner of the superior glenoid for anchor placement under the biceps root at its confluence with the superior labrum. For more posterior SLAP lesions, a second more posterior portal, the Port of Wilmington, is additionally required (see below). In addition to serving as a working portal, the anterosuperolateral portal is used as a secondary viewing portal during instability repair (anterior, posterior, multidirectional instability). This portal provides a panoramic view of the glenoid, particularly its anterior and posterior margins, making instability repair, joint balancing, and bone loss assessment more accurate. This portal is established through the rotator interval just anterior to the supraspinatus tendon and directly above the long head of the biceps (Fig. 2-10). The anterosuperolateral portal is also useful as a working portal during arthroscopic subscapularis repair. In this situation, the portal is established with particular attention to the angle of approach, which must allow the arthroscopic burr to approach the lesser tuberosity at a 5° to 10 ° angle for preparation of the bone bed.

The Port of Wilmington Portal

The Port of Wilmington portal is established approximately 1-cm anterior and 1-cm lateral to the posterolateral corner of the acromion. This portal is created while viewing through a posterior glenohumeral portal and it is placed to allow a 45° angle of approach to the posterosuperior glenoid. This portal is essential for anchor placement during repair of SLAP lesions with a large posterior component (see Fig. 2-10). For such cases, the anterosuperolateral portal affords too oblique an angle for successful anchor placement in the posterosuperior glenoid.

Posterolateral Portal

The posterolateral portal is established approximately 4- to 5-cm inferior to the posterolateral corner of the acromion and 4- to 6-cm lateral to the posterior portal. Although a standard posterior portal allows excellent visualization of the glenohumeral joint, this portal is inadequate for anchor placement in the posterior inferior glenoid because it is parallel to the glenoid surface. Instead, a posterolateral portal is essential for the proper angle of approach to the posterior labrum and posterior glenoid during posterior Bankart or multi-directional instability repairs. This portal allows an appropriate angle of approach for glenoid preparation and for anchor insertion in the posterior inferior glenoid (Fig. 2-11). To establish this portal, the glenohumeral joint is viewed through the anterosuperolateral portal and a spinal needle is used to establish the proper angle of approach.

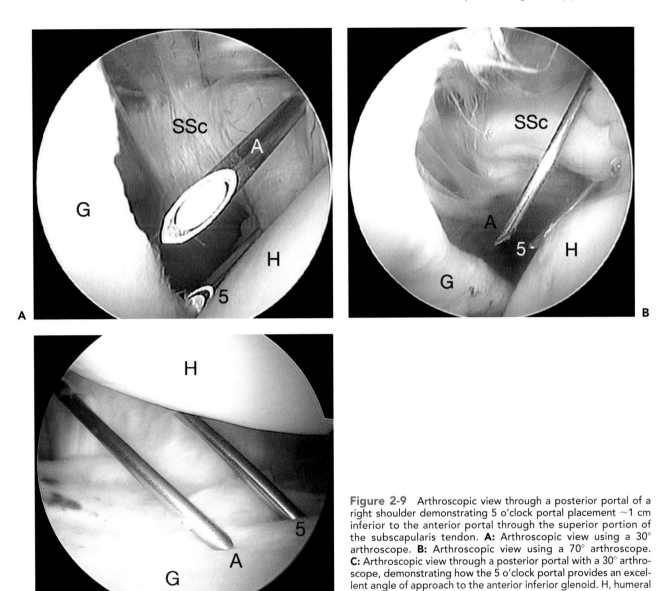

Figure 2-9 Arthroscopic view through a posterior portal of a right shoulder demonstrating 5 o'clock portal placement ~1 cm inferior to the anterior portal through the superior portion of the subscapularis tendon. **A:** Arthroscopic view using a 30° arthroscope. **B:** Arthroscopic view using a 70° arthroscope. **C:** Arthroscopic view through a posterior portal with a 30° arthroscope, demonstrating how the 5 o'clock portal provides an excellent angle of approach to the anterior inferior glenoid. H, humeral head; SSc, subscapularis tendon; G, glenoid; A, anterior portal; 5, 5 o'clock portal.

Subcromial Portals

The most commonly used subacromial portals are the posterior portal, lateral portal, anterior portal, modified Neviaser portal, and subclavian portal (Fig. 2-12).

Posterior Portal

The posterior subacromial portal is established through the same skin incision used to create the posterior glenohumeral portal. To establish this portal, the arthroscopy sheath and blunt trocar are directed superior to the glenohumeral joint, parallel to the undersurface of the acromion, and toward the anterolateral corner of the acromion. It is important when establishing this portal to penetrate the posterior "veil" or "curtain" of the subacro-

mial bursa (Fig. 2-13) to ensure adequate view of the subacromial bursa (i.e., "room with a view"). Remember, the actual subacromial "space" is located beneath the anterior half of the acromion. In cases where significant swelling has occurred before establishing this portal, it is helpful to use the blunt trocar and arthroscope sheath to palpate the posterior aspect of the acromion, and to penetrate the posterior deltoid muscle just inferior to this, paralleling the undersurface of the acromion. This is the initial portal used for subacromial bursoscopy.

Lateral Portal

The lateral subacromial portal is created approximately 4 cm lateral to the acromion in line with the posterior aspect of the clavicle while viewing through a posterior

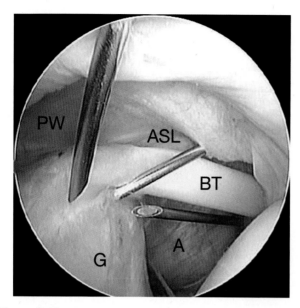

Figure 2-10 Arthroscopic view through a posterior viewing portal of a right shoulder, demonstrating positioning of the anterior, anterosuperolateral, and Port of Wilmington portals. The anterior portal provides an excellent angle of approach to prepare the bone bed on the superior glenoid neck. The anterosuperolateral portal is placed anterior to the supraspinatus tendon, posterior to the biceps tendon, and at a 45° angle to the superior glenoid, allowing an excellent angle of approach for anchor insertion and suture passage through the superior labrum. The Port of Wilmington portal is placed to allow a 45° angle of approach to the posterior aspect of the superior labrum and the posterosuperior glenoid for optimal anchor insertion into the posterosuperior glenoid. A, anterior portal; ASL, anterosuperolateral portal; PW, Port of Wilmington portal; H, humerus; G, glenoid; BT, biceps tendon.

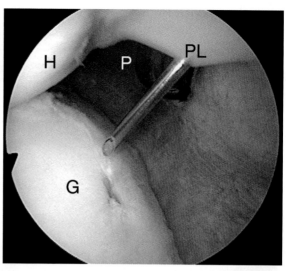

Figure 2-11 Arthroscopic view through an anterosuperolateral portal of a right shoulder, demonstrating portal placement for the posterior and posterolateral portals. Note: the posterolateral portal (marked by spinal needle in this photo) provides an appropriate angle of approach for anchor placement into the posterior inferior glenoid. P, posterior portal; PL, posterolateral portal; G, glenoid; H, humeral head.

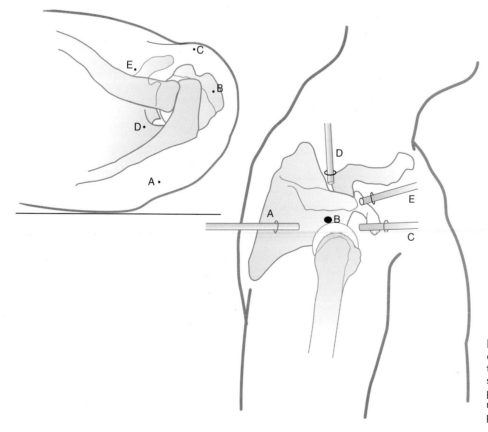

Figure 2-12 Schematic diagram demonstrating the relative positions of the most commonly used subacromial portals **(A)** posterior portal; **(B)** lateral portal; **(C)** anterior portal; **(D)** modified Neviaser portal; **(E)** subclavian portal.

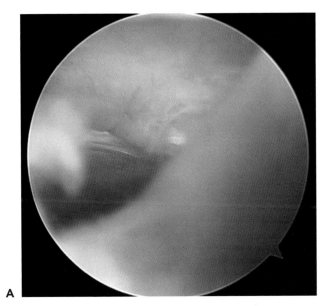
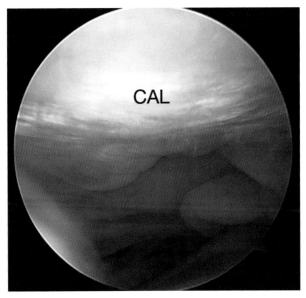

A   B

Figure 2-13 Arthroscopic view through a posterior subacromial portal of a right shoulder. **A:** The posterior subacromial "curtain" has not been penetrated and is obstructing visualization of the subacromial space. **B:** Once the subacromial curtain has been penetrated, the subacromial space is easily recognized. CAL, coracoacromial ligament.

subacromial portal. This portal is created parallel to the undersurface of the acromion (Fig. 2-14). During arthroscopic rotator cuff repair, this portal can be established while doing the intra-articular glenohumeral portion of the case because the defect in the cuff allows visualization into the lateral portion of the subacromial space. In this situation, a posterior glenohumeral viewing portal is used and the lateral portal is directed toward the apex of

the tear (Fig. 2-15A). This allows appropriate positioning of the portal relative to the rotator cuff tear for a "50 yard line" view (Fig. 2-15B). It is particularly helpful to establish this portal during glenohumeral arthroscopy if the lateral opening of the rotator cuff tear is small. In such cases, the footprint of the rotator cuff can be accurately and completely prepared all the way to the articular margin (Fig. 2-16) while viewing from an intra-articular perspective.

Anterior Portal

The anterior subacromial portal is established through the same skin incision used to create the anterior glenohumeral portal. To create this portal, the subacromial bursa is viewed through a posterior portal and the anterior subacromial portal is established by directing a switching stick superior toward the anterior acromion (Fig. 2-17). We generally use this portal for suture management or as a dedicated inflow cannula. In addition, it generally provides an excellent angle of approach as a working portal for distal clavicle excision.

Modified Neviaser Portal

The modified Neviaser portal can be used during arthroscopic rotator cuff repair, particularly when a "double row" or footprint restoration configuration is desired. It provides an excellent angle of approach to the central span of a large rotator cuff tear. This portal is created approximately 2 to 3 cm posteromedial to the acromioclavicular joint, in the "soft spot" bordered by the posterior clavicle, medial acromion, and the scapular spine

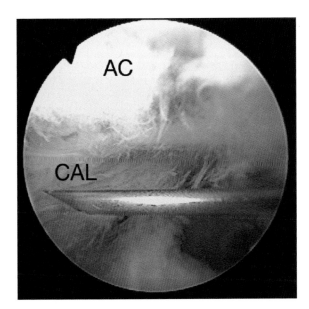

Figure 2-14 Arthroscopic view through a posterior subacromial portal, demonstrating the bursal position of the lateral subacromial portal. Note: The portal parallels the undersurface of the acromion. AC, acromion; CAL, coracoacromial ligament.

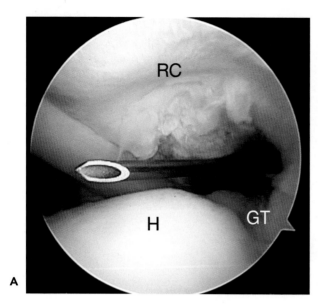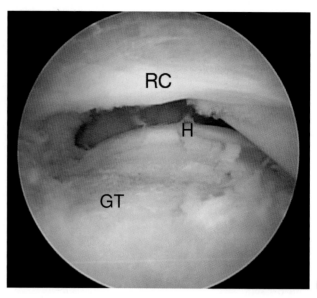

Figure 2-15   A: Arthroscopic view through a posterior glenohumeral portal demonstrating position of the lateral subacromial portal of a right shoulder. The portal is positioned toward the apex of the tear ensuring a "50 yard line" position of the lateral subacromial portal. **B:** Arthroscopic view through the same lateral subacromial portal demonstrating the 50 yard line position. H, humeral head; RC, rotator cuff.

(Fig. 2-18). While viewing from a lateral portal, we use a spinal needle as a guide to determine the proper position of the portal to allow an adequate angle of approach to the central rotator cuff (Fig. 2-19A). This portal is used only for suture passage. No cannula is necessary, because only a small (3-mm) skin puncture is required to accommodate suture-passing instruments. Using the needle as a guide, a suture-passing instrument

(Penetrator suture passer or Banana Lasso; Arthrex, Inc.; Naples, FL) can then be "walked" down the needle and its entry into the subacromial space can be visualized (Fig. 2-19B).

Subclavian Portal

The subclavian portal, as described by Nord et al. (2), is located 1 to 2 cm medial and inferior to the acromioclav-

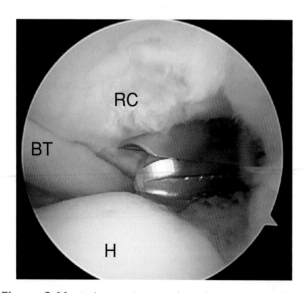

Figure 2-16 Arthroscopic view through a posterior glenohumeral portal of a right shoulder with a small rotator cuff tear, demonstrating débridement of the medial aspect of the footprint of the rotator cuff with a burr. Note: It is easier to visualize the medial aspect of the footprint of a small tear from an intra-articular perspective. H, humeral head; RC, rotator cuff; BT, biceps tendon.

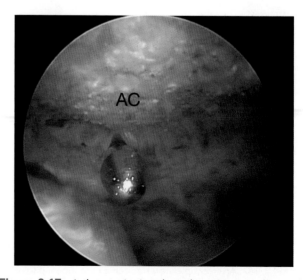

Figure 2-17 Arthroscopic view through a posterior subacromial portal of a right shoulder, demonstrating the position of the anterior subacromial portal. AC, acromion.

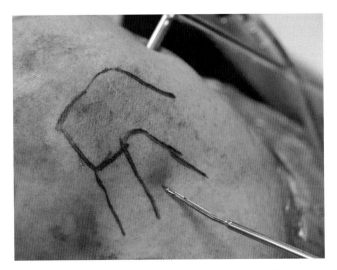

Figure 2-18 Clinical photo demonstrating the position of the modified Neviaser portal.

icular (AC) joint (Fig. 2-20). This portal can be useful during arthroscopic rotator cuff repair, particularly for suture passage through the anterior cuff. We create this portal while viewing through the lateral portal. This portal lies directly under the clavicle, and passes laterally just inferior to the AC joint toward the subacromial bursa (Fig. 2-21). We commonly create this portal following subacromial decompression, because a prominent anterior–inferior acromion can make passage of instruments and creation of the portal in the proper direction difficult.

Creating Portals

Once the initial posterior portal has been established, we create portals exclusively from an outside-in approach under direct vision. This method ensures the appropriate angle of approach is obtained to the area of interest, and we have found it a safe and effective method.

During portal placement using an outside-in method, a number of techniques can be used to ensure accurate portal placement and to minimize the risk of potential injury to the neurovascular structures. First, when initially determining the proper position of the portal, we commonly use an 18-gauge spinal needle as a guide (Fig. 2-22A). This can help in identifying where the skin incision should be made to ensure the appropriate angle of approach. Second, after the needle has located the appropriate angle and position, we always use a blunt-tipped switching stick placed parallel to the 18-gauge needle to bluntly tunnel through the soft tissues and enter the joint capsule (Fig. 2-22B). In this way, the soft tissues are spread apart and not disrupted by a sharp object. Finally, the portal is established by passing a smooth obturator and cannula over the switching stick (Fig. 2-22C). This avoids multiple punctures, thereby minimizing the risk of inadvertent neurovascular injury.

In contrast, when creating transrotator cuff portals (i.e., 5 o'clock portal, Port of Wilmington portal) or portals used exclusively for suture passage (modified Neviaser portal, subclavian portal), a cannula is rarely used, necessitating a different technique. These portals are generally used for anchor placement (e.g., 5 o'clock portal, Port of Wilmington portal) or suture passage only (modified

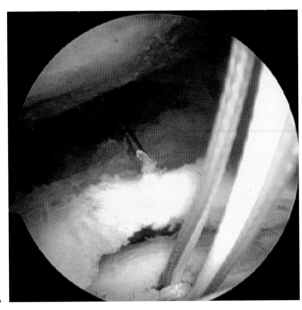

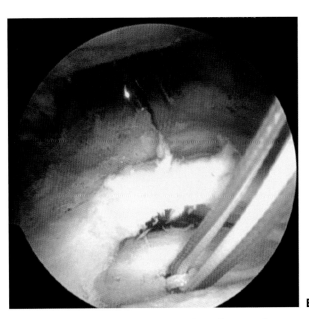

A   B

Figure 2-19 Arthroscopic view through a lateral subacromial portal of a right shoulder. **A:** A spinal needle is used as a guide to ensure proper position of the modified Neviaser portal. **B:** Using the spinal needle as a guide, a suture-passing instrument can then be "walked" down the needle parallel and adjacent to it for accurate insertion.

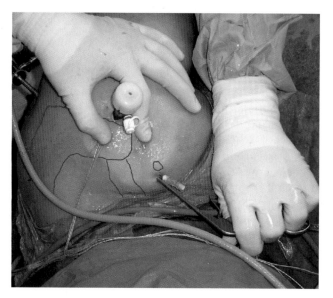

Figure 2-20 Clinical photo demonstrating the position of the subclavian portal relative to the acromioclavicular joint.

Neviaser portal, subclavian portal). When creating a 5 o'clock portal or Port of Wilmington portal, a spinal needle is initially used to locate the appropriate angle of approach to the anterior inferior glenoid or posterior superior glenoid, respectively (Fig. 2-23A). These portals are used for anchor placement only, so only a small (~3 mm) incision is required in the skin. We then use the 3-mm

BioSutureTak (Arthrex) sheath (or alternatively the BioFASTak sheath) with a sharp tipped trocar (Fig. 2-23B) to follow the same direction as the spinal needle and penetrate the rotator cuff toward the intended area (e.g., anterior–inferior glenoid or posterior superior glenoid) (Fig. 2-23C). Once the rotator cuff has been penetrated, then the sharp-tipped trocar is replaced with the standard drill (Fig. 2-23D) or punch to make the bone socket for the suture anchor. Similarly, when using the modified Neviaser portal, a Penetrator or Banana Lasso (Arthrex) is used to walk down the spinal needle toward the central portion of the rotator cuff.

WHEN TO USE A CANNULA AND WHICH ONE

Generally speaking, in the glenohumeral joint we use cannulas in portals that will require repeated usage (e.g., posterior, anterior, anterosuperolateral portals). This is to ensure a clear and consistent path through the deltoid muscle and rotator cuff into the glenohumeral joint. In the subacromial space, however, we do not often use cannulas, for a number of reasons. First, once the portal pathway has been used a couple of times, it is easy to remember and recreate the direction through the deltoid muscle to obtain access into the subacromial space. Second, in the subacromial space, cannulas commonly limit the direction of suture-passing instruments or the arthroscope, particularly

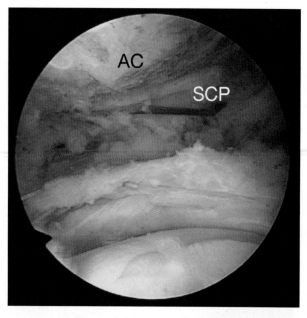
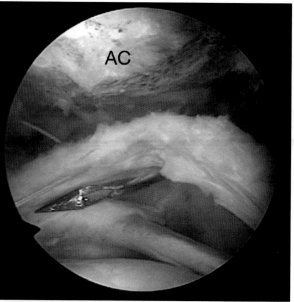

Figure 2-21 **A:** Arthroscopic view through a lateral subacromial portal of a right shoulder, demonstrating the bursal position of the subclavian portal (denoted by spinal needle). **B:** Note: This portal gives an excellent angle of approach for retrograde suture passage through the anterior rotator cuff. AC, acromion; SCP, subclavian portal.

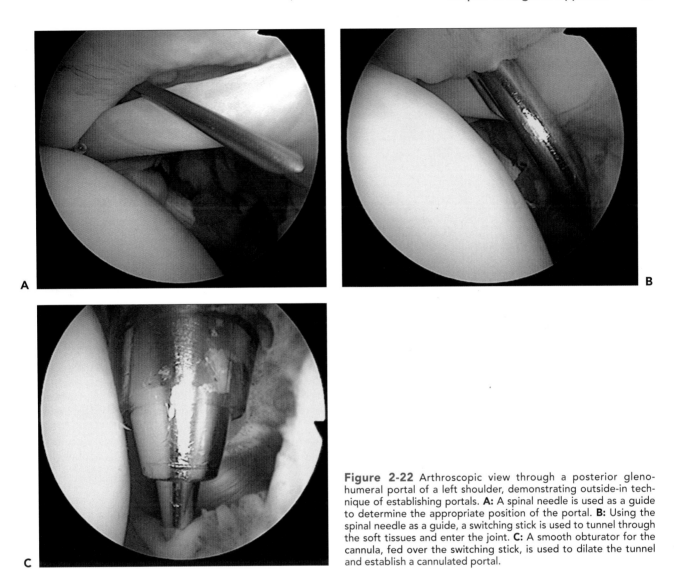

Figure 2-22 Arthroscopic view through a posterior gleno-humeral portal of a left shoulder, demonstrating outside-in technique of establishing portals. **A:** A spinal needle is used as a guide to determine the appropriate position of the portal. **B:** Using the spinal needle as a guide, a switching stick is used to tunnel through the soft tissues and enter the joint. **C:** A smooth obturator for the cannula, fed over the switching stick, is used to dilate the tunnel and establish a cannulated portal.

if using straight instruments (Fig. 2-24A). Removing the cannula increases the range of motion of an instrument, allowing greater access to all areas of the subacromial space (Fig. 2-24B). We, however, always tie knots through a cannulated portal to prevent the sutures from "fouling" on soft tissues.

Several cannulas are available to create cannulated portals. When choosing a cannula, it is important to have a clear understanding of what the cannula will be used for and which cannulas can accommodate certain suture-passing instruments. A smaller cannula might seem advantageous because it limits the disruption of the soft tissues and potentially limits swelling. Not all instruments, however, can fit through all cannulas. Furthermore, we have not seen any significant difference in cosmesis, pain, or return of function relative to cannula size. We generally use 5.5-mm, 7-mm, or 8.25-mm cannulas (Fig. 2-25). These are available with various

configurations to restrict backing out of the cannula (e.g., fully threaded, partially threaded, distal cleat). It is advantageous to use transparent or translucent cannulas (as opposed to opaque cannulas). These cannulas allow a clear view of the instruments as they pass in and out of the joint and increase the field of view. Furthermore, in cases of significant swelling, certain parts of the procedure can actually be performed within the cannula itself (Fig. 2-26).

INSTRUMENTATION

One of the greatest advances in shoulder arthroscopy over the last decade has been the explosion of procedure-specific instrumentation. This has allowed procedures that were previously considered "impossible" to be performed with relative ease. This, however, has also increased the

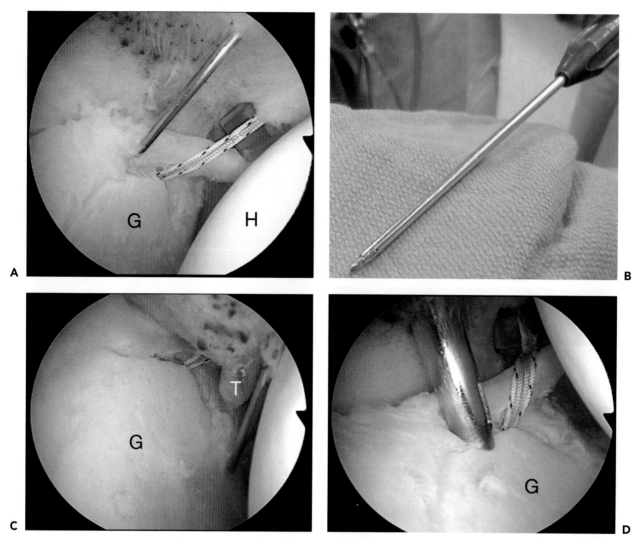

Figure 2-23 Technique for establishing the Port of Wilmington portal. **A:** Arthroscopic view through a posterior glenohumeral portal. A spinal needle is used initially to determine the appropriate position of the portal to approach the posterior superior quadrant of the superior labrum. **B:** Clinical photograph demonstrating the sharp-tipped trocar for the BioSutureTak (Arthrex, Inc.; Naples, FL) sheath used to penetrate soft tissues. **C:** Arthroscopic view through a posterior portal. Using the spinal needle as a guide, a BioSutureTak sheath with a sharp-tipped trocar is used to penetrate the rotator cuff. **D:** Arthroscopic view through a posterior portal. After the rotator cuff has been penetrated, the sharp-tipped trocar is replaced with a drill and the posterolateral glenoid is drilled. G, glenoid; H, humeral head; T, trocar for BioSutureTak sheath.

armamentarium of instruments that must be available to treat all pathology.

Suture-Passing Instruments

Retrograde Suture Passage

Retrograde suture-passing instruments are common and effective devices for suture passage. These instruments require penetration of the soft tissue structure first (Fig. 2-27A). The suture limb to be passed is then retrieved (Fig. 2-27B) and the instrument is withdrawn through the tissue and out the portal, effectively pass-

ing the suture limb through the soft tissue structure (Fig. 2-27C).

Because these instruments require retrieval of the suture after soft tissue penetration, it is important that the suture limb be relatively close to the area of soft tissue penetration. Otherwise, instrument manipulation during retrieval may inadvertently tear the tissue. It is also important to remember that, although many of these instruments are available in right, left, and multi-angled directions, pushing is the general motion involved when using these instruments. This limits the ability of these instruments to make large angled or

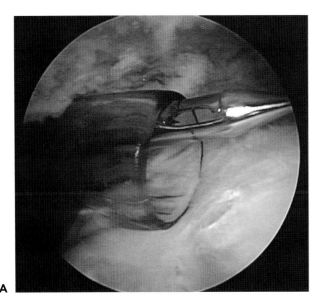 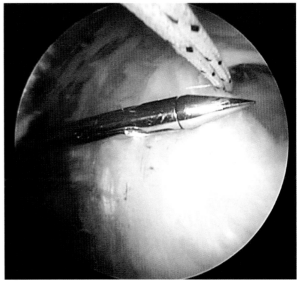

A   B

Figure 2-24 Arthroscopic view through a lateral portal. **A:** When instruments are introduced through a posterior cannulated portal, the cannula restricts the arc of motion of the Penetrator instrument (Arthrex, Inc.; Naples, FL). **B:** When instruments are introduced through the posterior portal without a cannula, the arc of motion of the Penetrator instrument is increased.

directional changes. Thus, when using these instruments, it is best to "line up the putt" before penetrating the soft tissue structure to ensure the instrument will end up close to the suture limb to be retrieved. This allows easy retrieval and subsequent suture passage.

Unlike antegrade suture-passing instruments, retrograde suture-passing instruments are advantageous because they are not limited to the depth of the "jaw" and large and thick "bites" of tissue can be incorporated into a repair. These instruments are particularly helpful in cases of multiple laminations in the tears to ensure that each layer is repaired.

BirdBeak

The BirdBeak (Arthrex) suture-passing instruments are available in 0°, 22.5°, and 45° angles (Fig. 2-28). The most commonly used are the 22.5° and 45° angles. These instruments are frequently used during passage of suture

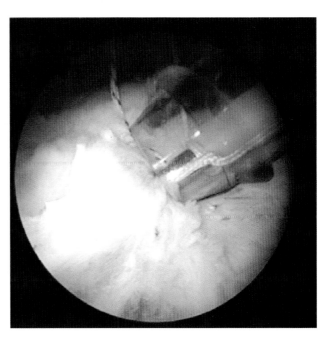

Figure 2-26 Arthroscopic view from a posterior subacromial portal of a right shoulder, demonstrating knot tying performed within a clear 8.25-mm cannula.

5.5-mm   7-mm   8.25-mm

Figure 2-25 Clinical photo demonstrating cannulas in sizes 5.5, 7, and 8.25-mm.

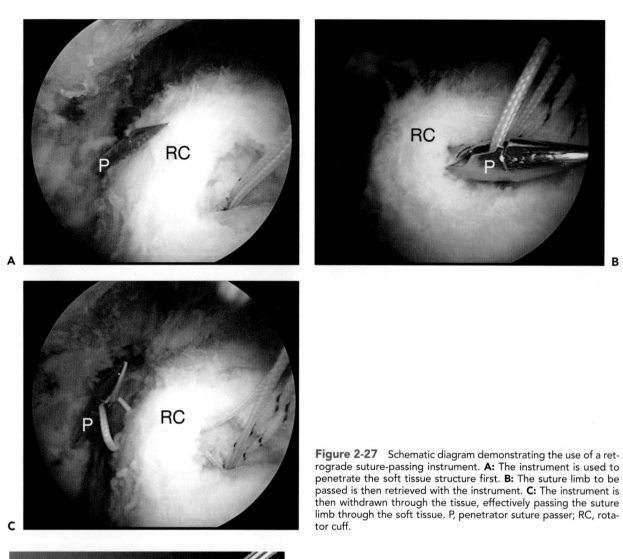

Figure 2-27 Schematic diagram demonstrating the use of a retrograde suture-passing instrument. **A:** The instrument is used to penetrate the soft tissue structure first. **B:** The suture limb to be passed is then retrieved with the instrument. **C:** The instrument is then withdrawn through the tissue, effectively passing the suture limb through the soft tissue. P, penetrator suture passer; RC, rotator cuff.

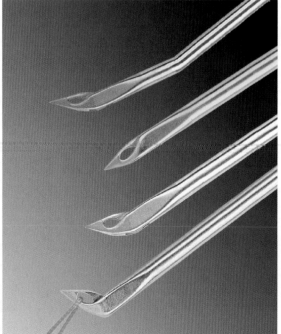

Figure 2-28 Clinical photo demonstrating the BirdBeak suture-passing instruments.

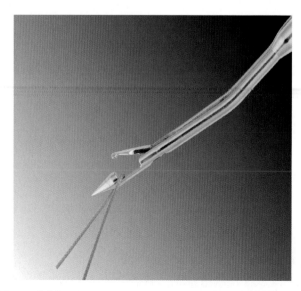

Figure 2-29 Clinical photo demonstrating a Penetrator suture-passing instrument.

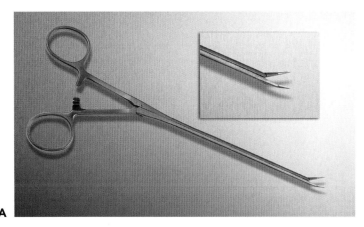

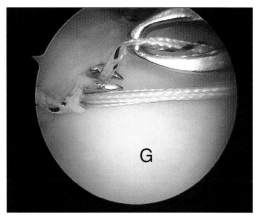

Figure 2-30 **A:** The Sidewinder suture-passing instrument. **B:** Arthroscopic view from an antero-superolateral photo, demonstrating suture passage through the anterior labrum of a right shoulder using the Sidewinder instrument. A suture retriever has been placed through the posterior portal "handing-off" the suture to the Sidewinder. G, glenoid.

through the labrum. The 45° angle of the BirdBeak allows the suture to be passed so that it encircles a robust piece of labrum rather than penetrating through a small portion of the labrum. Although these instruments can be useful for suture passage for Bankart or reverse Bankart repair, inadvertent tearing of the soft tissues can occur when a large shift is required or when passing suture in the anterior inferior labrum. Therefore, they are most useful during SLAP repairs, and for repair of the upper two thirds of the anterior labrum, and repair of the posterior labrum.

Penetrator

The Penetrator (Arthrex) suture-passing instruments are available in 0° or 15° angles (Fig. 2-29). This instrument is commonly used for retrograde suture passage through the rotator cuff. The Penetrator is a valuable instrument to use

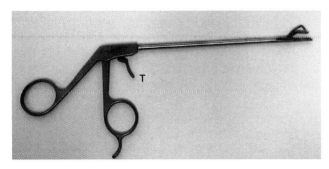

Figure 2-31 The Viper Suture Passer (Arthrex, Inc.; Naples, FL). The upper hooked jaw is used to penetrate the rotator cuff and draw the suture (from the lower jaw) through the tendon. The lower jaw holds the suture and, by using a separate trigger on the base of the handle, the suture can be positioned in an anterior or posterior position to activate suture transfer from the lower to the upper jaw. T, separate trigger for positioning the suture.

in the subacromial space. Its large "window" is helpful when retrieving sutures in the subacromial space. It is important to be careful not to lock the suture in the hinge of the jaw and inadvertently unload an anchor during retrograde passage.

Sidewinder

The Sidewinder (Arthrex) suture-passing instrument is available with angles of 45° and 90° at the tip of the instrument (Fig. 2-30A). This very strong stout instrument is used most commonly for suture passage through the labrum. It differs from the other retrograde suture-passing instruments in that the suture actually has to be grasped (rather than encircled) by the instrument, necessitating a hand-off technique (Fig. 2-30B).

Antegrade Suture Passage

Until recently, few antegrade suture-passing instruments were available. Now, however, several generations of antegrade suture-passing instruments are available, each with its own distinct advantage. These instruments are very intuitive because the suture is retrieved first, inserted into the instrument, and then passed through the tissue. This greatly simplifies suture passage, particularly through the rotator cuff. These antegrade instruments allow the arthroscopist to grasp the tissue, judge the proposed position, and deliver the suture through the tissue in one simple sequence of motion. The depth of "bite," however, is limited by the length of the jaws of the instrument.

Viper

The Viper (Arthrex) suture passer was one of the first antegrade suture-passing instruments available that did

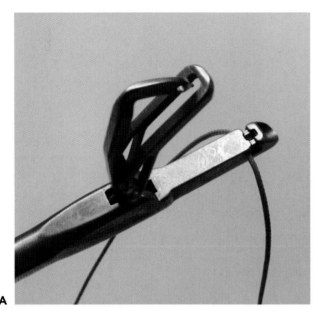
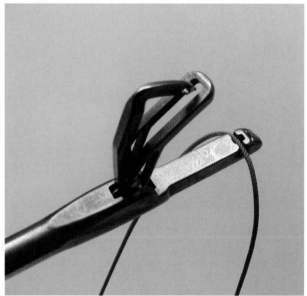

Figure 2-32   The Viper Suture Passer (Arthrex, Inc.; Naples, FL). **A:** The posterior suture position stows the suture safely away from the upper hook. **B:** The anterior suture position allows the suture to be engaged by the hook from the upper jaw by pushing the suture forward into the hook.

not require suture shuttling (Fig. 2-31). This invaluable instrument allows the surgeon to grasp the tissue, deliver the suture, and retrieve the suture in a single step. Furthermore, the tissue can be grasped and pulled toward the bone bed before stitch delivery to ensure that the proposed suture location is satisfactory. Because the Viper suture passer retrieves its own suture, a "blind" suture pass can be performed even without seeing the suture penetrate through the tissue.

This instrument is designed with a lower jaw, which holds the suture to be passed, and an upper hooked jaw, which penetrates the tissue and retrieves the suture from the lower jaw (Fig. 2-32). The lower jaw is constructed so that the suture can be held in an anterior or posterior position, which is controlled by a separate trigger on the handle of the instrument. In the posterior suture position, the suture is stowed safely out of reach of the upper hook (Fig. 2-32A). In the anterior position, the suture can be grasped by the upper jaw (Fig. 2-32B).

For suture passage, an 8.25-mm Twist-In, clear, threaded cannula (Arthrex) is usually used (in this case through the lateral portal) and a suture limb is retrieved from the suture anchor (Fig. 2-33A). The end of the suture is placed into the lower jaw of the Viper suture passer extracorporeally and loaded into the posterior position. The Viper is introduced through the cannula (Fig. 2-33B) as slack is eliminated by pulling on the opposite suture limb. Then, the instrument is used to grasp a portion of the rotator cuff (Fig. 2-33C). The tissue can then be tensioned or pulled to

ensure that suture placement is satisfactory. The suture is then moved into its anterior position using the separate trigger, and the jaws of the Viper instrument are opened, pulling the suture through the tissue and out the lateral portal (Fig. 2-33D,E,F). To help pass the suture through the tissue, it is easiest to "roll" the instrument sideways while opening the jaws rather than pushing forward and pulling back (Fig. 2-34). This rolling maneuver helps to prevent disengagement of the suture from the upper jaw after soft tissue penetration.

Scorpion

The Scorpion (Arthrex) suture-passing instrument is a recently introduced antegrade suture-passing instrument that has greatly simplified suture passage through the rotator cuff (Fig. 2-35). This instrument uses a specially constructed pointed, flat nitinol needle, which is loaded into the instrument and is used to penetrate the rotator cuff. A new nitinol flat needle should be used for each case.

This instrument is specially constructed with a two part grip with differential spring tensions. The anterior grip operates the jaws and allows the arthroscopist to grasp the tissue and judge its proposed position. The posterior grip advances the nitinol needle through the soft tissue. This unique grip allows easy passage through soft tissues without having to change hand position or assist with the other hand. The upper jaw of the instrument acts as a rigid open-section "backstop" that is

Text continues on page 28.

Chapter 2: Angle of Approach **25**

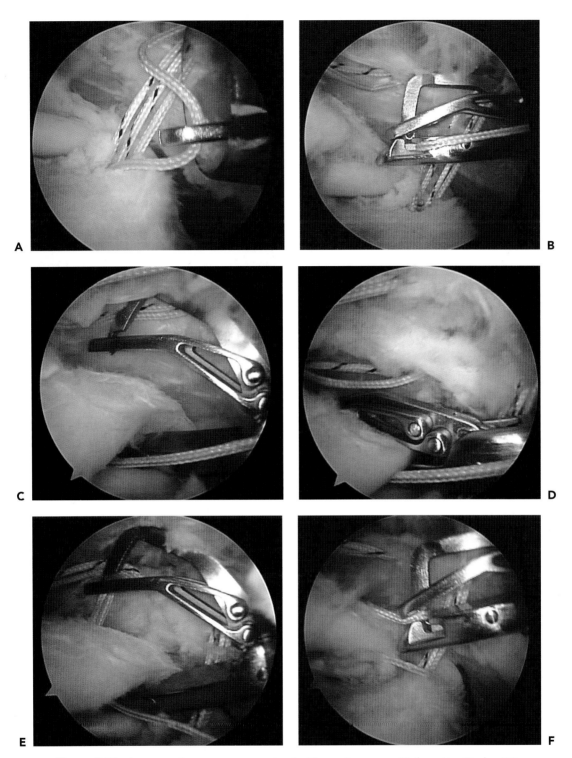

Figure 2-33 Anterograde suture passage using the Viper suture passer (Arthrex, Inc.; Naples, FL). Arthroscopic views through a posterior portal of a right shoulder. **A:** A 8.25-mm Twist-In instrument cannula (Arthrex) has been placed through the lateral portal and one limb of the suture from the anchor is retrieved through this cannula. **B:** The Viper has been loaded with the suture limb in the posterior position and introduced through the lateral cannula. **C:** The Viper jaws are opened and a portion of the rotator cuff is then grasped. **D:** The proposed suture placement is assessed. **E:** The suture is moved into the anterior position by activating the trigger; this pushes the FiberWire suture into the hook of the upper jaw. The jaws are then opened passing the suture through tendon. **F:** The suture is then pulled out the lateral portal.

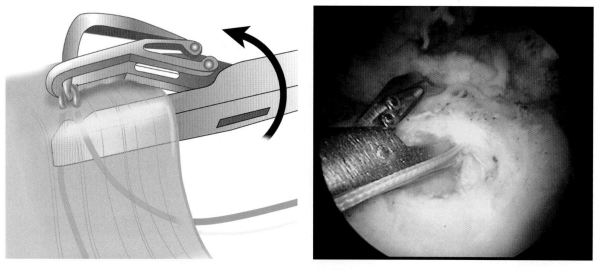

A   B

Figure 2-34   A: This illustration demonstrates the rolling maneuver of the Viper (Arthrex, Inc.; Naples, FL) instrument, which helps prevent disengagement of the suture from the upper jaw. **B:** Arthroscopic view of a left shoulder through a posterior portal using a 70° arthroscope, demonstrating rolling of the Viper suture passer for easy suture passage through the rotator cuff.

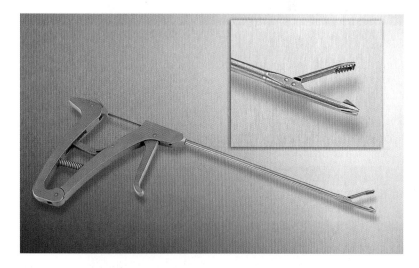

Figure 2-35 Clinical photo of the Scorpion (Arthrex, Inc.; Naples, FL) suture-passing instrument.

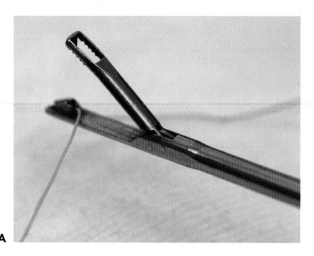
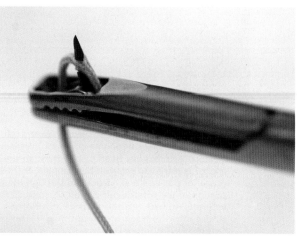

A   B

Figure 2-36 Clinical photos of the Scorpion suture-passing instrument (close-up of jaws). **A:** Photo demonstrating open jaws with suture. **B:** Photo with jaws closed, demonstrating penetration of the suture by the nitinol needle, which pushes the suture up through the soft tissue.

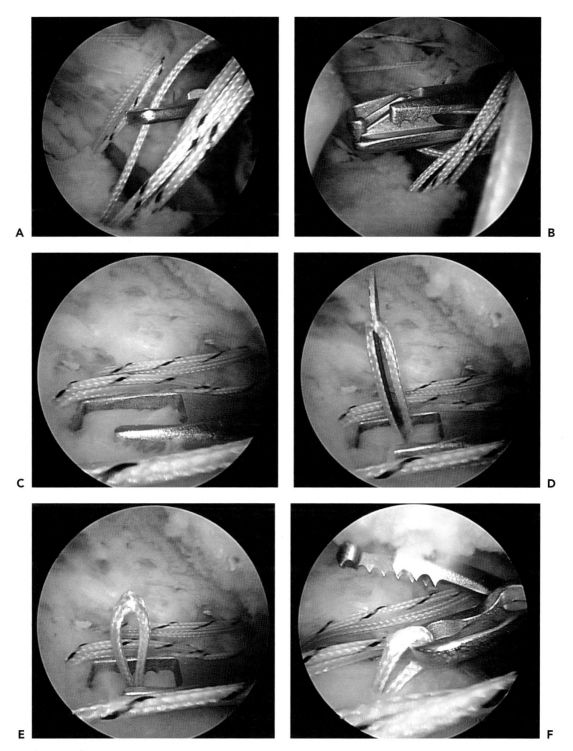

Figure 2-37 Arthroscopic view through a posterior subacromial portal demonstrating use of the Scorpion (Arthrex, Inc.; Naples, FL) suture passer. **A:** One limb of the suture is retrieved through the lateral portal. **B:** The suture limb is placed into the lower jaw of the Scorpion and the instrument is reintroduced through the lateral portal. **C:** The tissue is grasped, using the anterior grip, and the proposed suture position is assessed. **D:** The nitinol needle is then advanced, penetrating the suture and the tissue as the posterior grip is activated. **E:** Releasing the posterior grip retracts the nitinol needle, leaving the suture loop. **F:** The suture loop can then be retrieved, using a separate instrument through a different portal.

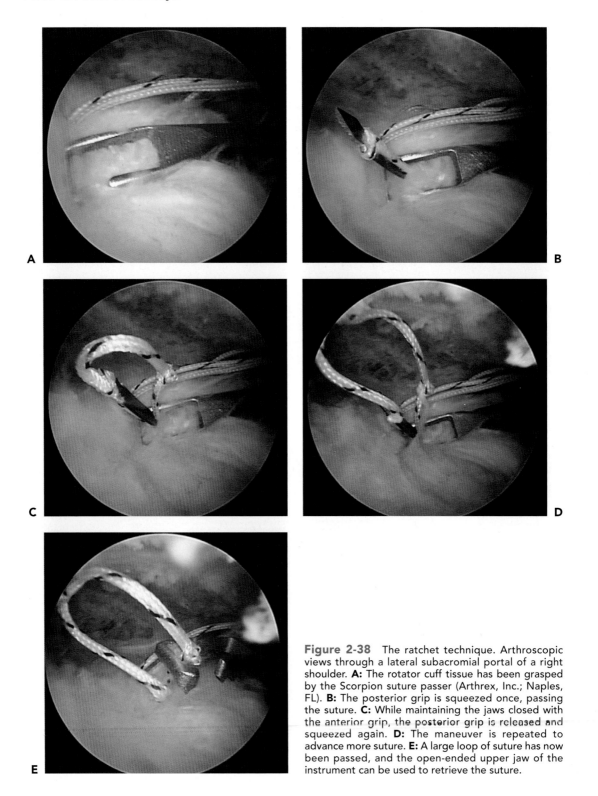

Figure 2-38 The ratchet technique. Arthroscopic views through a lateral subacromial portal of a right shoulder. **A:** The rotator cuff tissue has been grasped by the Scorpion suture passer (Arthrex, Inc.; Naples, FL). **B:** The posterior grip is squeezed once, passing the suture. **C:** While maintaining the jaws closed with the anterior grip, the posterior grip is released and squeezed again. **D:** The maneuver is repeated to advance more suture. **E:** A large loop of suture has now been passed, and the open-ended upper jaw of the instrument can be used to retrieve the suture.

used to hold the soft tissue as it is penetrated by the nitinol needle and suture (Fig. 2-36). The lower jaw of the instrument is used to hold the FiberWire (Arthrex) suture and deliver the nitinol needle. Advancing the needle causes its tip to penetrate the weave of the FiberWire (Arthrex)

suture in the lower jaw, pushing the suture through the tissue and through the profile of the upper jaw. A ratcheting maneuver of the posterior grip will push a progressively larger loop through. The Scorpion is next pulled laterally past the edge of the cuff, then pushed medially

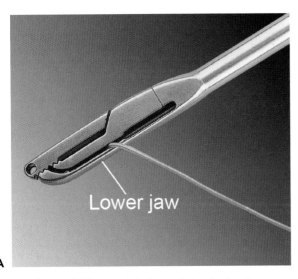
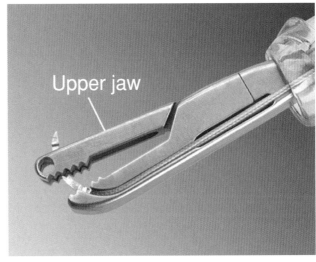

Upper jaw

Lower jaw

A   B

Figure 2-39 Clinical photo of Needle Punch (Arthrex, Inc.; Naples, FL) activation. **A:** Photo with needle in lower jaw. **B:** Photo with needle in upper jaw after activation.

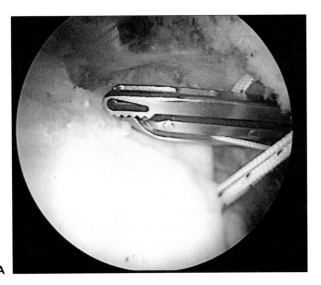
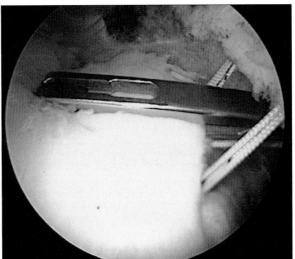

A   B

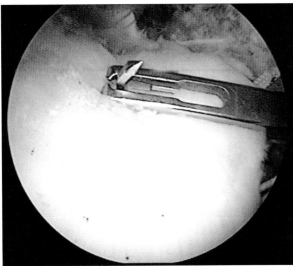

C

Figure 2-40 Arthroscopic view through a posterior subacromial portal of a right shoulder, demonstrating use of the Needle Punch (Arthrex) suture-passing instrument. **A:** The needle is loaded into the lower jaw of the instrument and introduced into the lateral cannula. **B:** The Needle Punch is used to grasp the tissue and the proposed suture placement is evaluated. **C:** The needle is then advanced through the tissue by squeezing the posterior grip. The needle is captured by a slot in the upper jaw.

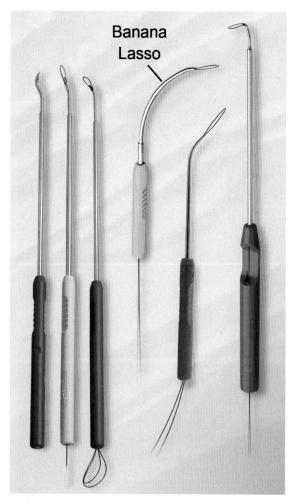

Banana
Lasso

Figure 2-41 Clinical photo of the Suture Lasso (at different angles) and the Banana Lasso (both instruments: Arthrex, Inc.; Naples, FL).

above the cuff to retrieve the loop of suture. Alternatively, the suture can be separately retrieved by a grasper introduced through a different portal. The depth of the bite is 15-mm, which makes it ideal for passing medial row sutures in a double-row repair.

Because of its low profile, a ≤7 mm cannula can be used. One limb of the suture is retrieved through the cannula (in this case a lateral portal) (Fig. 2-37A). The suture limb is then placed into the lower jaw (Fig. 2-37B). The Scorpion is introduced through the cannula and the tissue grasped using the anterior grip (Fig. 2-37C). The proposed position is evaluated and tensioned. The posterior grip is then used to advance the needle and suture through the tissue (Fig. 2-37D). Releasing the posterior grip retracts the nitinol needle, leaving the suture loop (Fig. 2-37E). The Scorpion jaws are then opened by releasing the anterior grip and the suture is retrieved (Fig. 2-37F).

To retrieve the suture loop using the upper jaw of the Scorpion, it is easiest to ratchet a larger loop through the tissue before hooking the suture loop with the open upper jaw (Fig. 2-38).

In using the Scorpion, we try to limit needle activation to 15 times per needle to avoid potential fatigue fracture or breakage of the nitinol needle. It is important to be cognizant of the number of times the needle has been activated by ratcheting.

Needle Punch

The Needle Punch (Arthrex) requires the use of a special suture that has a malleable needle tip, which is used to penetrate the soft tissue. The needle tip, which is loaded into the lower jaw of the instrument, is controlled by a separate posterior grip on the back of the instrument similar to the Scorpion handle. The anterior grip controls closure of the jaws. The posterior grip is used to push the needle through the tissue (Fig. 2-39). The needle is then captured in a slot in the upper jaw, allowing self-retrieval of the needle and suture. The needle can only be used for a single passage. The depth of bite is 10 mm or 15 mm, depending on whether the standard needle punch or the long-jaw version is being used.

Previously the needle was only available on separate sutures, necessitating suture shuttling. Needle tips are now available preloaded on suture anchors, eliminating the need for shuttling sutures if a simple suture construct is used.

When using the Needle Punch, a 7-mm cannula can be used (in this case through a lateral portal). A 5-mm BioCorkscrew or BioCorkscrew-FT (Arthrex) suture anchor with needle-tipped suture will have already been placed. Then, one limb of the suture is retrieved through the lateral portal. The needle is loaded into the lower jaw of the instrument (Fig. 2-40A) and introduced through the lateral cannula. The needle punch is used to grasp the tissue and the proposed suture placement is evaluated (Fig. 2-40B). The needle is then advanced through the tissues by squeezing the posterior grip (Fig. 2-40C). The needle self-locks into the upper jaw, the jaw is opened and the suture is retrieved through the cannula.

Helpful Hint

When using the Viper or the Needle Punch suture-passing instruments, it is helpful to pull the other limb of the suture to remove any slack in the system. This limits potential suture tangling during suture passage. Do not hold on to the suture or place too much tension into the system, however, because excess tension or pulling on the other limb can prevent the suture from actually passing through the tissue. When using the Scorpion, do not pull all the slack

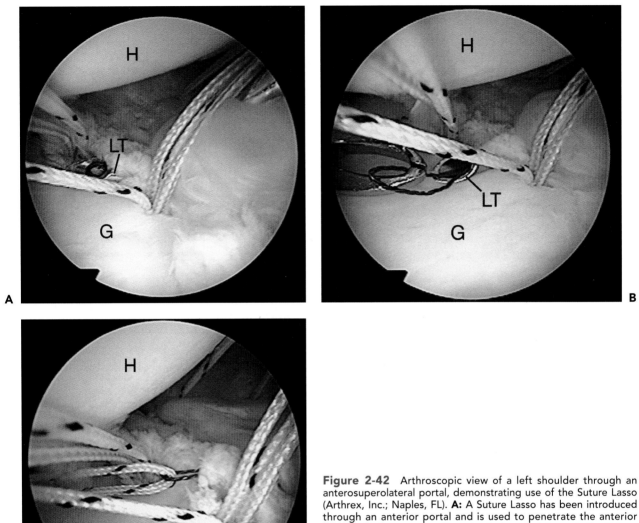

Figure 2-42 Arthroscopic view of a left shoulder through an anterosuperolateral portal, demonstrating use of the Suture Lasso (Arthrex, Inc.; Naples, FL). **A:** A Suture Lasso has been introduced through an anterior portal and is used to penetrate the anterior labrum. **B:** A suture-passing wire is then fed through the Suture Lasso, and the suture-passing wire and the suture limb to be passed are retrieved through the posterior portal. **C:** The suture limb is then fed through the loop of the suture-passing wire extracorporeally and the suture-passing wire is then pulled back through the soft tissues. The suture is thereby shuttled through the soft tissues and out the anterior cannula. G, glenoid; H, humeral head; LT, lasso tip.

out of the suture limb, or else the excess tension will cause the nitinol needle to bend excessively and the suture will not pass.

Shuttling Instruments

Shuttling instruments include the Suture Lasso (Arthrex) and the Banana Lasso. These instruments are available in a number of angles and directions to ensure a proper angle of approach (Fig. 2-41). These instruments require that they penetrate through the soft tissue structure first, (Fig. 2-42A), followed by passage of a suture-passing

wire or loop (Fig. 2-42B). The suture-passing wire and a suture limb are then retrieved through a separate portal and the suture limb is then fed through the loop of the suture-passing wire extracorporeally. By pulling on the suture-passing wire, the suture limb is then pulled back into the joint (Fig. 2-42C) and "shuttled" through the soft tissue and out the other cannula. When shuttling sutures, it is easiest to do this with only one suture limb in the cannula to avoid suture tangling. In addition, shuttling through a suture the same cannula and back on itself (i.e., 360° shuttle) can be difficult because of increased friction.

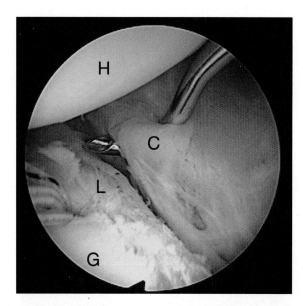

Figure 2-43 Arthroscopic view of a left shoulder through an anterosuperolateral portal demonstrating a suture anchor-based plication of the capsule to the labrum using the Suture Lasso (Arthrex, Inc.; Naples, FL) through an anterior portal. G, glenoid; H, humeral head; L, labrum, C, capsule.

Although these instruments can be universally used for all reconstructive procedures in the shoulder requiring suture passage, we find the Suture Lasso most useful during repair of the labrum and the Banana Lasso useful during rotator cuff repairs. The disadvantage of these instruments is that an extra step must be used (the shuttle) to pass the suture. These fine-tipped instruments are advantageous when performing procedures requiring "pinpoint" accuracy with minimal disruption to the soft tissue, however, because of their small-diameter tips. Furthermore, these instruments are advantageous when performing tissue repairs that require a significant change in the direction of the instrument, particularly if not in line with the cannula. Because of this feature, they are particularly useful in performing capsular plication of the capsule to the labrum (Fig. 2-43).

REFERENCES

1. Lo IK, Lind CC, Burkhart SS. Glenohumeral arthroscopy portals established using an outside-in technique: neurovascular anatomy at risk. *Arthroscopy.* 2004;20(6):596–602.
2. Nord KD, Mauck BM. The new subclavian portal and modified Neviaser portal for arthroscopic rotator cuff repair. *Arthroscopy.* 2003;19(9):1030–1034.

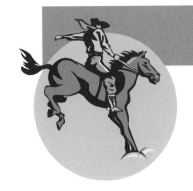

Creating a Stable Construct

3

COWBOY PRINCIPLE 3

A wishbone ain't no substitute for a backbone.

It has been said that there are two ways to do things—the easy way and the cowboy way. The cowboy way demands attention to detail and an emphasis on durability. After all, the cowboy's corrals have to securely hold 1,200-pound Longhorn steers. Building such structures on the woodless prairie with basic tools requires innovation, craftsmanship, conviction, perseverance, and a strong work ethic. The cowboy refers to this combination of traits as backbone, the quality that makes the cowboy as strong as the things he builds.

GENERAL PRINCIPLES

Most reconstructive shoulder procedures require a method of securing soft tissue to bone to create a stable construct. The future holds promise in augmenting and enhancing the soft tissue healing process biologically. However, it is essential that reconstructive surgery maximize the mechanical stability of the construct to allow biology to succeed. To accomplish the goal of optimized stability, a myriad of factors need to be considered. These are outlined below.

Bone Tunnels versus Suture Anchors

Traditional open surgical management of rotator cuff or Bankart repairs have relied on transosseous tunnels for secure soft tissue fixation to bone. Although historically this method has provided adequate fixation during open repairs, more recent studies suggest that failure through bone tunnels can occur, particular during rotator cuff repair. Mechanical studies by Burkhart et al. (1,2) demonstrated that, under cyclic loads, transosseous rotator cuff repair constructs failed at low cycles by cutting of the suture through bone. This failure was particularly common when the distal bone holes of transosseous tunnels exited through weak metaphyseal bone and not through thick, cortical bone (1–3).

In contrast, under cyclic loading, rotator cuff repair constructs secured using suture anchors did not fail by cutting of the suture through bone but by cutting of the suture through the tendon (1). Importantly, these failures occurred on average at higher cycles than similar transosseous repairs. Thus, by using suture anchors, the weak link was effectively transferred from the bone to the rotator cuff tendon (1,2).

Although using suture anchors increased the number of cycles to failure of rotator cuff repair constructs, all constructs did eventually fail. These constructs failed by a consistent pattern where the central portion of the cuff failed first, followed by the peripheral portions of the repair. In these constructs, the repair portion under greatest tension was the central portion of the tear and, thus, this area of the repair failed first because of tension overload (Fig. 3-1). Thus, when repairing a crescent-shaped tear, the bone bed should be prepared and the anchors placed so that minimal tension will be placed on the repair by respecting the crescent-shaped margin of the tear. This is particularly important if only a single row of suture anchors can be placed (Fig. 3-2).

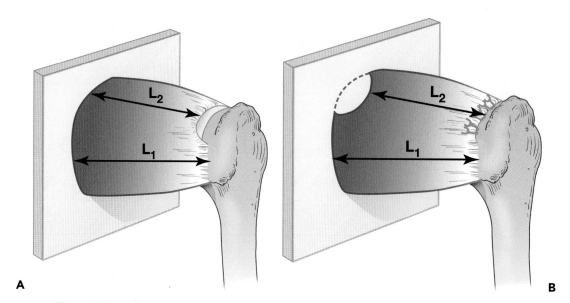

Figure 3-1 **A:** Diagrammatic representation of a rotator cuff tear. Muscle-tendon units are referenced to an arbitrary plane of origin through the medial scapula. The undisturbed muscle–tendon unit has a length L_1. The shortened muscle–tendon unit at the apex of the cuff tear has a length L_2, which is less than L_1. **B:** Repair of the rotator cuff defect in a straight line along the articular margin can only be accomplished by releasing the origin of the muscle–tendon units that comprise the defect and repairing the defect without undue tension, or by closing the defect under tension, thereby creating a "tension mismatch" between L_1 fibers and L_2 fibers.

Minimizing Soft Tissue Suture Cut Out: Distributing Load through Multiple Fixation Points

As stated above, suture anchor repair constructs under cyclic loading commonly fail by cutting of the suture through tendon. To minimize such an occurrence, various techniques have been used, including various "grasping type" sutures. Studies by Gerber et al. (4) suggest that a modified Mason Allen stitch secured the rotator cuff tendon to a bone trough better than other stitch configurations.

Complex "weaving" sutures (e.g., a modified Mason Allen stitch) may be predisposed to early failure during cyclic loading. This occurs secondary to "cinching" or tightening of the suture weave through the tendon as the cyclic loads are applied. As the suture weave tightens with each successive load, the suture loop, in fact, enlarges (i.e., loss of loop security) and the tendon begins to pull away from bone. An *in vitro* study by Petit et al. (5) has confirmed this failure mechanism whereby rotator cuff repair constructs that were secured using modified Mason Allen stitches failed by cinching of the complex weave and

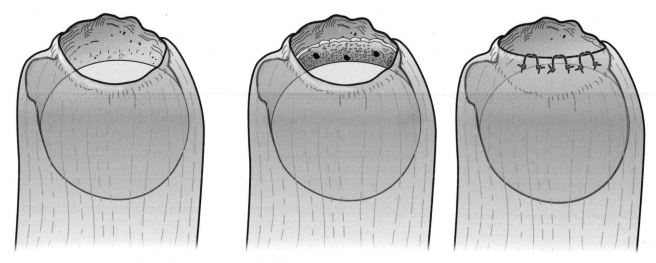

Figure 3-2 The bone bed of a crescent-shaped tear should be prepared so that the rotator cuff is repaired under minimal or no tension, by respecting to some extent the crescent-shaped margin of the tear. This is particularly important in single-row repairs.

pulling away of the tendon from bone. This failure occurred at fewer cycles to failure than those of constructs secured with simple stitches. Intuitively, this makes sense because to minimize the effect of cinching of a suture loop, the most efficient loop should be used—a simple stitch. Newer stitch configurations (e.g., the "Mac" stitch) may help minimize this cinching effect while maintaining the load-bearing capacity of the stitch (6).

One simple method of minimizing suture cut out through tendon is to increase the number of fixation points in the repair construct. This occurs because, with multiple fixation points, the load per fixation point is decreased and, thus, the load the soft tissue must resist to prevent cut out is similarly decreased. Because the number of suture anchors that can be placed in bone is limited by the size of the bone bed (and the size of the anchor), the best way to increase the number of fixation points in the repair constructs is to increase the number of sutures (7). This can be easily accomplished by using double-loaded suture anchors.

For example, consider the case of a 4-cm (in anterior to posterior length) crescent-shaped rotator cuff tear that subtends the rotator crescent and is subjected to a maximal muscle force contraction. Because the average cross-sectional area of the supraspinatus and infraspinatus muscles is 8.8-cm^2 and the maximal contraction of muscle per unit area is 3.5-kg/cm^2, the maximal muscle contraction force across the rotator cuff tear is 302 N (8,9). Suppose the rotator cuff tear is repaired by three suture anchors, 1 cm apart. If each anchor has one suture, then there are a total of five fixation points (three by suture, two by tendon-to-bone insertions) that equally share the load of 302 N (Fig. 3-3A). In this case, each suture–rotator cuff interface must resist a load of 60.4 N. If each anchor is double loaded with two sutures, however, eight fixation points exist (six by suture, two by tendon-to-bone insertions) to share the load (Fig. 3-3B). In this situation, each suture–rotator cuff interface needs only to resist a 37.7 N load, clearly a more advantageous situation. This enhanced load resistance is particularly relevant in rotator cuff repairs where tendon tissue can be significantly weakened by degeneration. Furthermore, not only does double-loading suture anchors decrease the risk of suture cutting through tendon, it also minimizes failure of suture loop constructs by knot slippage or knot breakage (7).

CHOOSING AN ANCHOR: DIFFERENTIATING CHARACTERISTICS

On the market today are an endless number of anchors for soft tissue fixation to bone, making choosing an anchor a difficult and perplexing task. In addition, because most anchors have sufficient pull-out strength (superior to the maximal failure force of other points along the construct [e.g., suture strength, tendon strength]) for clinical usage, particularly when placed at an appropriate deadman angle (see below), pull-out strength alone is not an adequate criterion for choosing an anchor (10,11). As long as the anchors are double loaded or can accept at least two sutures, then what characteristic is to be used to differentiate and discriminate between anchors?

Recently, the effect of suture anchor design on suture abrasion has been studied by Bardana et al. (12) and ourselves (13). Our interest in suture abrasion was precipitated by the occurrence of suture breakage, both experimentally and clinically, during rotator cuff repair (1). Despite the fact that the most commonly used suture, #2 Ethibond (Ethicon, Somerville, NJ), should be strong enough to resist predicted *in vivo* forces (mean ultimate tensile strength = 128 N) (14), breakage of Ethibond suture commonly continues to occur, even during the repair itself.

One possible explanation for this inconsistency is abrasive wear (with partial fiber failure) of the suture during arthroscopic surgery, which decreases the suture's breaking strength. Suture abrasion can occur during suture passage (e.g., inadvertent suture damage by sharp instruments) or during arthroscopic knot tying. During arthroscopic knot tying, abrasion can occur as the result of suture sliding through the anchor eyelet, suture abrading against bone, suture sliding through the knot pusher, or at the actual knot site.

Suture abrasion by the anchor eyelet can be particularly magnified during tying of arthroscopic sliding knots. After tying an arthroscopic sliding knot extracorporeally, the post limb is pulled to draw the sliding knot into the joint. To accomplish this, however, the suture must slide through the anchor eyelet and, therefore, can be subjected to abrasion.

To investigate the potential role of suture abrasion, Bardana et al. (12) and Lo et al. (13) cycled #2 Ethibond suture under load through various suture anchor eyelets until the suture catastrophically failed (Fig. 3-4). Both these studies consistently observed that metal anchors

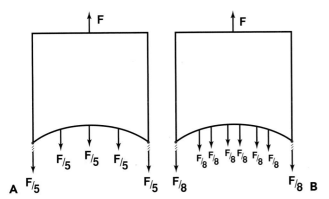

Figure 3-3 **A:** With one suture per anchor there are five fixation points for a three-anchor construct. **B:** With two sutures per anchor there are eight fixation points for a three-anchor construct.

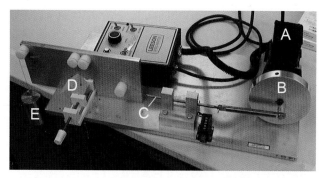

Figure 3-4 Abrasion testing apparatus. Electronically controlled motor *(A)*, wheel *(B)*, plunger *(C)*, polyurethane block containing anchor *(D)*, and weight *(E)*. Note: The construct is being tested at a 45° suture–anchor angle.

produced significantly more suture abrasion than polymer biodegradable anchors. Furthermore, orienting the metal anchor eyelet at an angle to the suture (e.g., a 45° angle between the suture and suture anchor) or rotating the anchor eyelet (e.g., rotating the anchor 90° to the suture) produced significantly more suture abrasion and decreased the number of cycles to failure to worrisome levels (e.g., #2 Ethibond mean cycle to failure using Corkscrew anchor [Arthrex, Inc.; Naples, FL] angled 45°: 7.4 cycles; range: 3–17 cycles; Fig. 3-5).

When using biodegradable anchors, however, the results (12,13) were different and were related to the design of the suture eyelet itself. For example, the 5.0-mm Corkscrew anchor contains a standard metallic suture eyelet. The 5.0-mm BioCorkscrew (Arthrex) suture anchor eyelet, however, is distinctly different. This anchor is

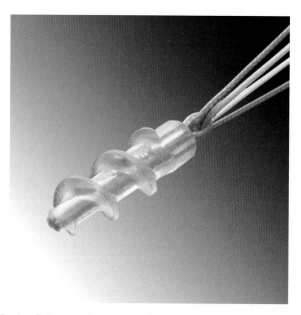

Figure 3-6 A 5.0-mm BioCorkscrew suture anchor (Arthrex, Inc.; Naples, FL). Note: The eyelet, which consists of #5 polyester suture insert molded into the anchor, can accommodate two sutures.

designed with an eyelet consisting of a flexible loop of #5 polyester suture that is insert-molded into the body of the anchor (Fig. 3-6). This design, theoretically, should decrease abrasion in comparison to metallic suture eyelets because the flexible loop should not be affected by anchor angle or rotation. This hypothesis was confirmed in both studies where the BioCorkscrew anchor demonstrated no significant differences with respect to orientation

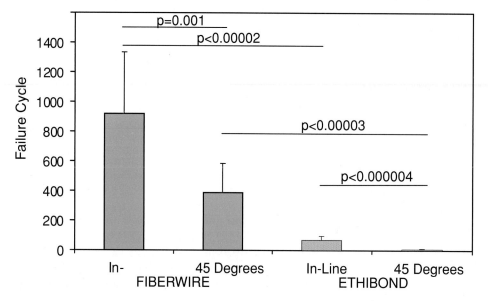

Figure 3-5 Abrasion resistance of #2 FiberWire (■) Arthrex and #2 Ethibond (■) (Ethicon, Inc.) using the 5.0-mm Corkscrew anchor (Arthrex) at different suture-anchor angles. Note: Lines denote significant differences between groups.

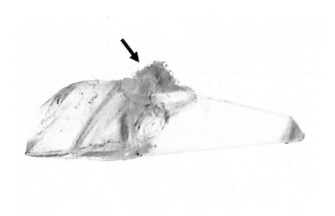

Figure 3-7 Photograph of the failure mechanism during abrasion testing of the Panalok RC-suture construct by cutting of the suture through the biodegradable anchor eyelet (*arrow*), which is a hole in the body of the anchor.

and the suture failed at significantly higher cycles when compared with similar metallic anchors (12,13). More recently, we have been using the fully threaded (BioCorkscrew-FT; Arthrex, Inc.), which has the added advantage of greater pullout because the threads extend from the top to the bottom of the anchor.

Other biodegradable anchor designs did not fare as well. One common method of biodegradable anchor design incorporates a hole through the polymer body of the anchor to form the suture eyelet. This design is a feature of the Panalok RC anchor (Mitex, Inc.), the 3.5-mm Panalok anchor, and other anchors. Surprisingly, in all cases of this design that we tested, these constructs failed by cutting of the Ethibond suture through the suture eyelet (12,13) (Fig. 3-7) and at low cycles (Panalok RC mean cycle to failure: 11.2; 3.5-mm Panalok mean cycle to failure: 12.5) (13), suggesting that the polymer was the weakest part of the construct.

The suture loop eyelet is advantageous because it is strong (i.e., stronger than comparable eyelets made through polymer), causes less suture abrasion than metal anchors, is unaffected by eyelet orientation or rotation, and clinically causes less fouling of sutures even though it is double loaded. For these reasons we prefer to use the BioCorkscrew-FT, BioFASTak, and BioSutureTak suture anchors (Arthrex).

CHOOSING A SUTURE

Once an anchor has been chosen, the suture to be loaded on the anchor needs to be considered. Many anchors come preloaded with suture material produced by the manufacturer of the anchor. In many cases, the suture provided may be an inferior product. When considering the suture type to be used, it is important to consider various characteristics, including whether permanent or resorbable suture will be used, suture size, suture abrasion effect, tying ease, and the suture's effect on knot performance.

Although resorbable suture has been used by others (e.g., polydiaxanone suture), we prefer to simulate an open reconstruction and use permanent suture when performing reconstructive shoulder arthroscopy. Furthermore, the routine reliance on rates of suture absorption is worrisome, particularly when considering rotator cuff repair healing rates and potential complications of synovitis, chondrolysis, and capsulitis. To avoid these concerns, we use #2 FiberWire (Arthrex) permanent sutures.

Although #2 Ethibond was previously our suture of choice, a recent explosion of interest has occurred in the use of suture formed in part by polyethylene. The first polyethylene suture available to the arthroscopist was FiberWire. This composite suture is formed by a core of polyethylene that provides the major strength characteristics of the suture and an outer sleeve of polyester that provides the "feel" and tying characteristics of the suture. This suture is available in both #2 and #5 sizes. More recently, other sutures have become available on the market including OrthoCord (DePuy Mitek; polydiaxanone and polyethylene), Herculine (Linvatec, ultra high molecular weight polyethylene), MaxBraid (Arthrotek; ultra high molecular weight polyethylene), UltraBraid (Smith & Nephew; polyethylene with and without a monofilament polypropylene marker), and ForceFiber (Stryker; ultra high molecular weight polyethylene). The last four suture types are essentially the same because they are all produced from Dyneema, a braided ultra high molecular weight polyethylene, which is highly oriented and highly crystalline. These last four suture types are merely marketed differently through various companies. All the new generation sutures are considered advantageous because they have strength characteristics that far surpass those of Ethibond.

Recently, we (13) studied the effect of suture type on various characteristics, including suture abrasion and knot characteristics. We compared the most commonly used standard suture, #2 Ethibond with #2 FiberWire. Interestingly, #2 FiberWire failed at significantly higher cycles when compared with #2 Ethibond under all tested abrasion conditions even when using metallic anchors (see Fig. 3-5). In fact, #2 FiberWire failed at cycles 5 to 51 times greater than #2 Ethibond (Fig. 3-8). These cycles were so high that it is likely that when using #2 FiberWire, abrasion from the suture eyelet is clinically irrelevant (Fig. 3-9).

Furthermore, tying sliding knots (e.g., Roeder knot) secured with three reversing half-hitches on alternating posts (RHAP) or a surgeon's knot (see below for a complete description and discussion of various arthroscopic knots), using #2 FiberWire significantly increased the maximal force to failure when compared with the same knot tied with #2 Ethibond (range: 24.4% to 92.0% increase; $p < 0.01$), suggesting that in addition to superior abrasion resistance, #2 FiberWire also enhances knot security (for a

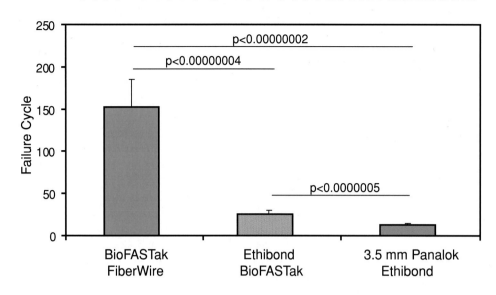

Figure 3-8 Abrasion resistance of #2 FiberWire (■)(Arthrex Inc.; Naples, FL) and #2 Ethibond (■) (Ethicon, Inc.) using the 3.0-mm BioFASTak anchor (Arthrex) and the 3.5-mm Panalok anchor (■)(Mitek, Inc.). Note: Lines denote significant differences between groups.

complete discussion of knot security and tying knots, see the discussion below) (14). When comparing FiberWire with other newer polyethylene sutures (e.g., OrthoCord, Herculine, MaxBraid, UltraBraid), # 2 FiberWire still outperformed all other sutures with superior maximal force to failure ($p < 0.001$) (Fig. 3-10) and comparable loop circumference ($p > 0.05$)(when tying a static surgeon's knot, Roeder knot, or Weston knot) (Fig. 3-11) (15).

For these reasons we continue to use #2 FiberWire double loaded on the BioFASTak, BioSutureTak, BioCorkscrew, or BioCorkscrew-FT suture anchors for all of our arthroscopic shoulder reconstructions.

ANCHOR INSERTION

Maximizing Pullout: The Deadman Analogy

A suture anchor should be inserted into bone at the optimal angle to maximize its pull-out strength. Suture anchors used for shoulder reconstruction function in the same way that a "deadman" functions to support a corner fence post on a South Texas ranch (16). A deadman is a large rock that is buried approximately 3 feet under the ground. Attached to this rock is a wire that extends through the ground to the top of the post and serves to support the

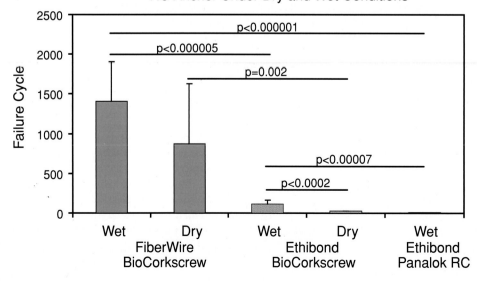

Figure 3-9 Abrasion resistance of #2 FiberWire (■) (Arthrex, Inc.; Naples, FL) and #2 Ethibond (■) (Ethicon, Inc.) using the 5.0-mm BioCorkscrew anchor (Arthrex) and the Panalok RC anchor (Mitek, Inc.) under dry and wet conditions. Note: Lines denote significant differences between groups.

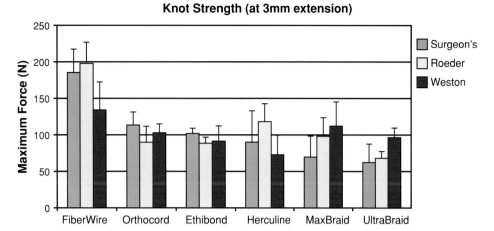

Figure 3-10 Maximal force to failure of three different arthroscopic knots tied with various #2 suture types. FiberWire (Arthrex, Inc.; Naples, FL) provided the maximal force to failure when tying the surgeon's knot ($p <$ 0.001) and the Roeder knot (p <0.001) when compared with all other suture types. When tying a Weston knot, only #2 FiberWire was significantly greater than Herculine ($p = 0.001$).

corner fence post as a guywire. In the deadman analogy, the suture anchor is represented by the rock, the suture is represented by the guywire, and the soft tissue (in this case the compressed rotator cuff tissue beneath the suture) is represented by the corner fence post (Fig. 3-12).

When placing a corner fence post, all good ranchers know that there is an ideal angle that the guywire must make with the ground. This angle is ≤45°. If the "deadman" angle is >45°, the corner fence post will lean. Similarly, the optimal suture insertion angle can be determined. In this situation, two angles must be considered: the angle that the suture makes with the perpendicular to the anchor (Θ_1, the pull-out angle) and the angle that the suture makes with the direction of pull of the rotator cuff (Θ_2, the tension-reduction angle) (Fig. 3-13).

Thus, Θ_1 (defined as the angle that the suture makes with the perpendicular to the anchor) is the pull-out angle of the anchor. Intuitively, the more acute the angle Θ_1, the more difficult it will be to pull out the anchor. Furthermore, as Θ_2 decreases, so does the tension in the suture. A low Θ_2 angle, therefore, is also advantageous by protecting against suture breakage because it lowers the tension in the suture when compared with a high Θ_2 angle. Clinically, these theoretical findings suggest that suture anchors should be inserted at an angle toward the free margin of the rotator cuff and that the suture

from the anchor should make an acute angle with the direction of pull of the rotator cuff.

TYING A SECURE ARTHROSCOPIC KNOT

After inserting the anchor and passing the sutures, a method must be used to close the loop. Despite recent advances in knotless technology and suture welding, tissue fixation by tying an arthroscopic knot is, and likely will remain, the most common method of soft tissue fixation. Arthroscopic knots are generally formed outside the joint with the suture already having been passed through the anchoring device and tissue to be repaired. The difficulty for most novice arthroscopic surgeons is the endless selection of knot configurations that can be tied, and choosing a knot generally has been based on surgeon preference rather than scientific investigation. This overabundance of choice has confused and complicated an already confusing topic.

UNDERSTANDING ARTHROSCOPIC KNOTS

When tying an arthroscopic knot, there are two limbs of the suture called the post limb and the wrapping limb. The post

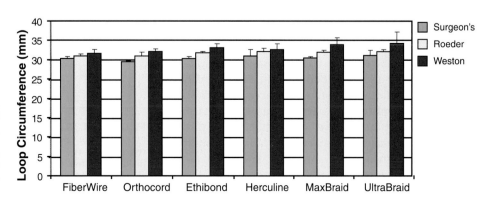

Figure 3-11 Loop circumference of three different types of arthroscopic knots tied with various #2 suture types. FiberWire (Arthrex, Inc.; Naples, FL) had comparable loop circumference to the other high-strength sutures, and had significantly better knot security.

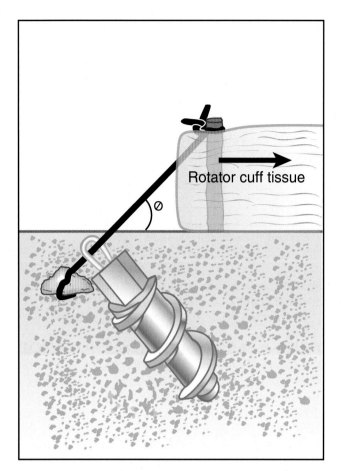

Figure 3-12 Analogy of the deadman system to the suture–anchor rotator cuff system. The deadman is analogous to the suture anchor; the deadman wire is analogous to the suture; the pull of the fence wire on the corner post is analogous to the pull of the rotator cuff; and the fence post is analogous to the compressed rotator cuff tissue between the suture and the bone (Θ, deadman angle).

the complex "weave" of the two suture limbs relative to one another, can be increased by increasing the complexity of the weave and increasing the length of contact between the suture limbs. Slack between throws decreases knot security. Slack between throws can be decreased by removing any twists between the two suture limbs before seating a half-hitch (Fig. 3-16) and by past pointing (Fig. 3-17). Loop security is the ability to maintain a tight suture loop as a knot is tied (7,17). Thus, it is possible for any tied knot to have good knot security but poor loop security (e.g., a loose suture loop) and, therefore, be ineffective in approximating the tissue edges to be repaired, creating an unstable construct (Fig. 3-18).

Knot Classification

Knots are generally classified into nonsliding (static) knots and sliding knots. Nonsliding knots are generally

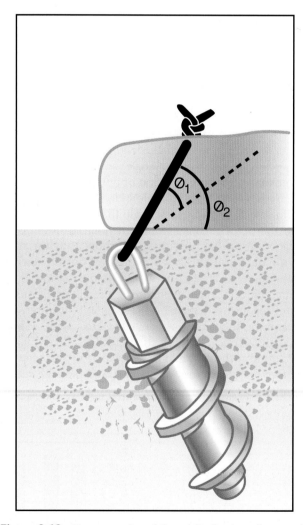

Figure 3-13 Representation of Θ_1 and Θ_2. Θ_1, the pull-out angle for the anchor (angle the suture makes with the perpendicular to the anchor); Θ_2, the tension-reduction angle (angle the suture makes with the rotator cuff pull direction). Ideally, Θ_1 and Θ_2 should both be ≤45°.

limb is the straight portion of the suture and this limb is purely defined as the suture limb that is under the most tension (Fig. 3-14). Because arthroscopic knots are formed outside the body, they are generally slid along the straight post limb. The wrapping limb is the portion of the other suture limb that wraps around the post limb, creating the knot.

A knot consists of two portions: the knot proper and the loop. The knot proper is composed of the wrappings and the post that is contained within the wrappings, whereas the loop is defined as the loop portion of the suture distal to the knot proper that encircles the soft tissue (Fig. 3-15).

For a knot to be effective, it must possess the attributes of both knot security and loop security. Knot security is defined as the effectiveness of the knot at resisting slippage when load is applied and is dependent on three factors: friction, internal interference, and slack between throws (7). Friction is greater for knots tied with braided multifilament suture than for comparable knots tied with monofilament suture. Internal interference, which refers to

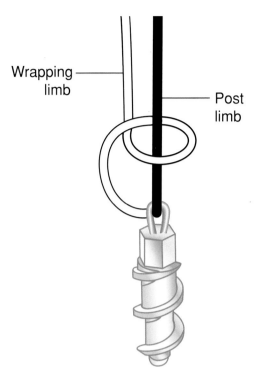

Figure 3-14   Schematic diagram representing a half-hitch with a post limb and wrapping limb.

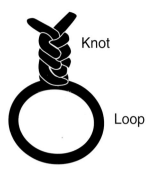

Figure 3-15   Schematic diagram representing a knot with a loop that would encircle tissue.

composed of a stack of half-hitches and are the only knots that can be used in situations when the suture does not slide through the tissue and anchoring device. A nonsliding knot can always be tied, however, whether the suture slides or not because tying a nonsliding knot avoids the theoretic disadvantages of suture abrasion, anchor abrasion, or damaging the soft tissue. The most commonly used nonsliding knots are the Revo knot as popularized by Snyder and the 6-throw surgeon's knot, the knot we prefer to tie (Fig. 3-19).

Sliding knots can only be used when the suture slides easily through the anchoring device and tissue. These knots are preferred by some surgeons because the complete knot is tied extracoporeally and the knot can be slid down the post limb without unraveling or jamming prematurely, in most cases. Commonly used sliding knots include the Duncan loop, Tennessee slider, Nicky's knot, Roeder knot, SMC (Samsung Medical Center) knot, and the Weston knot (Fig. 3-20).

Half-Hitches

The half-hitch, which is the simplest of all knots to tie, is formed by wrapping the suture limb once around the post. Two basic types of half-hitches (i.e., over-under and under-over) are used, which are named according to the position of the wrapping limb relative to the post limb as viewed by the surgeon during knot tying (Fig. 3-21). Although only two basic half-hitch configurations exist, when tying successive half-hitches several more variables can be introduced.

The simplest way to tie successive half-hitches is to throw a half-hitch in the same direction along the same

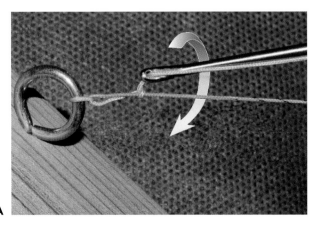
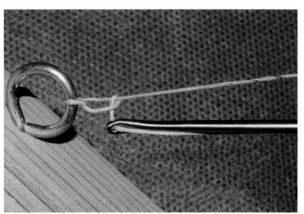

A   B

Figure 3-16   Clinical photo with a single-diameter knot pusher. Twists between throws **(A)** should be removed by looping the tip of the knot pusher around the post suture, so that the knot will lay flat **(B)**.

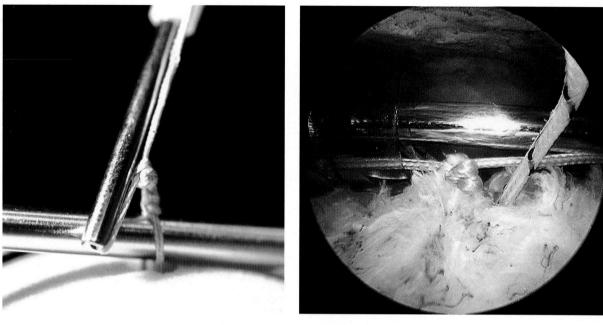

Figure 3-17 **A:** Clinical photo demonstrating past pointing. **B:** Arthroscopic photo demonstrating past pointing.

suture limb as the post (Fig. 3-22A). Because the two half-hitches are in the same direction, they will not "lock" and act as a sliding knot. By changing the direction of the half-hitch (i.e., over-under to under-over), called reversing the half-hitch, the knot will now not easily slide because of increased internal interference of the knot (Fig. 3-22B). In addition, the same-direction half-hitch can be thrown, but the other suture limb is used as the post (this is called alternating the post or flipping the post) (Fig. 3-22C) or the half-hitch can be reversed and serve as an alternating post for the next throw (Fig. 3-22D). The more convoluted the weave of suture, the greater the internal interference and the greater the knot security. Thus, it is common to secure

or lock any arthroscopic knot with a series of three RHAP (reversing half-hitches on alternating posts) (Fig. 3-23). In fact, locking any base knot (sliding or nonsliding) with three RHAP has been shown to change a knot's mode of failure from knot slippage to suture breakage (when using monofilament or Ethibond suture), demonstrating that knot security in the construct has been maximized.

Tying Stacked Half-Hitches
The drawback to tying stacked half-hitches with a standard single-diameter knot pusher is that the first half-hitch has a tendency to loosen while the second half-hitch is being thrown (Fig. 3-24A). This can be particularly concerning if

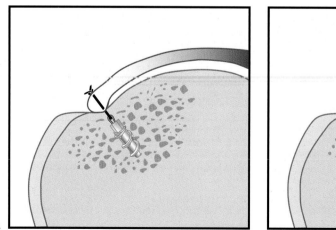
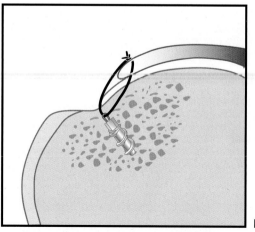

Figure 3-18   Loop security. **A:** A tight suture loop holds the soft tissue tightly apposed to the prepared bone bed. **B:** A loose loop allows the soft tissue to pull away from the prepared bone bed, regardless of how securely the knot is tied.

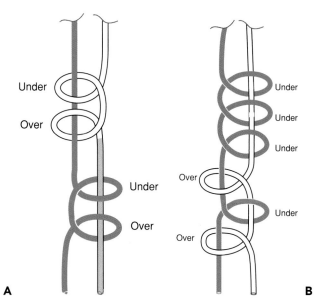

Figure 3-19 Schematic drawing demonstrating Revo knot **(A)** and surgeon's knot **(B)**.

the second half-hitch is on the opposite post because the knot could lock prematurely, resulting in a loose loop and loss of loop security (Fig. 3-24B). One way to minimize the chance of loosening of the loop is to stack three half-hitches on the same post initially as a base knot so that sufficient internal interference prevents the loop from loosening as the three RHAP are applied on top of the base knot to lock it.

Another method of tying stacked half-hitches is to use a double-diameter knot pusher [Surgeon's Sixth Finger (Arthrex)]. This instrument is formed by an inner metal knot pusher and an outer plastic sleeve (Fig. 3-25). When using this instrument to tie half-hitches, the suture (usually the suture limb on the tissue side) is threaded through the cannulated inner metal knot pusher and out the proximal portion of the instrument (Fig. 3-26A). Any excess suture is wrapped around the fingers of one hand (Fig. 3-26B) to apply any needed tension (Fig. 3-26C) when tying the knot. The free hand is used to throw successive half-hitches around the knot pusher. We prefer using the dominant hand to throw these half-hitches (Fig. 3-26D). With this knot pusher, the outer plastic sleeve is used to push the half-hitch into the shoulder. After the initial half-hitch has been placed, the inner metal knot pusher is used to hold the first half-hitch in place as subsequent half-hitches are thrown and pushed into the joint using the outer plastic sleeve (Fig. 3-26E). In addition, to remove twists using the Surgeon's Sixth Finger, the outer plastic sleeve and the inner metal tube are rotated so that the knot will lay flat without any slack between throws (Fig. 3-27). Thus, the use of the Surgeon's Sixth Finger can maximize both loop and knot security.

Using the Surgeon's Sixth Finger knot pusher does require dedicated practice. Once mastered, however, it is an easy, reproducible and incredibly quick method of tying secure half-hitches. When mastered, this method is so

effective that mechanical studies have demonstrated superior loop security in comparison to comparable knots tied with a single-diameter knot pusher, or even hand-tied knots (Fig. 3-28) (17).

Reversing the Half-Hitch and Alternating Posts without Rethreading

Every knot, whether a stacked half-hitch knot or a sliding knot, should be locked with a series of three reversing half-hitches on alternating posts. One method to do this is to rethread the knot pusher after each throw. This can be a time-consuming process, however. Instead, the half-hitch can be reversed and the post alternated by tensioning the wrapping limb, thereby flipping the post and reversing the throw (Fig. 3-29) (see Chapter 8, *Gaining Speed and Tricks of the Trade*, for a complete discussion of reversing the half-hitch and alternating the post without rethreading).

Sliding Knots

The most common sliding knots are the Duncan loop, Nicky's knot, Tennessee slider, Roeder knot, SMC knot, and Weston knot (see Fig. 3-20). These knots can be further divided into nonlocking sliding knots (Duncan loop) (Fig. 3-30A), and locking sliding knots (Nicky's knot, Tennessee slider, Roeder knot, SMC knot, Weston knot) (Fig. 3-30B-C). Locking knots are advantageous because they can be flipped or locked to prevent backing off of the knot, whereas nonlocking knots can back off if the repair is under tension. Locking is performed by pulling on the wrapping limb, which kinks the post and prevents the knot from backing off. Locking knots can be further divided into proximal locking, middle locking, and distal locking knots, according to where within the suture weave the post is kinked during locking. Proximal locking knots include the Nicky's knot (see Fig. 3-30B), middle locking knots (where locking occurs halfway between the proximal and distal ends of the knot) include the Tennessee slider and SMC knot, and distal locking knots include the Roeder knot and Weston knot (see Fig. 3-30C). Nonlocking knots (Duncan loop) resist slippage by the tight grip of the wrappings around the post (see Fig. 3-30A).

When tying a sliding knot, the post should be kept short and the wrapping limb, as seen extracorpoteally, should be kept approximately half the total length of the suture. This is done so that the two limbs will be approximately equal in length when the sliding knot is delivered into the joint. This equalization of suture limb length occurs because as the knot slides into the joint, the knot takes the wrapping limb with it, shortening it while the post limb lengthens.

Choosing a Knot: Optimizing Loop Security and Knot Security

For a knot to be effective, it must possess the attributes of both knot security and loop security. The security of various

Text continues on page 48.

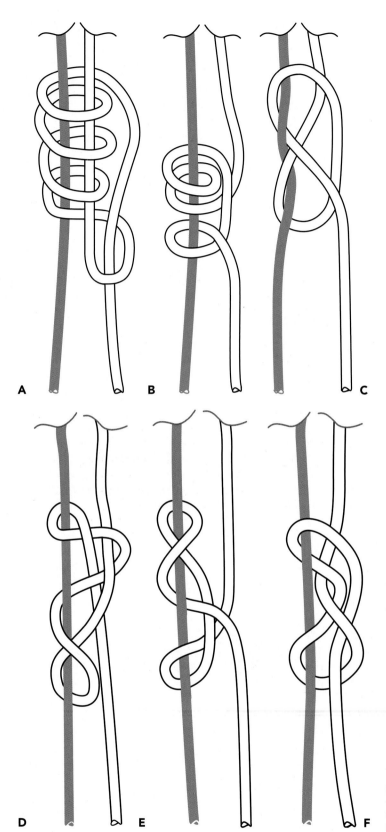

Figure 3-20 Schematic drawing demonstrating modified Duncan loop **(A)**, Nicky's knot **(B)**, Tennessee slider **(C)**, Roeder knot **(D)**, SMC (Samsung Medical Center) knot **(E)**, and Weston knot **(F)**.

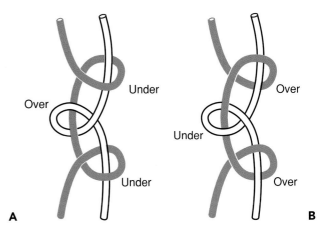

Figure 3-21 Schematic drawing demonstrating half-hitches: over-under **(A)** and under-over **(B)**.

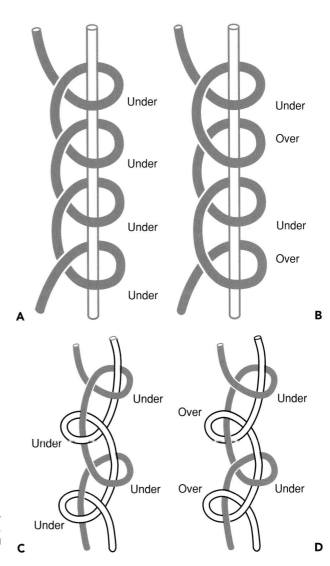

Figure 3-22 Schematic drawing demonstrating successive half-hitches. Same throw, same post **(A)**, reverse throw, same post **(B)**, same throw, alternating post **(C)**, and reverse throw, alternating post **(D)**.

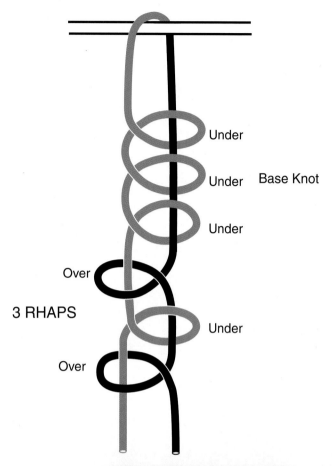

Under

Under   Base Knot

Under

Over

3 RHAPS

Under

Over

Figure 3-23 Schematic drawing of base arthroscopic knot locked with three reversing half-hitches on alternating posts (RHAP).

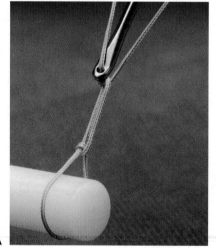

A

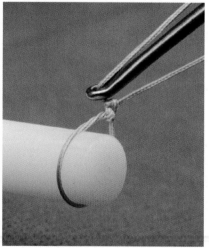

B

Figure 3-24 Clinical photo demonstrating serial half-hitches tied with a single diameter knot pusher. **A:** As the second half-hitch is being thrown, the first half-hitch has a tendency to back off, causing loss of loop security. **B:** A second half-hitch can prematurely lock the knot, resulting in a loose loop and loss of loop security.

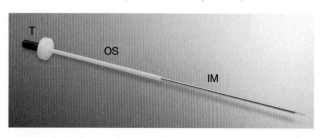

T

OS

IM

Figure 3-25 Clinical photo of the Surgeon's Sixth Finger (Arthrex, Inc.; Naples, FL) double-diameter knot pusher. Note: The inner metal knot pusher with an outer plastic sleeve. The inner metal knot pusher is cannulated. T, threader; OS, outer sleeve; IM, inner metal knot pusher.

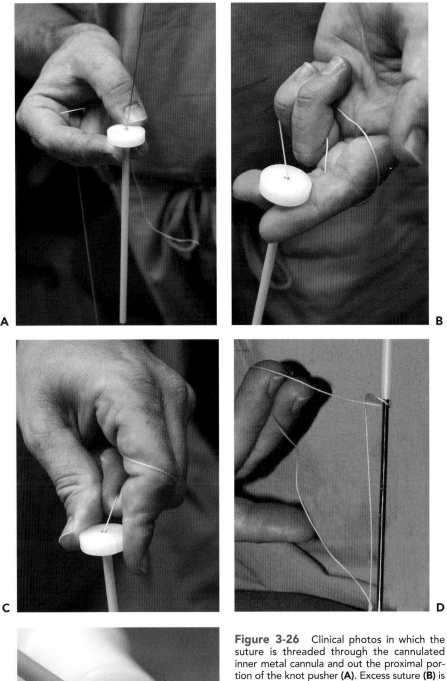

Figure 3-26 Clinical photos in which the suture is threaded through the cannulated inner metal cannula and out the proximal portion of the knot pusher (**A**). Excess suture (**B**) is wrapped around the fingers of one hand (**C**) to apply and release tension by pulling or pushing against the plastic disk at the proximal end of the knot pusher. The middle finger acts as a "pulley" to increase or decrease tension in the post suture. The opposite hand is used to throw successive half-hitches around the inner metal knot pusher (**D**). As the plastic sleeve is used to push successive half-hitches down the inner metal tube of the knot pusher, the tip of the inner metal tube is used to hold the initial half-hitch securely while the left hand maintains tension in the post suture (**E**). This ensures a tight loop and maximizes loop security.

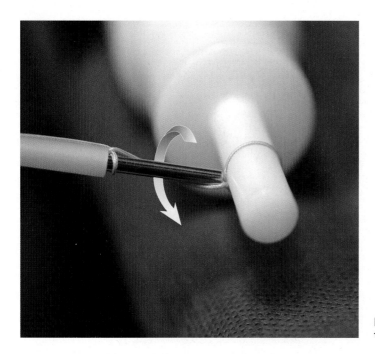

Figure 3-27   Clinical photo demonstrating untwisting of the half-hitch by rotating the two parts of the knot pusher.

arthroscopic knots has previously been investigated extensively. To determine the optimal knot configuration to be tied, it is important to consider both loop security and knot security. A recent study (14) by the authors evaluated a static surgeon's knot and six commonly used arthroscopic sliding knots (Duncan loop, Nicky's knot, Tennessee slider, Roeder knot, SMC knot, Weston knot) with and without a series of three RHAP. All knots were tied using #2 Ethibond over a 30-mm circumference post to create a suture loop of ~30 mm.

Using a previously validated protocol, each knot was mounted on an MTS (Material Testing System) machine and loop security was defined by the suture loop circumference at a 5 N preload. Because all knots were tied over a 30-mm circumference post, the closer the loop circumference was to 30 mm, the better the loop security. Knot security was measured as the maximal force to failure at 3 mm of crosshead displacement.

The results of the study are summarized in Figures 3-31 and 3-32. These figures demonstrate that both loop security and knot security were important criteria in determining the optimal knot configuration. The static surgeon's knot provided the highest force to failure and the tightest loop circumference (102.8 N ± 11.5 N; 30.51 ± 0.17 mm) and, thus, was the optimal knot in comparison to all the combinations of knots tested.

In choosing to tie a sliding knot, the other sliding knots must be considered. As can be seen in Figures 3-31 and 3-32, all sliding knots tied without RHAP demonstrated low force to failure (all force to failures <74.1 N) and loose suture loops (all loops >32.5 mm). Our conclusion is that sliding knots should not be tied without RHAP.

The addition of three RHAP improved knot security (range: 46.3% to 1,689.5 % increase; all p <0.0001) and, in most cases, improved loop security of sliding knots (four of six knots; p <0.03) (see Figs 3-31 and 3-32). Although several of these sliding knots with RHAP had adequate knot security for clinical usage, the Roeder knot with RHAP demonstrated the best balance of loop security and knot security (99.5 N ± 9.7 N; 30.66 ± 0.42 mm) and was similar to the surgeon's knot. The Roeder knot was considered the optimal sliding knot to be tied.

Interestingly, tying sliding knots with RHAPs or a surgeon's knot using #2 FiberWire significantly increased the maximal force to failure when compared with the same

Text continues on page 52.

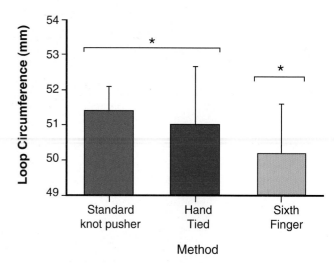

Figure 3-28   Bar graph shows that the Surgeon's Sixth Finger knot pusher forms a loop that is significantly smaller than those formed by a standard single-hole knot pusher or by hand. This smaller loop circumference is a measure of improved loop security. Groups under the same line are not significantly different. (p >0.05).

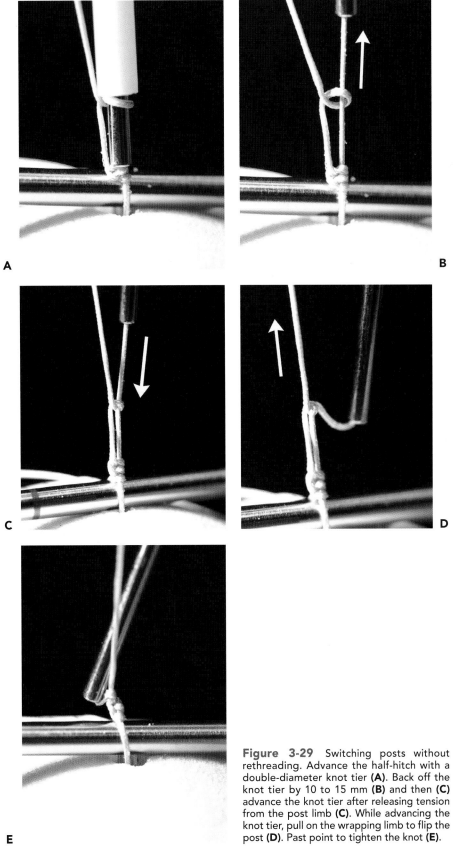

Figure 3-29 Switching posts without rethreading. Advance the half-hitch with a double-diameter knot tier **(A)**. Back off the knot tier by 10 to 15 mm **(B)** and then **(C)** advance the knot tier after releasing tension from the post limb **(C)**. While advancing the knot tier, pull on the wrapping limb to flip the post **(D)**. Past point to tighten the knot **(E)**.

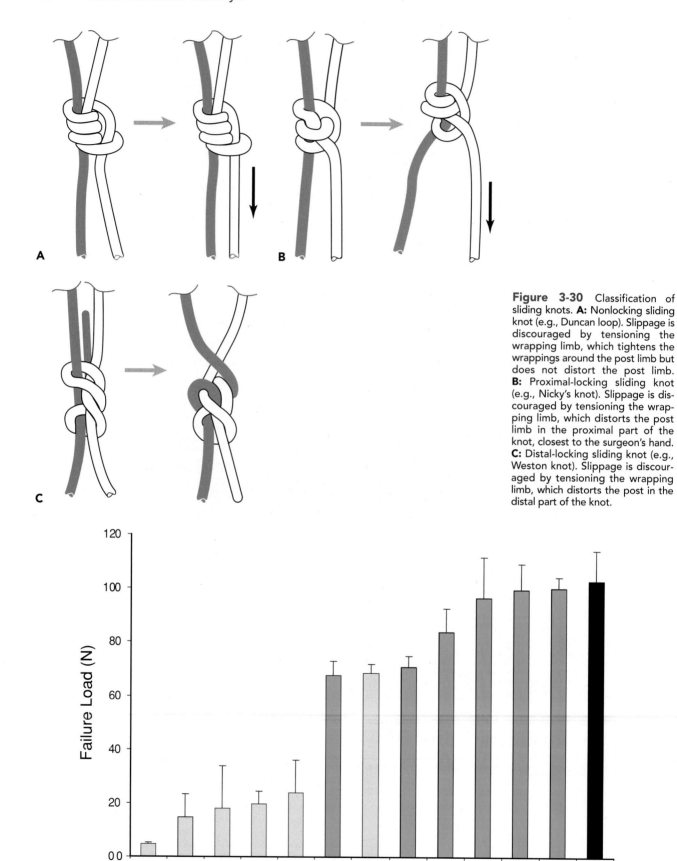

Figure 3-30 Classification of sliding knots. **A:** Nonlocking sliding knot (e.g., Duncan loop). Slippage is discouraged by tensioning the wrapping limb, which tightens the wrappings around the post limb but does not distort the post limb. **B:** Proximal-locking sliding knot (e.g., Nicky's knot). Slippage is discouraged by tensioning the wrapping limb, which distorts the post limb in the proximal part of the knot, closest to the surgeon's hand. **C:** Distal-locking sliding knot (e.g., Weston knot). Slippage is discouraged by tensioning the wrapping limb, which distorts the post in the distal part of the knot.

Figure 3-31 Maximal force to failure of sliding knots with (■) and without (□) reversing half-hitches on alternating posts (RHAP) and the surgeon's knot (■) using #2 Ethibond (Arthrex, Inc.; Naples, FL). Tenn, Tennessee slider; SMC, Samsung Medical Center knot.

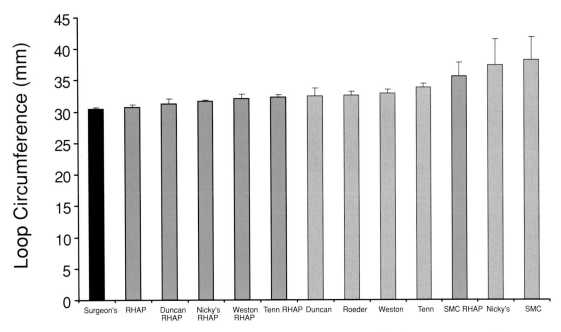

Figure 3-32 Loop circumference of sliding knots tied with (■) and without (▨) reversing half-hitches on alternating posts (RHAP) and the surgeon's knot (■) using #2 Ethibond (Arthrex, Inc.; Naples, FL). Tenn, Tennessee slider; SMC, Samsung Medical Center.

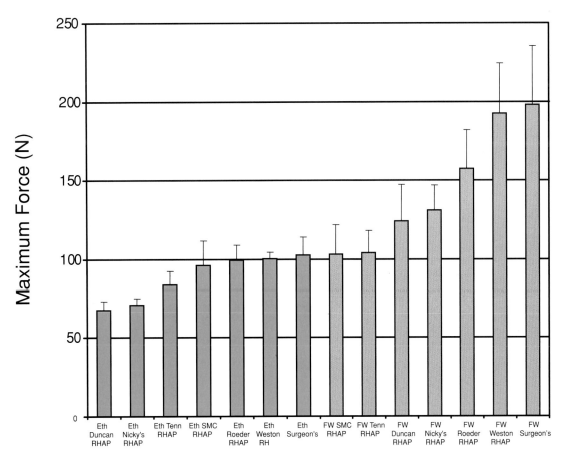

Figure 3-33 Maximal force to failure of sliding knots secured with three reversing half-hitches on alternating posts (RHAP) and the surgeon's knot using #2 Ethibond (■) and #2 FiberWire (Arthrex, Inc.; Naples, FL) (▨) Tenn, Tennessee slider; Eth, Ethibond.

Figure 3-34 Expansion of the suture loop with locking of the sliding knot. **A:** A Nicky's knot (proximal-locking knot) has been tied to a 30-mm circumferential post and close apposition of the suture to the post is demonstrated. **A:** Locking the knot by tensioning the wrapping limb "flips" the knot and prevents the knot from slipping backward but also enlarges the suture loop. Note: See how the suture loop is pulled away from the 30-mm circumferential post.

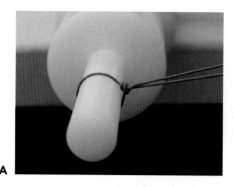 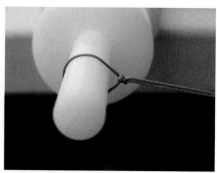

knot tied with #2 Ethibond (range: 24.4% to 92.0% increase; $p < 0.01$) (Fig. 3-33).

In this study, we also noted a common mechanism of suture loop enlargement (i.e., loss of loop security) during tying of sliding knots. When a sliding knot is tied, locking of the knot is commonly performed by tensioning the wrapping limb and "flipping" the knot to prevent the knot from sliding back. Locking the sliding knot, however, also caused expansion of the suture loop (Fig. 3-34). This effect was seen in all the sliding knots, which required a flipping maneuver to be locked. Expansion of the suture loop was related to the locking mechanism of each type of sliding knot (i.e., both proximal locking and distal locking knots). Thus, this factor must also be considered when tying and choosing an arthroscopic knot. One way to minimize this effect is to resist the knot from backing off with the knot pusher when flipping the knot (Fig. 3-35).

Based on our biomechanical studies, when performing arthroscopic shoulder reconstructive procedures, we prefer to use the 3-mm BioFASTak or BioSutureTak suture anchor (e.g., for labral repair), 5-mm BioCorkscrew or BioCorkscrew-FT suture anchor (e.g., for rotator cuff repair), or the 6.5-mm BioCorkscrew suture anchor (e.g., for rotator cuff repair in poor bone), all double loaded with #2 FiberWire and secured with a six-throw static surgeon's knot tied with a Surgeon's Sixth Finger knot pusher.

REFERENCES

1. Burkhart SS, Diaz-Pagan JL, Wirth MA, et al. Cyclic loading of anchor-based rotator cuff repairs: confirmation of the tension overload phenomenon and comparison of suture anchor fixation with transosseous fixation. *Arthroscopy.* 1997;13:720–724.
2. Burkhart SS, Johnson TC, Wirth MA, et al. Cyclic loading of transosseous rotator cuff repairs: tension overload as a possible cause of failure. *Arthroscopy.* 1997;13:172–176.
3. Caldwell GL, Warner JP, Miller MD, et al. Strength of fixation with transosseous sutures in rotator cuff repair. *J Bone Joint Surg Am.* 1997;79:1064–1068.
4. Gerber C, Schneeberger AG, Beck M, et al. Mechanical strength of repairs of the rotator cuff. *J Bone Joint Surg Br.* 1994;76:371–380.
5. Petit CJ, Boswell R, Mahar, A, et al. Biomechanical evaluation of a new technique for rotator cuff repair. *Am J Sports Med.* 2003;31(6):849–853.
6. MacGillivray JD, Ma CB. An arthroscopic stitch for massive rotator cuff tears: the Mac stitch. *Arthroscopy.* 2004;20(6):669–671.
7. Burkhart SS, Wirth MA, Simonich M, et al. Knot security in simple sliding knots and its relationship to rotator cuff repair: how secure must the knot be? *Arthroscopy.* 2000;16:202–207.
8. Bassett RW, Browne AL, Morrey BF, et al. Glenohumeral muscle force and mechanics in a position of shoulder instability. *J Biomech.* 1990;23:405–408.
9. Ikai M, Fukunaga T. Calculation of muscle strength per unit of cross-sectional area of human muscle. *Int Z Angelwandte Physiol Arbeitphysiol.* 1968;26:26–30.
10. Barber FA, Herbert MA, Click JN. The ultimate strength of suture anchors. *Arthroscopy.* 1995;11:21–28.
11. Barber FA, Herbert MA, Click JN. Internal fixation strength of suture anchors: update 1999. *Arthroscopy.* 1999;13:355–362.
12. Bardana DD, Burks RT, West JR, et al. The effect of suture anchor design and orientation on suture abrasion: an in vitro study. *Arthroscopy.* 2003;19(3):274–281.
13. Lo IK, Burkhart SS, Athanasiou K. Abrasion resistance of two types of nonabsorbable braided suture. *Arthroscopy.* 2004;20(4):435–441.
14. Lo IK, Burkhart SS, Chan KC, et al. Arthroscopic knots: determining the optimal balance of loop security and knot security. *Arthroscopy.* 2004;20(5):489–502.
15. Lo IK, Burkhart SS. A biomechanical analysis of arthroscopic knots tied with polyethylene suture material. *Arthroscopy,* 2006. In Press.
16. Burkhart SS. The deadman theory of suture anchors: observations along a South Texas fence line. *Arthroscopy.* 1995;11:119–123.
17. Burkhart SS, Wirth MA, Simonich M, et al. Loop security as a determinant of tissue fixation security. *Arthroscopy.* 1998;14:773–776.

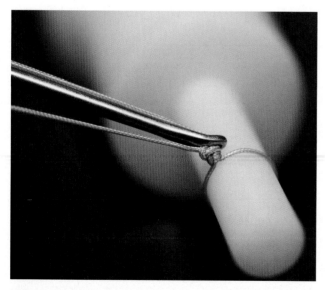

Figure 3-35 Clinical photo demonstrating locking of a knot by holding the knot down with a knot pusher, thereby resisting loop expansion.

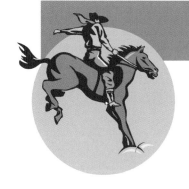

Understanding and Recognizing Pathology

TEARS OF THE GLENOID LABRUM

Normal Anatomy and Variants

The labrum is a ringlike fibrocartilaginous structure that circumferentially surrounds the *cavitas glenoidalis*, commonly called the "glenoid" (Fig. 4-1). In addition to increasing the depth and surface area of the glenoid, the labrum acts as a chock-block or wedge, preventing the humeral head from "rolling" off the glenoid (Fig. 4-2). The circumferential nature of the labrum is important also. It allows the rotator cuff to compress the humeral head into a congruent, articulating glenoid, providing an important component of the concavity–compression function of the rotator cuff (Fig. 4-3). Finally the labrum provides the attachment site for the glenohumeral ligaments. These ligamentous structures function at the extremes of rotation and their relative importance is dependent on the position of the arm and

the force applied (Fig. 4-4). In general, the inferior glenohumeral ligament is the primary ligamentous restraint against anterior, posterior, and inferior translation with the glenohumeral joint between 45° and 90° of elevation, whereas the superior and middle glenohumeral ligaments limit anterior, posterior, and inferior translation with the arm in adduction.

The glenoid labrum is normally well attached to the glenoid. In the superior half of the glenoid, however, the labral anatomy can vary significantly. This applies to both the anterior and superior labrum. The sublabral hole or sublabral foramen is a normal anatomic variant, with detachment of the anterior superior labrum above the midglenoid producing a communication with the subscapularis recess. This is not pathologic (Fig. 4-5). Another anatomic variant is the Buford complex (1) composed of a cordlike middle glenohumeral ligament that attaches superiorly to the superior labrum at a point just anterior to the base of biceps tendon, in association with absence of the anterior labrum above the midglenoid notch (Fig. 4-6).

ANTERIOR LABRAL LESIONS

The Bankart lesion is usually referred to as a disruption of the anterior inferior aspect of the labrum from the glenoid below the equator of the glenoid (Fig. 4-7). This results in loss of the normal chock-block effect of the labrum, affects the concavity compression mechanism of the rotator cuff, and disrupts the continuity of the inferior glenohumeral ligament. These lesions can be diagnosed using a posterior glenohumeral portal (Fig. 4-7A) or an anterosuperolateral portal (Fig. 4-7B). We prefer, however, to evaluate the ante-

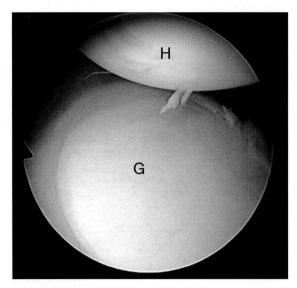

Figure 4-1 Arthroscopic view from an anterosuperolateral portal of a left shoulder. G, glenoid; H, humeral head.

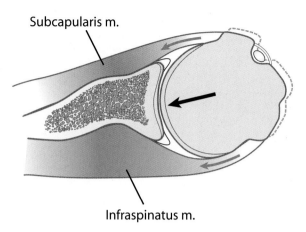

Subcapularis m.

Infraspinatus m.

Figure 4-3 One dynamic stabilizing function of the rotator cuff is to compress the humeral head into the glenoid and glenoid labrum.

rior, inferior, and posterior labrums through an anterosuperolateral portal. This provides an *en face* view of the glenoid that allows simultaneous evaluation of all the labrum below the equator of the glenoid. With this view, an accurate assessment can be made of the extent of labral tearing, particularly if the tear extends posterior to the 6 o'clock position. Furthermore, during repair, this view is superior for "balancing" the glenohumeral joint and ensuring recentering of the humeral head (Fig. 4-8).

Occasionally, the anterior labrum initially appears to have healed back to the glenoid neck in an anatomic position and that no disruption of the labrum exists. Simple pal-

pation with a probe or manipulation with an elevator, however, may reveal inadequate healing and fixation (Fig. 4-9). In some patients, the labrum initially will appear "absent" (Fig. 4-10A). In most cases, however, the labrum can be found in a medialized position, scarred to the anterior aspect of the glenoid neck, the so-called "ALPSA" lesion (anterior labrum periosteal sleeve avulsion) (Fig. 4-10B). In this situation, the labroligamentous complex must be elevated and mobilized from the glenoid neck (Fig. 4-10C)

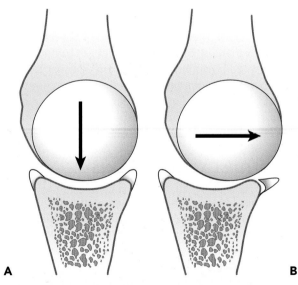

Figure 4-2   A: The glenoid labrum acts as a chock-block or wedge to prevent the humeral head from rolling off the glenoid. **B:** In order for a soft-tissue Bankart lesion to occur, the humerus must translate over the wedge of the anterior glenoid.

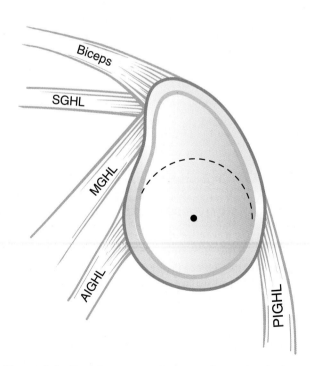

Figure 4-4 The labrum serves as an attachment for the biceps tendon but also as the attachment point of various stabilizing ligaments, including the superior glenoid humeral ligament (*SGHL*), the middle glenohumeral ligament (*MGHL*), the inferior glenohumeral ligament (*IGHL*) and its bands, the anterior band of the inferior glenohumeral ligament (*AIGHL*) and the posterior band of the inferior glenohumeral ligament (*PIGHL*).

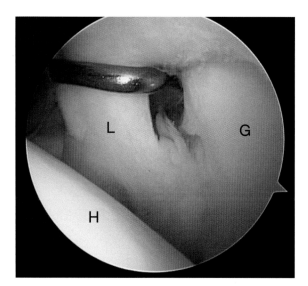

Figure 4-5 Arthroscopic view through a posterior glenohumeral portal of a left shoulder in a beach chair orientation, demonstrating a sublabral foramen. Note the detachment of the labrum above the midglenoid notch anteriorly and the smooth edges of the labrum as it crosses the sublabral foramen. G, glenoid; H, humeral head; L, glenoid labrum.

until the complex floats up to the glenoid (Fig. 4-10D). This allows for a tension-free repair to the glenoid face (Fig. 4-10E).

POSTERIOR LABRAL LESIONS

Posterior labral tears are less common than anterior labral tears. These tears can be associated with pain, posterior

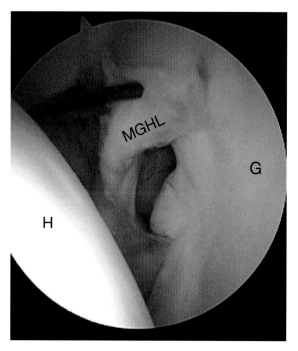

Figure 4-6 Arthroscopic view through a posterior glenohumeral portal of a left shoulder demonstrating a Buford complex. Note the cordlike middle glenohumeral ligament (MGHL) and the absence of the anterior labrum above the midglenoid notch. G, glenoid; H, humeral head.

instability, or both. Posterior labral tears are easiest to diagnose through an anterosuperolateral viewing portal. These usually demonstrate disruption of the labrum from the glenoid (Fig. 4-11). They are usually minimally displaced, however, and it is rare to have an ALPSA equivalent posteriorly.

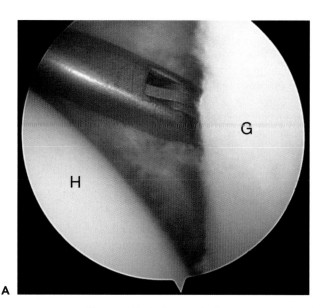

A

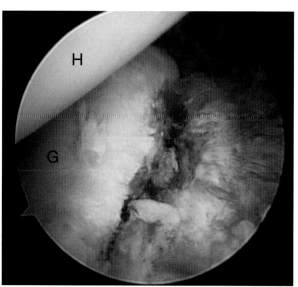

B

Figure 4-7 Arthroscopic views demonstrating Bankart lesions of the left shoulder **(A)** posterior portal view and **(B)** anterosuperolateral portal view. H, humeral head; G, glenoid.

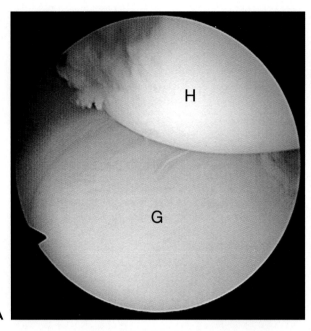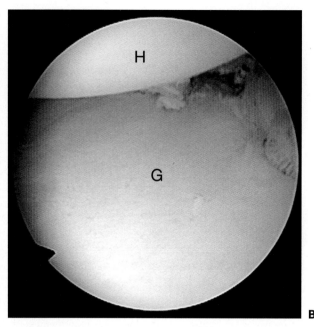

A   B

Figure 4-8 Arthroscopic views through an anterosuperolateral portal of a left shoulder demonstrating position of the humeral head relative to the glenoid. **A:** Before repair, demonstrating a Bankart lesion with subluxation of the humeral head anteroinferiorly. **B:** After Bankart repair, demonstrating centering of the humeral head above the glenoid. G, glenoid; H, humeral head.

SUPERIOR LABRUM TEARS

In 1985, Andrews et al. (2) were the first to report tears of the anterosuperior glenoid labrum in throwing athletes. They treated these patients with arthroscopic débridement. Not until Snyder et al. (3) in 1990 coined the term "SLAP"

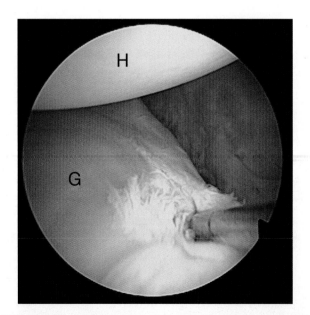

Figure 4-9 Arthroscopic view through an anterosuperolateral portal demonstrating a partially "healed" Bankart lesion. Simple palpation with a probe demonstrates the labrum is poorly attached to the glenoid. G, glenoid; H, humeral head.

lesions (superior labrum anterior and posterior) in the general population did the diagnosis and treatment became popularized. They classified SLAP lesions into four types (Fig. 4-12): Type I SLAP lesions (Fig. 4-13) involve fraying or degeneration of the superior labrum; type II (Fig. 4-14) involve detachment of the superior labrum and bicep anchor from the glenoid rim; type III (Fig. 4-15) involve bucket-handle tearing of the superior labrum with the remaining superior labral tissue and biceps anchored to superior glenoid; and type IV (Fig. 4-16) are bucket-handle tears of the superior labrum, with extension of the tear into the long head of the biceps tendon. Subsequently, several other types of SLAP lesions have been described, although the Snyder et al. (3) classification is the one most commonly used.

Since the description of SLAP lesions in 1990, significant controversy has developed over the pathoanatomy, biomechanics, and diagnosis of SLAP lesions. In particular, the relationship of type II SLAP lesions to the disabled throwing shoulder has been the subject of controversy.

Patient Population

In our experience, SLAP lesions generally occur in two major groups of patients. One group consists of patients who do not have a prodrome of shoulder symptoms and experience a traction-countertraction load. These include patients who have an eccentric contraction of the biceps muscle (e.g., fall off ladder while holding on) (Fig 4-17), a fall on an outstretched arm, or a rear-end motor vehicle

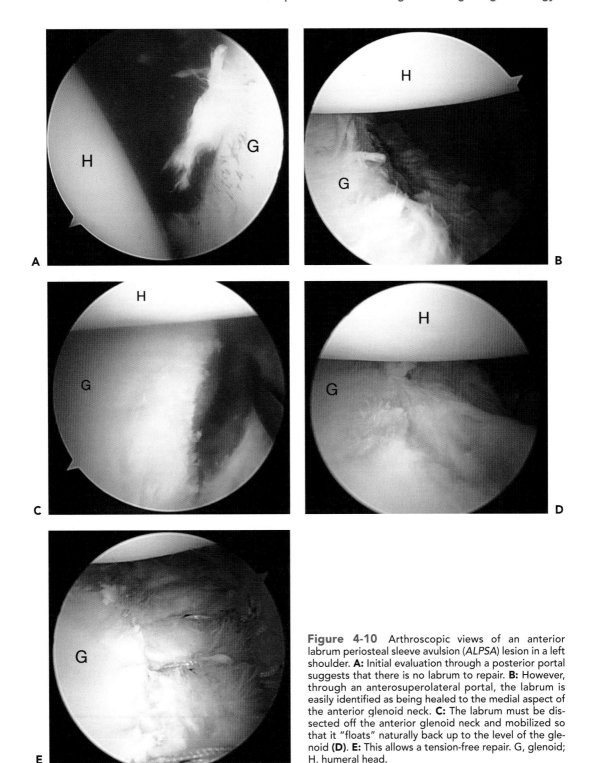

Figure 4-10 Arthroscopic views of an anterior labrum periosteal sleeve avulsion (*ALPSA*) lesion in a left shoulder. **A:** Initial evaluation through a posterior portal suggests that there is no labrum to repair. **B:** However, through an anterosuperolateral portal, the labrum is easily identified as being healed to the medial aspect of the anterior glenoid neck. **C:** The labrum must be dissected off the anterior glenoid neck and mobilized so that it "floats" naturally back up to the level of the glenoid **(D). E:** This allows a tension-free repair. G, glenoid; H, humeral head.

accident while bracing against the wheel. The other patient population is the overhead athlete. As described below, these patients generally have a prodrome of symptomatology; they develop a glenohumeral internal rotation deficit and, eventually, an inability to perform overhead athletic activity effectively (Fig. 4-18). This patient population is unique and the relation of type II SLAP lesions to the "dead-arm syndrome" continues to evolve.

The Overhead Athlete and the Dead Arm Syndrome

In North America and abroad, the overhead athlete continues to fascinate and capture the imagination of the general

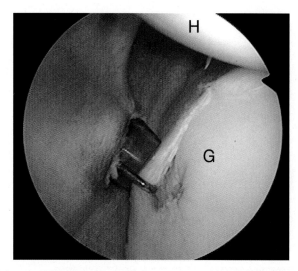

Figure 4-11 Arthroscopic view through an anterosuperolateral portal of a left shoulder demonstrating a posterior Bankart lesion. G, glenoid; H, humeral head.

public. The inherent ability to throw a ball in excess of 90 miles per hour with pinpoint accuracy and control is an athletic feat few can master. The sudden loss of this ability, termed the "dead-arm syndrome," has become a relatively common occurrence. We define the dead-arm syndrome as any pathologic shoulder condition where the overhead athlete is unable to throw the ball at preinjury velocity and control because of pain or the subjective feeling of unease in the shoulder.

Most throwing athletes complain of pain or discomfort in the late cocking or early acceleration phase of the throwing motion, as the arm begins to move anteriorly. With this discomfort, the throwing athlete is unable to throw the ball at maximal velocity with control and the arm goes "dead."

Historically, the cause of the dead-arm syndrome was enigmatic and included almost every conceivable shoulder pathology, including subacromial impingement, acromial osteophytes, rotator cuff disease, biceps tendinitis, acromioclavicular joint derangement, posterior glenoid calcifications, microinstability, internal impingement, SLAP lesions, and psychopathology. Initially, the most popular model for the dead-arm syndrome was internal impingement and microinstability.

Internal impingement, or posterosuperior glenohumeral impingement, was initially described by Walch et al. (4) as a pinching of the posterosuperior rotator cuff between the posterosuperior glenoid labrum and the greater tuberosity (Fig. 4-19). Walch et al. (4) described this as a normal finding that occurred in all shoulders at 90° of abduction and 90° of external rotation. Jobe (5) extrapolated this concept to the overhead athlete. He hypothesized that internal impingement would be particularly exacerbated in throwers with progressive stretching of the anterior ligamentous structures (i.e., microinstability)

with repetitive throwing. This theory supported the practice of performing an open anterior capsulolabral reconstruction to treat microinstability—internal impingement overlap in the throwing shoulder. The results of this procedure, however, were unpredictable for returning athletes to their preinjury level of throwing. Furthermore, the hypothesis of anterior instability exacerbating internal impingement was refuted by Halbrecht et al. (6), who demonstrated that anterior instability, in fact, would alleviate internal impingement. Not until Burkhart, Morgan, and Kibler. (7) reported on their collective experience and unified theory of the disabled throwing shoulder was it recognized that type II SLAP lesions were the major pathology associated with the dead-arm syndrome (7–9).

Development of SLAP Lesions in the Throwing Athlete: Posteroinferior Capsular Contracture, Glenohumeral Rotation Deficit, and Type II SLAP Lesions

It has been well documented that the throwing shoulder acquires progressively more external rotation in abduction over time (5,10–14). Some authors interpreted this increased external rotation as evidence of repetitive microtrauma to the anterior capsule of the shoulder in the late cocking phase of throwing (5,10–14). By this theory, microtrauma would progress to symptomatic anterior instability and shoulder dysfunction (5,10–14). Although anterior capsular stretching can occur as a late tertiary problem, symptomatic throwers often initially demonstrate severe loss of internal rotation in abduction. In the symptomatic throwing shoulder, the loss of internal rotation in abduction far exceeds any external rotation gain.

Glenohumeral internal rotation deficit (GIRD) is defined as the loss of glenohumeral internal rotation in the throwing shoulder as compared to the nonthrowing shoulder (7). This is easiest to measure using a goniometer with the patient supine and the scapula stabilized while the arm is abducted 90° (Fig. 4-20). In 1991, Verna (15) was the first to document the relationship between GIRD and shoulder dysfunction in the throwing athlete. He reported on 39 professional pitchers who had GIRD of ≥35°. Of these pitchers, 60% subsequently developed shoulder problems during the study period. Furthermore, the relationship of type II SLAP lesions and GIRD has been documented. Burkhart, Morgan, and Kibler (7), in a series of 124 baseball pitchers with type II SLAP lesions, reported that the mean GIRD was 53°, whereas a mean GIRD of 33° was found in overhead athletes with type II SLAP lesions.

The value and effectiveness of stretching to minimize GIRD has also been demonstrated. Over a 2-year period, Kibler (16) prospectively evaluated two groups of high-level tennis players. One group performed daily stretching exercises to minimize GIRD, whereas the other group did not. Over the study period, those who stretched had significantly increased their internal rotation (and total

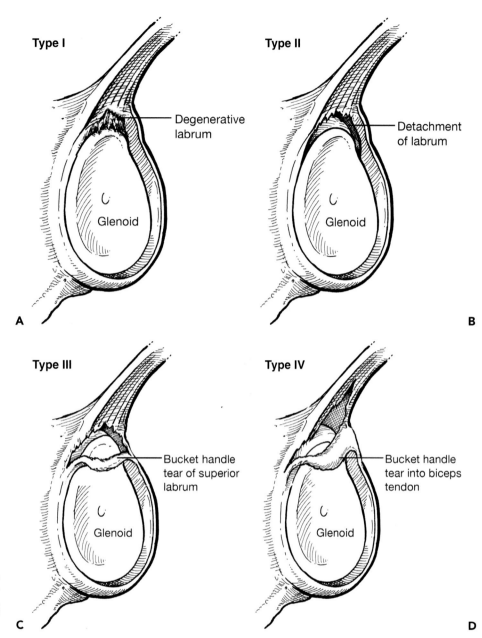

Figure 4-12 A: Type I superior labrum anterior and posterior (SLAP) lesion. **B:** Type II SLAP lesion. **C:** Type III SLAP lesion. **D:** Type IV SLAP lesion.

rotation) and had a 38% decreased incidence of shoulder problems compared with those who did not stretch. In addition, Cooper stretched 22 major league baseball pitchers daily to minimize GIRD to ≤20° over a 3-year period (P Donley, J Cooper, personal communication, November, 2000). Over this time period, he reported no innings lost, no intra-articular shoulder problems, and no surgical procedures required for this group. Collectively, these reports demonstrate the importance of a posteroinferior capsular stretching program in minimizing GIRD and in preventing secondary intra-articular shoulder problems (i.e., type II SLAP lesions).

In general, most symptomatic throwers with GIRD (>25°) will respond to a posteroinferior capsular stretch-

ing program with reduction of GIRD to an acceptable level (GIRD of <20°, or <10% difference in total rotation between the two shoulders) over a 2- to 6-week period. The key feature is incorporating sleeper stretches into a dedicated daily stretching program (Fig. 4-21). Approximately 10% of throwers do not respond to a posteroinferior capsular stretching program. This usually occurs in high-level throwers who have been throwing for years, with severe and chronic GIRD. These throwers are also more likely to have a type II SLAP lesion. In throwers who are resistant to a dedicated stretching program, selective arthroscopic capsular release with type II SLAP lesion repair (if a SLAP lesion is present) should be considered (Fig. 4-22). These patients will usually demonstrate a severely contracted and

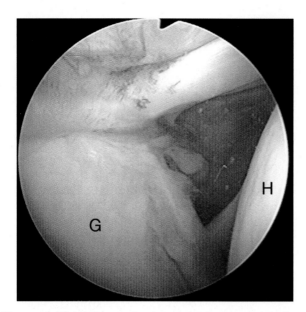

Figure 4-13 Arthroscopic view through a posterior glenohumeral portal of a left shoulder demonstrating a type I superior labrum anterior and posterior (SLAP) lesion. G, glenoid; H, humeral head.

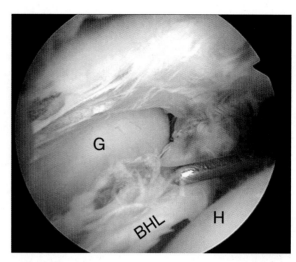

Figure 4-15 Arthroscopic view through a posterior glenohumeral portal of a left shoulder demonstrating a type III superior labrum anterior and posterior (SLAP) lesion. G, glenoid; H, humeral head; BHL, bucket-handle fragment of superior labrum.

thickened posteroinferior capsule. Selective release of the posteroinferior capsule should result in an immediate 65° to 75° of glenohumeral internal rotation (Fig. 4-23).

How does contracture of the posteroinferior capsule result in a type II SLAP lesion? Several sequential events are pivotal to this pathologic cascade. First, when a tight posteroinferior capsular contracture occurs, a posterosuperior shift of the glenohumeral contact point ensues as the arm is brought into abduction and external rotation (Fig. 4-24). This occurs because, in abduction and external rotation, the posterior inferior glenohumeral ligament is positioned

beneath the anteroinferior aspect of the humeral head, causing a shift of the glenohumeral rotation point posterosuperiorly (Fig. 4-25). This consequence has been demonstrated mechanically in the laboratory (17,18). This shift is accentuated because the biceps force vector changes to a posterior direction. Second, with a posterosuperior shift of the glenohumeral contact point, further external rotation of the shoulder is gained because this shift allows the greater tuberosity to clear the glenoid rim through a greater arc of external rotation before internal impingement occurs. The contact point shift also minimizes the cam

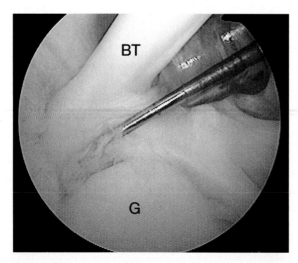

Figure 4-14 Arthroscopic view through a posterior glenohumeral portal of a left shoulder demonstrating a type II superior labrum anterior and posterior (SLAP) lesion. G, glenoid; BT, biceps tendon.

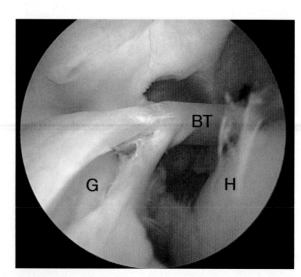

Figure 4-16 Arthroscopic view through a posterior glenohumeral portal of a left shoulder demonstrating a type IV superior labrum anterior and posterior (SLAP) lesion. H, humeral head; G, glenoid; BT, biceps tendon.

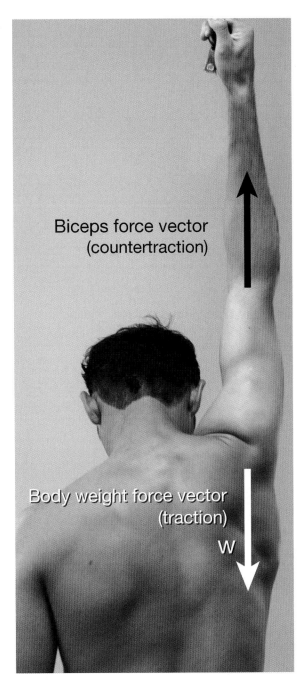

Biceps force vector
(countertraction)

Body weight force vector
(traction)

W

Figure 4-17 The traction-countertraction mechanism of injury for type II superior labrum anterior and posterior (SLAP) lesions. In this photo, a person who is falling from a height will grab a stationary object to set up the traction-countertraction mechanism. W, body weight.

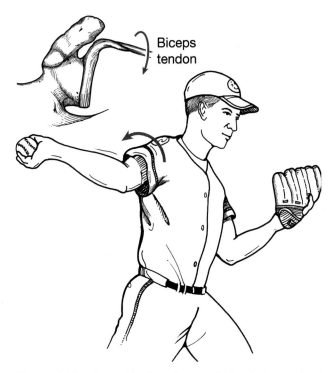

Biceps
tendon

Figure 4-18 The peel-back mechanism of injury in the overhead athlete for type II superior labrum anterior and posterior (SLAP) lesions.

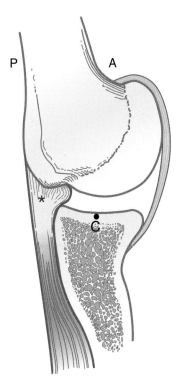

P   A

*

C

Figure 4-19 In abduction and external rotation of the shoulder, the greater tuberosity abuts against the posterosuperior glenoid, entrapping the rotator cuff between the two bones (*). This has been dubbed "internal impingement. A, anterior; P, posterior; C, glenohumeral center of rotation.

effect of the proximal humerus on the anteroinferior capsule, allowing further external rotation (Fig. 4-26). This allows throwers to externally rotate beyond their normal set point in the late cocking position. Third, because of this new glenohumeral contact point, as the shoulder abducts and excessively externally rotates, both shear and torsional forces at the biceps anchor and the posterosuperior labral attachment increases. The biceps anchor and posterosupe-

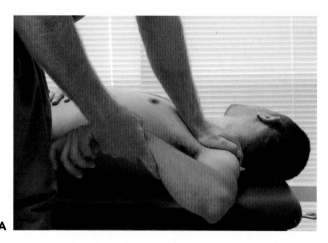
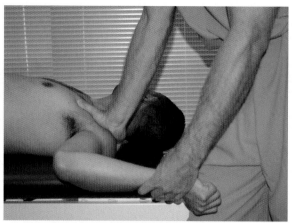

A   **B**

Figure 4-20   **A:** Internal rotation is measured with the patient's shoulder in 90° of abduction and the elbow in 90° of flexion while the examiner stabilizes the scapula against the examination table. The endpoint of internal rotation is taken as the point at which the superior border of the scapula begins to rotate off the examination table. **B:** External rotation is also measured while stabilizing the scapula. Note: The neutral position (0°) is that in which the forearm is perpendicular to the patient's body (12 o'clock position in the supine patient). All measurements should be made with a goniometer.

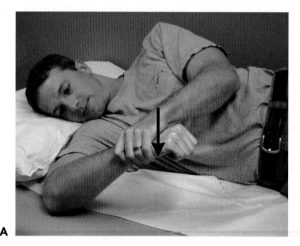
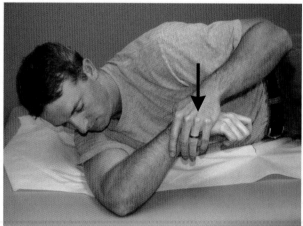

A   **B**

Figure 4-21   Focused posterior inferior capsular stretches. **A:** In the sleeper stretch, the patient is side lying with the scapula stabilized against the examination table, the shoulder flexed 90°, and the elbow flexed 90°. Passive internal rotation is applied to the arm by the nondominant arm to the dominant wrist. **B:** The roll-over sleeper stretch is the same as the sleeper stretch, except that the patient rolls forward 30° to 40° from vertical side-lying position.

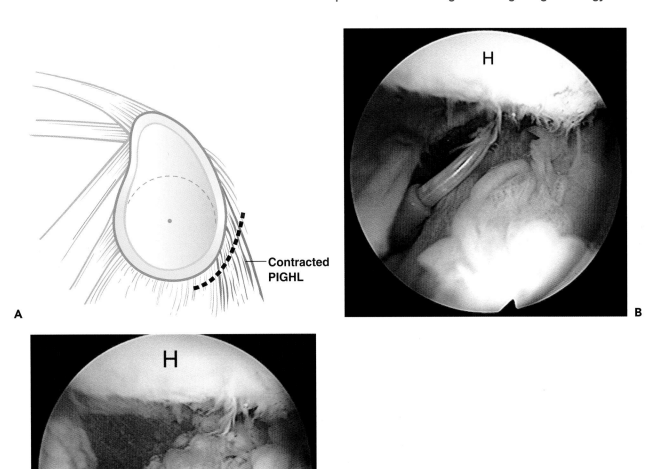

Contracted PIGHL

A

B

C

Figure 4-22 Selective posteroinferior capsulotomy. **A:** The capsular contracture is located in the posteroinferior quadrant of the capsule in the zone of the posterior band of the inferior glenohumeral ligament *(IGHL)* complex. The capsulotomy is made ¼ inch away from the labrum and extends from the 9 or 3 o'clock position to the 6:30 and 5:30 positions respectively. **B:** Arthroscopic view through an anterosuperolateral portal of a left shoulder. A hooked electrocautery probe is introduced through a posterior portal and a capsulotomy is made. **C:** Completed posteroinferior release. H, humeral head.

rior labrum then begin to fail via the peel-back mechanism (see below) producing a type II SLAP lesion.

Hyper-External Rotation of the Humerus: Delayed Internal Impingement

In simplistic terms, the most effective way to gain velocity in throwing is to increase the arc of rotation through which the arm gains angular velocity. Pitchers who possess the ability to throw particularly hard invariably have marked hyperexternal rotation of the humerus, often beyond 130°, with the arm abducted to 90°. Because of the posterosuperior shift of the glenohumeral contact point, internal impingement of the greater tuberosity against the glenoid rim does not occur in the normal location in the posterosuperior quadrant of the glenoid, but is "delayed" until a

later point of hyperexternal rotation in the posteroinferior quadrant (Fig. 4-27). At that point, internal impingement occurs. Jobe suggested that the abrasion effect of the rotator cuff against the glenoid caused by internal impingement also caused undersurface rotator cuff damage (5). The cuff, however, is also subjected to repetitive hypertwist of its fiber bundles at their insertion points because of the hyperexternal rotation of the humerus (Fig. 4-28). The magnitude of these torsional forces (and hence their ability to damage the rotator cuff) is much greater than that of the relatively small abrasion forces, and must be considered the major factor causing rotator cuff damage. Therefore, we conclude that internal impingement (with relatively low-grade abrasion forces on the cuff) is not the primary cause of cuff damage in the thrower. Instead, it is

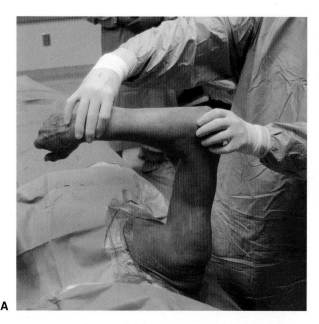
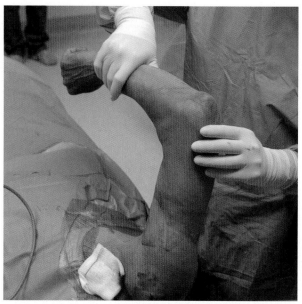

A   B

Figure 4-23 Right-handed baseball pitcher with a type II superior labrum anterior and posterior (SLAP) lesion and severe glenohumeral internal rotation deficit (GIRD) that was nonresponsive to stretch. Examination under anesthesia revealed no (0°) internal rotation before arthroscopy, and 75° of internal rotation after a selective posteroinferior capsulotomy and type II SLAP lesion repair.

the *delay* of internal impingement that occurs with hyperexternal rotation of the humerus that is pathologic, causing high-grade torsional forces that damage the rotator cuff.

Peel-Back Mechanism of Posterior and Combined Anteroposterior SLAP Lesions

The peel-back mechanism of SLAP lesions occurs in the late cocking phase of throwing with the arm in abduction

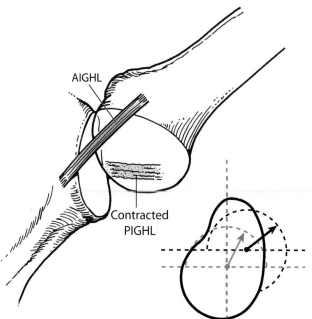

Figure 4-24 When the posterior capsule shortens (contracted posterior band), the glenohumeral contact point shifts posterosuperiorly and the allowable arc of external rotation (before the greater tuberosity contacts the posterior glenoid) significantly increases (*dotted lines*).

and external rotation. As the arm is brought up into this position, a dynamic angle change occurs in the biceps tendon to a more posterior position, in addition to a twist at the base of the biceps tendon (Fig. 4-29). This twist is transmitted as a torsional force to the posterior superior labrum. In a normal shoulder with a well-fixed superior labrum, what is observed arthroscopically is purely an angular and torsional change at the biceps root, and the superior labrum remains well fixed to the superior glenoid.

If, however, the superior labrum is unstable (i.e., a type II SLAP lesion) when the arm is brought into abduction and external rotation, the superior labrum will rotate medially over the corner of the superior glenoid onto the scapular neck and shift the biceps root medial to the supraglenoid tubercle (a positive peel-back sign). This phenomenon will occur in type II SLAP lesions involving the posterior superior labrum or combined anteroposterior superior labral tears (Fig. 4-30). Pure anterior SLAP lesions without extension into the posterosuperior quadrant, however, will generally not demonstrate a positive peel-back test. A throwing athlete who has a SLAP lesion will usually demonstrate a positive peel-back sign with extension of the type II SLAP lesion into the posterosuperior quadrant.

As seems apparent, the throwing athlete with a tight posteroinferior capsule is a "set-up" for injury and failure. With the arm in abduction and external rotation, the tight posteroinferior capsule shifts the glenohumeral contact point posterosuperiorly, creating maximal shear forces exactly when peel-back forces are also at their greatest. In addition, the late cocking phase (i.e., with the arm in abduction and external rotation) is also the point in the throwing cycle and in the kinetic chain at which energy

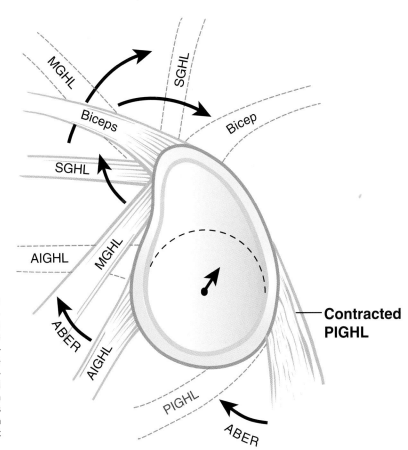

Figure 4-25 This diagram shows the shift in position that occurs in the major tendon and capsuloligamentous structures of the glenohumeral joint between the resting position (*solid lines*) and the abducted externally rotated (ABER) position (*dotted lines*). In abduction and external rotation, the bowstrung posterior band of the inferior glenohumeral ligament (*PIGHL*) is beneath the humeral head, causing a shift in the glenohumeral rotation point; and the biceps vector shifts posteriorly as the peel-back forces are maximized. The result is a posterosuperior shift of the glenohumeral contact point.

from the trunk is being funneled to the shoulder to accelerate the arm, making it particularly vulnerable. Thus, maximal shear meets maximal torsion meets maximal peel-back forces meets maximal acceleration forces, and the shoulder at risk becomes the victim.

TYPE II SLAP LESIONS: DIAGNOSIS

Physical Examination

In our experience, no physical examination test has proved infallible in diagnosing SLAP lesions. This may be because certain test results are related to the anatomic location of the type II SLAP lesion (19). It appears that the Speed test (Fig. 4-31) and O'Brien test (Fig. 4-32) are more specific for anterior type II SLAP lesions. In contrast, the modified Jobe relocation test is more specific for posterior SLAP lesions, and is typically positive in throwing athletes with posterior or combined anteroposterior SLAP lesions. In performing the modified Jobe relocation test, once the arm is brought into abduction and external rotation, the patient usually complains of pain in the posterosuperior aspect of the shoulder along the posterosuperior joint line (Fig. 4-33). When a posteriorly directed force is applied to the proximal humerus, the discomfort is relieved.

In viewing this test dynamically via arthroscopy with the arm in the initial position of abduction and external rotation, a positive peel-back sign is demonstrated. By applying a posteriorly directed force, however, the biceps tendon is subjected to a tensile traction force and the subluxed labrum and biceps root are reduced back onto the superior glenoid (see Fig. 4-33). We believe that the reversal of the peel-back sign, with reduction of the labral subluxation, is what results in pain relief with the modified Jobe relocation test.

Despite these clinical findings, we continue to believe that the diagnosis of a type II SLAP lesion remains an arthroscopic diagnosis.

Arthroscopic Findings

We base our diagnosis of a type II SLAP lesion on four arthroscopic findings. These are

1. A superior sublabral sulcus >5-mm in depth
2. A bare superior labral footprint
3. A displaceable biceps root
4. A positive peel-back sign.

One or more of these arthroscopic findings in a shoulder should strongly suggest a SLAP lesion.

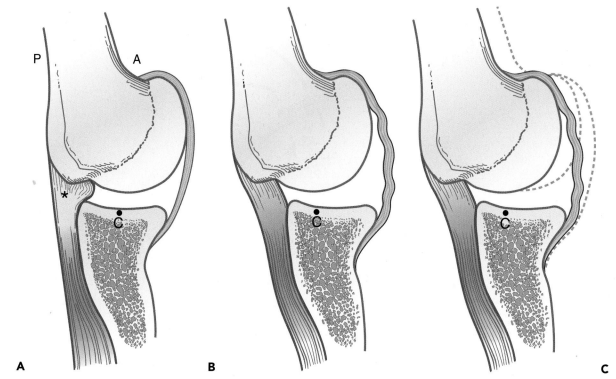

Figure 4-26   A: With the arm in a position of abduction and external rotation, the humeral head and the proximal curvature of the humeral calcar produce a significant cam effect of the anteroinferior capsule, tensioning the capsule by the space-occupying effect. **B:** With a posterosuperior shift of the glenohumeral contact point, the space-occupying effect of the proximal humerus on the anteroinferior capsule is reduced (reduction of the cam effect). This creates a relative redundancy in the anteroinferior capsule that has probably been misinterpreted in the past as microinstability. **C:** Superimposed neutral position (*dotted line*) shows the magnitude of the capsular redundancy that occurs as a result of the shift in the glenohumeral contact point.* rotator cuff as it is pinched in the internal impingment position; A, anterior; P, posterior; C, glenohumeral contact point.

Superior Sublabral Sulcus

A normal superior sulcus of up to 5-mm can be demonstrated beneath the superior labrum. This sulcus is usually covered with articular cartilage and appears as a smooth transition from labrum to superior glenoid (Fig. 4-34A). A sublabral sulcus that is >5-mm or labral attachments that appear tenuous, however, suggests a SLAP lesion (Fig. 4-34B). We have seen interstitial SLAP lesions in which poor quality labral tissue is loosely attached to the labral footprint, yet the peel-back test is positive. Such interstitial SLAP lesions are pathologic and should be repaired. The sulcus is easiest to evaluate while viewing through a posterior glenohumeral portal and introducing an angled probe through an anterior portal.

Bare Superior Labral Footprint

A normal sublabral sulcus, even if large, is usually covered with a smooth cartilaginous surface. If, however, a bare labral footprint with exposed bone (Fig. 4-35) is seen or if evidence exists of fiber failure to the superior labral attachment to bone, a SLAP lesion is present and should be repaired.

Displaceable Biceps Root

While viewing through the posterior portal and using a probe through an anterior portal, assess the stability of the biceps root. A displaceable biceps root and superior labrum can be easily manipulated and pushed medially onto the glenoid neck, as if no direct interconnection of fibers existed between the biceps root and the superior glenoid neck (Fig. 4-36).

Peel-Back Sign

To perform a peel-back test, place the arthroscope in the posterior portal and view the superior labrum with the glenoid horizontal and parallel to the floor. Have an assistant then position the arm in 90° of abduction and slowly externally rotate the arm 90°. In patients with SLAP lesions involving the posterior superior quadrant, as the arm is brought into the position of 90° abduction combined with 90° of external rotation; the superior labrum or biceps anchor will drop medially over the corner of the glenoid (Fig. 4-37). Patients with pure anterosuperior quadrant SLAP lesions may not have a positive peel-back sign, but will demonstrate other signs of a SLAP lesion. Patients with normal superior labra

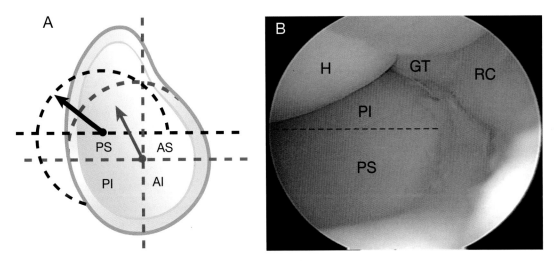

Figure 4-27 A: The glenoid has four quadrants: anterosuperior (*AS*), anteroinferior (*AI*), postero-superior (*PS*), and posteroinferior (*PI*). Ordinarily, internal impingement in which the greater tuberosity of the humerus abuts the glenoid occurs in the posterosuperior quadrant. A posterosuperior shift of the contact point can "delay" internal impingement so that it occurs in the posteroinferior quadrant. **B:** Right shoulder of a 20-year-old baseball pitcher, from an anterosuperolateral viewing portal. Posterosuperior shift of the glenohumeral contact point delays internal impingement of the greater tuberosity against the glenoid rim from the normal location in the posterosuperior quadrant to the posteroinferior quadrant (as we see in this patient with hyperexternal rotation).

(or pure anterosuperior quadrant SLAP lesions) will only demonstrate an angular change of the biceps tendon (without peel-back) with the arm in 90° of abduction and 90° of external rotation. The posterior labral attachments must be disrupted for the peel-back test to be positive.

Drive-through Sign

Although the drive-through sign was initially described as a sign of instability, it is also usually positive in patients with SLAP lesions. The drive-through test is performed by sweeping the arthroscope (from a posterior portal) from superior to inferior between the glenoid and humeral head. An arthroscope that can be easily "driven through" the joint is said to have a positive drive-through sign.

Surgery for the Refractory Disabled Throwing Shoulder

At this point, we will depart somewhat from our format for this chapter by explaining our surgical rationale and intra-operative decision-making for the refractory throwing shoulder. We do this now because the decision-making in this group of patients is so integrally related to the patho-logic findings on arthroscopic examination.

Assume that a right-handed overhead athlete has been refractory to nonoperative treatment and has signs and symptoms of a dead arm. A preoperative magnetic reso-nance imaging (MRI) study is suggestive of a possible SLAP lesion and also shows tendinosis of the rotator cuff. The patient is taken to the operating room. Examination under anesthesia demonstrates marked hyperexternal rotation and loss of internal rotation (GIRD). In fact, with the arm at 90° abduction, the patient has 140° of external rotation and only 15° of internal rotation on the dominant side. The patient has GIRD, presumably because of a tight pos-teroinferior capsule that has not responded to a stretching program.

Furthermore, the patient has hyperexternal rotation that is exacerbated by factors (decrease in the cam effect; shift in

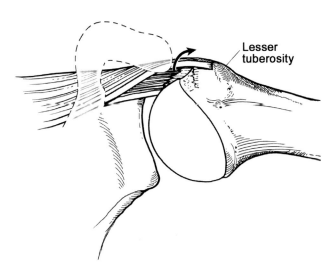

Figure 4-28 Torsional overload with repetitive hypertwisting of rotator cuff fibers occurs on the articular surface of the rotator cuff, the most common location of cuff failure in the thrower.

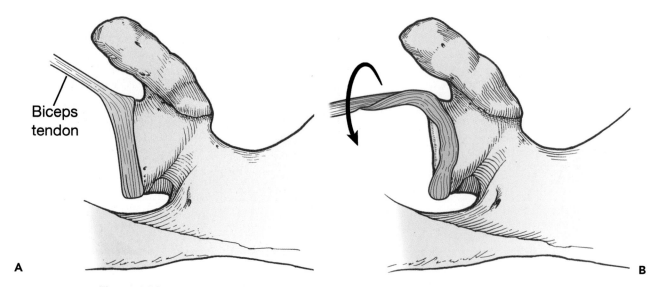

Figure 4-29   A: Superior view of the biceps-superior labral complex of a left shoulder in a resting position. **B:** Superior view of the biceps-superior labral complex of a left shoulder in the abducted, externally rotated position, showing peel-back mechanism as the biceps vector shifts posteriorly.

the glenohumeral rotation contact point) related to GIRD and its role in shift of the glenohumeral contact point. Finally, the patient's rotator cuff tendinosis is related to the hypertwist of the cuff fibers because of hyperexternal rotation.

Our assessment before placing the scope in the joint is that the major pathologic components that will require correction and repair are

1. SLAP lesion
2. Tight posteroinferior capsule
3. Hyperexternal rotation.

We then proceed with arthroscopy and we find that the patient has a positive peel-back test and a positive drive-through sign. Also an unequivocal SLAP lesion is found on arthroscopic inspection, with a bare sublabral footprint and a displaceable biceps root. Next, we place our scope in an anterosuperolateral viewing portal and observe the

glenohumeral joint with the arm in 90° abduction. Then, we progressively externally rotate the arm while it is maintained in 90° abduction. In this way, we can define the point at which internal impingement occurs—the point at which the greater tuberosity and rotator cuff abut against the glenoid rim. In most patients, this internal impingement occurs in the posterosuperior quadrant. In this patient, however, internal impingement does not occur until the patient's arm has rotated all the way to the posteroinferior quadrant, a situation in which "delayed" internal impingement has occurred. The patient has some scuffing of the posteroinferior labrum from frictional contact, but no frank posteroinferior labral tear. We suspect that the rotator cuff tendinosis is caused mainly by the large torsional forces to which the cuff is subjected because of hyperexternal rotation, with hypertwist of the cuff fibers.

The surgery that we will perform and the rationale on which it is based is as follows:

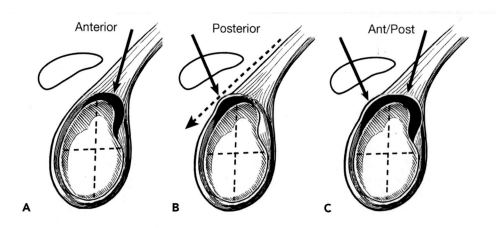

Figure 4-30 Three subtypes of type II superior labrum anterior and posterior (SLAP) lesions, designated by anatomic location: anterior (**A**), posterior (**B**), and combined anteroposterior (**C**).

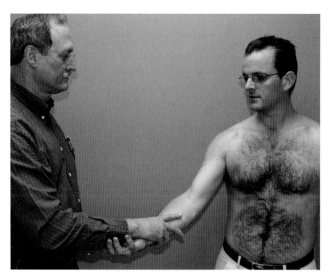

Figure 4-31 The Speed test. A positive test reproduces pain with resisted forward flexion with the arm in supination.

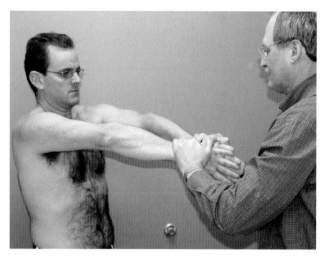

Figure 4-32 The O'Brien test. A positive test reproduces pain with resisted forward flexion with the arm in adduction, internal rotation, and pronation.

1. SLAP repair. In throwers, this usually requires two double-loaded suture anchors.
2. Posterior capsular release from 9 o'clock to 6:30 to allow increased internal rotation and shift of the glenohumeral contact point back to its normal location.
3. Anterior miniplication. This portion of the procedure is done not to treat instability, but to somewhat reduce (without excessively reducing) hyperexternal rotation. By placing two or three sutures to plicate the middle glenohumeral ligament to the anterior band of the inferior glenohumeral ligament, we will generally restrict external rotation by 10° to 15°. In this patient, that would mean external rotation of 125° or so with the arm abducted 90°.

It would be a mistake to infer, after seeing the posteroinferior labral scuffing, that the posteroinferior labrum needs to be repaired. If this were to be done, it would actually make the situation worse by tightening the posteroinferior capsule even further, which would make the GIRD worse. It would also be a mistake to do an open capsulolabral repair, because this would dramatically reduce compliance of the anterior capsule (which is necessary in throwers) and would probably reduce external rotation (at 90° abduction) to such a level that the athlete would never regain throwing velocity.

TRIPLE LABRAL LESIONS

Triple labral lesions represent an uncommon complex of lesions to the labrum, including injury to the anterior (Bankart lesion), posterior (reverse Bankart lesion), and superior (SLAP lesion) labrum. In our experience, this triad of labral injury represents approximately 2.5% of all labral lesions treated arthroscopically. Despite the fact that distinct lesions occur to the anterior (Fig. 4-38A), posterior (Fig. 4-38B), and superior (Fig. 4-38C) labra, most patients with such lesions will complain primarily of anterior instability and pain. These symptoms are generally confirmed on physical examination with apprehension in abduction and external rotation, which is relieved with the modified Jobe relocation maneuver. Although patients may demonstrate posterior translational laxity, they rarely complain of symptomatic posterior instability. SLAP lesion tests are generally equivocal.

Triple labral lesions are easy to diagnose with appropriate diagnostic arthroscopy. Careful evaluation of all parts of the labrum, capsule, and humeral insertions is performed. In particular, viewing through an anterosuperolateral portal is essential because this provides an *en face* view of the glenoid and labrum for appropriate assessment of the anterior, inferior, and posterior labrum. A clear view of the entire inferior labrum must be obtained.

Why these triple labral lesions occur is unclear. Warren and his associates (20–25) have introduced the "circle" concept as a mechanism for capsular and labral dysfunction in instability. This concept has been supported by a number of biomechanical studies (20–25). In particular, it has been demonstrated in cadaveric studies that a simulated anterior Bankart lesion increases the anterior translation of the humeral head only minimally (25) and, for a complete dislocation to occur, damage to the anterior and posterior sides of the capsule is necessary (20–23). The circle concept predicts that, for an anterior dislocation to occur, a significant secondary injury to the posterior aspect of the glenohumeral stabilizing structures must occur.

Recently, a trend among some surgeons has shifted toward arthroscopically addressing the presumed posterior capsular injury in patients with primary anterior instability. That is, in patients with anterior instability

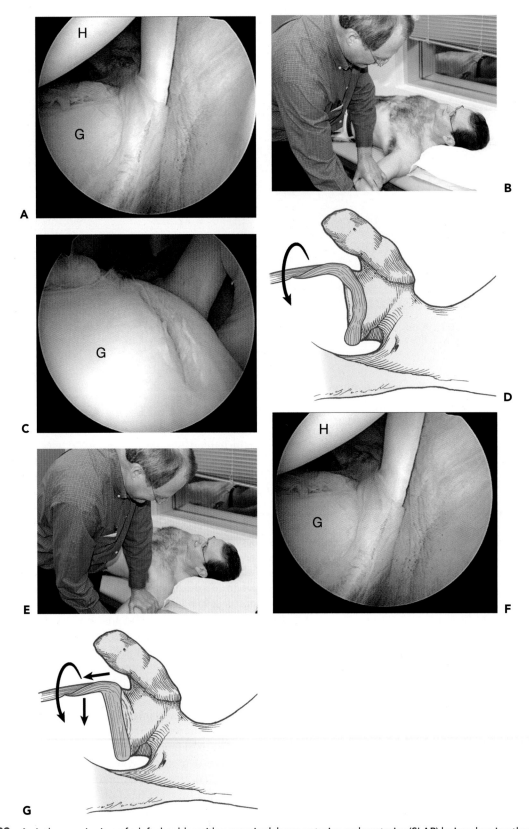

Figure 4-33 **A:** Arthroscopic view of a left shoulder with a superior labrum anterior and posterior (SLAP) lesion showing the normal location of the superior labrum with the arm at the side. **B:** Provocative modified Jobe relocation maneuver of forced passive abduction and external rotation causes posterosuperior shoulder pain (not apprehension) in a patient with a posterior SLAP lesion. **C:** Arthroscopic view of the pathologic anatomy in a left shoulder during the provocative Jobe maneuver showing a positive peel-back test, with medial subluxation of the bicep-superior labral complex. **D:** Diagrammatic representation of the peel-back, with subluxed superior labrum. **E:** Posteriorly directed force on the proximal humerus relieves the pain that was caused by the provocative Jobe maneuver. **F:** Arthroscopic view of the pathoanatomy during the application of the posterior force during the Jobe test (same patient as in **A** and **C**). The force on the proximal humerus creates a tensile force in the biceps tendon, which reduces the subluxed labrum, thereby relieving the pain. **G:** Diagrammatic depiction of the biceps tensile force produced by the Jobe relocation maneuver, which reduces the subluxed labrum to its anatomic position. G, glenoid; H, humeral head.

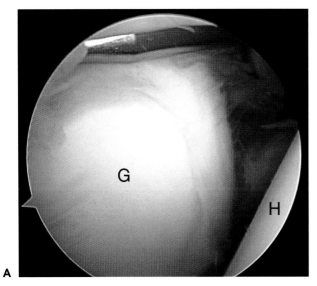
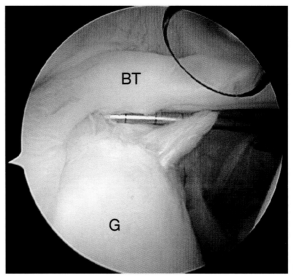

A   B

Figure 4-34 Arthroscopic view through a posterior glenohumeral portal of a right shoulder demonstrating **(A)** a normal sublabral sulcus; **(B)** a sublabral sulcus of >5-mm. G, glenoid; H, humerus; BT, biceps tendon.

and an anterior Bankart lesion, Snyder and Wolf (personal communication) have separately recommended a posterior capsular plication in patients with evidence of an enlarged posterior capsule. Although the rationale is to effectively balance effectively the shoulder, the utility of routine plication of the posterior capsule remains to be determined. In general, we only do posterior repairs for posterior labral disruption or demonstrable capsular damage.

"Contrecoup" lesions (i.e., a posterior capsulolabral lesion in an anterior instability patient), however, can manifest as either capsular injuries, labral injuries, or both. Although it is unclear whether a posterior capsular injury,

in a patient with an anterior instability, will heal without surgical intervention (although we believe this to be true in most cases), labral detachment lesions generally do not heal and, may continue to contribute to instability of the shoulder and persistent symptoms. Thus, we routinely repair posterior labral lesions to restore effectively the static supporting role of the labrum (i.e., increase glenoid socket depth, chock-block effect, surface area) and, more importantly, to restore the continuity of the glenohumeral ligaments that attach to it. We similarly repair type II SLAP lesions because detachment of the superior labrum has been associated with an increase in anteroposterior and superoinferior translation of the humeral head (24). By repairing the anterior, posterior, and superior labra, we restore the "circle" of stability.

HUMERAL AVULSION OF THE GLENOHUMERAL LIGAMENTS (HAGL) AND REVERSE HUMERAL AVULSION OF THE GLENOHUMERAL LIGAMENTS (RHAGL) LESIONS

Humeral avulsion of the glenohumeral ligaments (HAGL) is a pathologic lesion associated with anterior glenohumeral instability (Fig. 4-39). These lesions occur less commonly than capsulolabral disruptions or classic Bankart lesions. Their low incidence, however, may be related to their mechanisms of injury. For example, the general incidence of reported HAGL lesions has ranged from 2% to 9.3% (26,27). Thus, whereas the incidence of HAGL lesions in the Western world relatively seem low, Bokor et al. (28) reported on a large series of 41

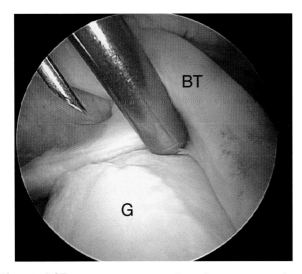

Figure 4-35 Arthroscopic view through a posterior glenohumeral portal of a left shoulder demonstrating a bare labral superior footprint with exposed bone. G, glenoid; BT, biceps tendon.

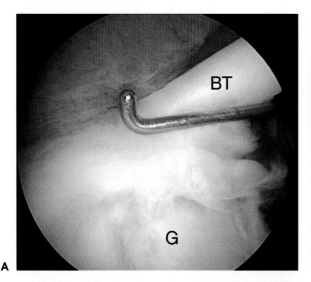 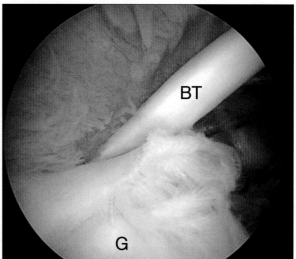

A   B

Figure 4-36   A: Arthroscopic view through a posterior glenohumeral portal of a right shoulder demonstrating an unstable biceps root. **B:** The biceps root is easily displaceable medially with a probe. (The probe is barely out of view at the base of the biceps.) G, glenoid; BT, biceps tendon.

cases of traumatic HAGL lesions. Most of these lesions were produced by violent rugby injuries. Furthermore, it is important to recognize that the diagnosis of HAGL lesions has likely been previously underreported. In particular, these lesions are likely missed during standard open stabilization with a subscapularis take-down, where the capsule is disrupted from bone just below the subscapularis take-down and may not be recognized as a traumatic disruption.

Reverse HAGL (RHAGL) lesions have previously been described by Snyder. These lesions generally occur with posterior instability and similarly demonstrate avulsion of the posterior inferior glenohumeral ligaments from the humeral head (Fig. 4-40).

Any patient with shoulder instability should be assessed for HAGL lesions. Both HAGL and RHAGL lesions can occur with other associated pathology, including Bankart lesions and Hill-Sachs lesions and their corresponding posterior instability pathologies; thus, all possible pathologies should be assessed during diagnostic arthroscopy. In some situations, a 70° arthroscope will be required to assess the humeral insertion of the ligaments and may be required for precise repair (Fig. 4-41).

ROTATOR INTERVAL AND CAPSULAR LAXITY

A discussion on the significance of the rotator interval and capsular laxity in shoulder instability must be separated into distinct diagnoses. Although recently significant attention has focused on the involvement of the

rotator interval and capsular laxity in contributing to anterior shoulder instability (including traumatic anterior shoulder instability), the classic pathology of a "widened" rotator interval and a "patulous" inferior capsule is synonymous with true multidirectional instability. The term multidirectional instability has likely been overused, however, and cases of symptomatic capsular laxity likely have been inappropriately categorized as multidirectional instability.

We prefer the term multidirectional instability in the classic sense to include only patients with symptomatic instability in at least two directions. This type of instability is characterized pathologically by a grossly patulous and redundant capsule. It is important to recognize, that the most important features of multidirectional instability are clinical (i.e., symptoms and signs) and are only confirmed by pathologic findings at surgery. Thus, we never make the diagnosis of multidirectional instability based on findings at arthroscopy alone (Fig. 4-42). In our hands, multidirectional instability is clearly a preoperative diagnosis. It is treated after confirmation of pathology at arthroscopy. Surgical reconstruction should include closure of the rotator interval (Fig. 4-43A) and capsulolabral reconstruction or plication (Fig. 4-43B).

Recently, various pathologies associated with unidirectional instability have been implicated as factors contributing to ongoing or recurrent instability. These include associated superior labral tears, bone lesions (both glenoid and humeral), and capsular redundancy. In particular, failure to treat capsular laxity has been implicated as a reason for failure of arthroscopic Bankart repair by some authors who believe that capsular laxity occurs secondary to stretching

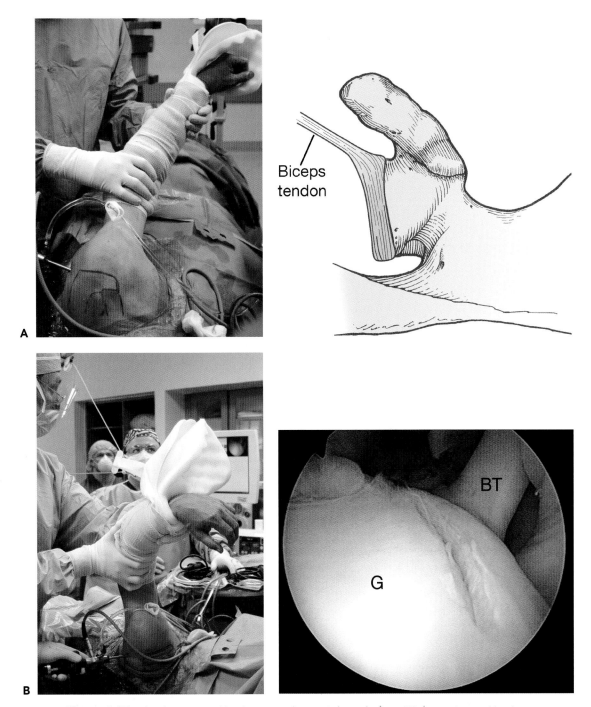

Biceps tendon

Figure 4-37   The dynamic peel-back test. As the arm is brought from (A) the resting position into (B) 90° of abduction and 90° external rotation, the biceps-superior labral complex displaces medially over the edge of the glenoid, confirming a posterior superior labrum anterior and posterior (SLAP) lesion. G, glenoid; BT, biceps tendon.

or plastic deformation of the ligaments from repetitive load (i.e., instability).

This zeal for soft tissue plication escalated to the point that various authors now recommend both anterior capsular plication (with Bankart repair) and posterior capsular plication for routine traumatic unidirectional anterior

instability to "balance" the shoulder. Although we agree that superior labral tears and significant bone lesions should be appropriately treated, we do not routinely treat presumed "capsular laxity or redundancy" in cases of traumatic unidirectional instability. We believe that most cases of capsular laxity or injury on the coup and contrecoup

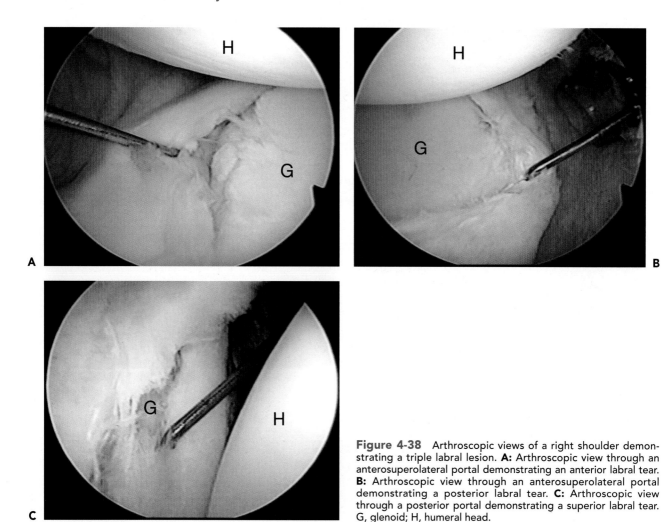

Figure 4-38 Arthroscopic views of a right shoulder demonstrating a triple labral lesion. **A:** Arthroscopic view through an anterosuperolateral portal demonstrating an anterior labral tear. **B:** Arthroscopic view through an anterosuperolateral portal demonstrating a posterior labral tear. **C:** Arthroscopic view through a posterior portal demonstrating a superior labral tear. G, glenoid; H, humeral head.

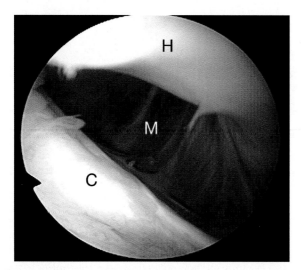

Figure 4-39 Arthroscopic view through a posterior portal of a right shoulder demonstrating a humeral avulsion of the glenohumeral ligament (HAGL). Note: The muscle is visible deep to the retracted capsular margin. H, humeral head; C, avulsed edge of the anteroinferior capsule; M, underlying muscle.

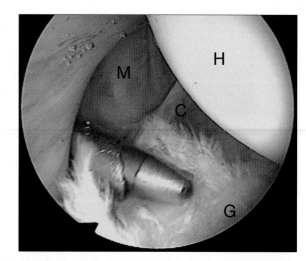

Figure 4-40 Arthroscopic view through an anterosuperolateral portal of a left shoulder demonstrating a reverse humeral avulsion of the glenohumeral ligament (RHAGL). The posterior cannula has been introduced through the defect of the RHAGL lesion. G, glenoid; H, humeral head; C, avulsed capsule margin; M, underlying muscle.

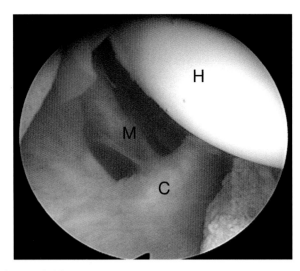

Figure 4-41 Arthroscopic view of a humeral avulsion of the glenohumeral ligament (HAGL) lesion through a posterior portal of a right shoulder using a 70° arthroscope. H, humeral head; C, avulsed capsule margin; M, underlying muscle.

sides of instability (as described above) probably heal and do not require routine repair.

In contrast, it has been our experience that unrecognized bone deficiencies account for most failures following soft tissue repair for instability and that capsular laxity is rarely the primary reason for failure (see Chapter 7: *Insurmountable Problems—Bone Deficiency*, for a complete discussion of bone lesions and instability). The results of Bankart repair in patients with minimal or no bone lesions have approached the results of open Bankart repair (i.e., 4% recurrence rate) (29).

Furthermore, we find it difficult to determine

1. What is normal capsular laxity in the shoulder?
2. What is a normal rotator interval in the shoulder?
3. What is abnormal capsular laxity in the shoulder?
4. What is a widened rotator interval in the shoulder?

Therefore, we find it difficult to determine

1. How much capsular laxity to plicate?
2. How much rotator interval to close?

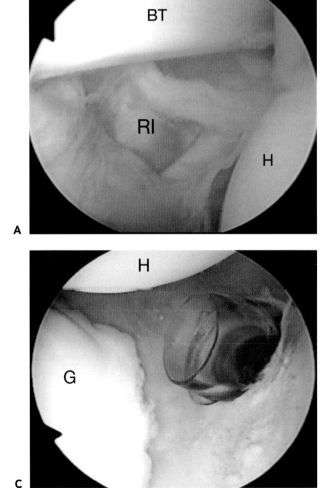

Figure 4-42 Arthroscopic view through a posterior glenohumeral portal of a right shoulder in a patient with a clinical diagnosis of multidirectional instability demonstrating **(A)** a wide rotator interval and **(B)** a patulous axillary recess. Arthroscopic view through an anterosuperolateral portal demonstrating a patulous posterior capsule **(C)**. BT, biceps tendon; G, glenoid; H, humeral head; RI, rotator interval; AR, axillary recess.

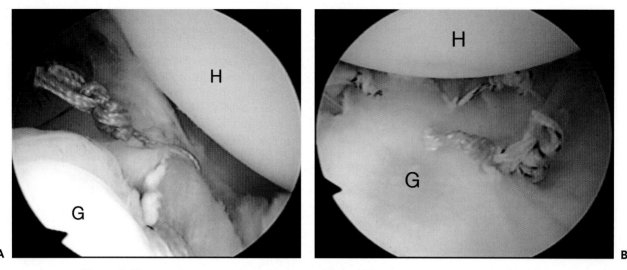

Figure 4-43 **A:** Arthroscopic view through a posterior portal demonstrating closure of the rotator interval. **B:** Arthroscopic view through an anterosuperolateral portal demonstrating anterior and posterior capsular plication. G, glenoid; H, humeral head. Same patient as in Figure 4-42.

This is not to say that we never close the rotator interval or perform a capsular plication in patients with anterior instability or superior labral tears. Closure of the rotator cuff interval is considered in the rare case of a patient with traumatic unidirectional anterior instability, with a significant sulcus sign that does not reduce with the arm in maximal external rotation. In addition, in patients with a significant drive-through sign that does not reduce following SLAP repair, then anterior mini-plication is considered. These patients are often older overhead athletes. Patients with refractory symptomatic global multidirectional instability will be treated with arthroscopic capsular plication with suture anchors in the inferior half of the shoulder.

MEASURING AND CLASSIFYING BONE DEFICIENCY

When assessing patients with glenohumeral instability, bone deficiency can occur on the glenoid or humeral sides. This can result in defects, including the engaging Hill-Sachs lesion, the nonengaging Hill-Sachs lesion, and the inverted pear glenoid. Significant bone lesions (i.e., engaging Hill-Sachs lesion, inverted pear glenoid) are relative contraindications to isolated arthroscopic Bankart repair because the recurrence rate in the presence of such bone lesions is unacceptably high. It is more appropriate to treat these lesions with a bone-grafting procedure (see Chapter 7, for a complete discussion of bone defects and bone grafting procedures).

An engaging Hill-Sachs lesion is a humeral head defect that engages or "locks into" the anterior glenoid rim when the arm is brought into a position of athletic function (i.e., 90° of abduction, 90° of external rotation). Even with a secure Bankart repair, an engaging Hill-Sachs

lesion can be symptomatic as the arm is rotated and the defect begins to articulate with the glenoid rim and anterior capsulolabral structures. In contrast, a nonengaging Hill-Sachs lesion is one where the humeral head defect does not engage or lock into the glenoid rim when the arm is brought into a position of athletic function. The nonengaging Hill-Sachs lesion is oriented at an angle to the anterior glenoid rim such that it does not engage when the arm is brought into a position of athletic function. These lesions only engage when the arm is brought into a nonfunctional position of extension or abduction of <70°.

To determine whether the Hill-Sachs lesion is engaging or nonengaging, it is easiest to view it through a posterior glenohumeral portal. Initially, the Hill-Sachs lesion, unless exceptionally large, will not be seen (Fig. 4-44A). Then, the arm is taken out of the traction boom and brought into a position of 90° of abduction (Fig. 4-44B). The arm is then slowly externally rotated until the Hill-Sachs lesion is presented to the anterior glenoid rim (Fig. 4-44C). Engaging Hill-Sachs lesions are large with the Hill-Sachs lesion oriented parallel to the anterior glenoid rim with the arm in a position of athletic function. These lesions will engage or lock out with rotation (Fig. 4-44D). In contrast, the nonengaging Hill-Sachs lesion is usually smaller and oriented nonparallel to the anterior glenoid rim with the arm in athletic function and it will not lock out (Fig. 4-44E).

An inverted pear glenoid configuration is one that has lost significant bone in the anterior inferior aspect of the glenoid. Normally, when viewed *en face*, the glenoid appears pear-shaped, with the inferior glenoid wider than the superior glenoid (Fig. 4-45). If, however, significant bone loss has occurred to the inferior glenoid secondary

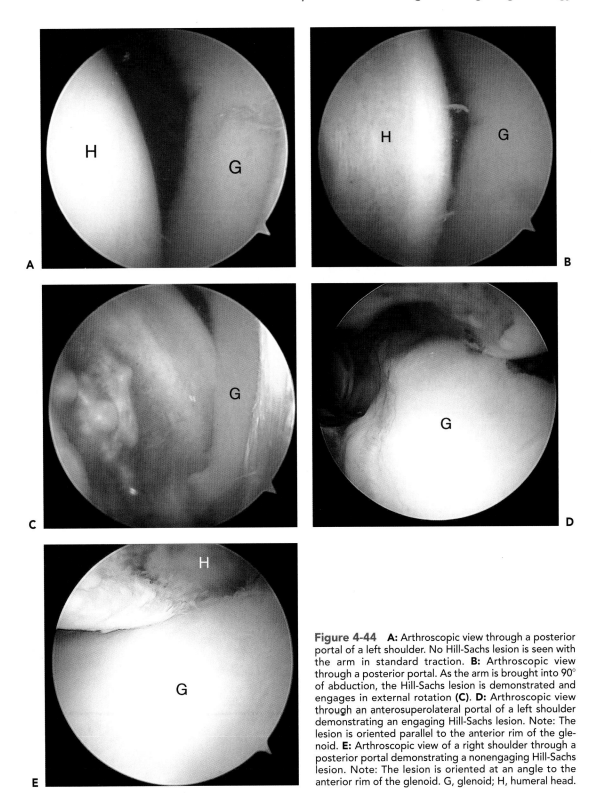

Figure 4-44 **A:** Arthroscopic view through a posterior portal of a left shoulder. No Hill-Sachs lesion is seen with the arm in standard traction. **B:** Arthroscopic view through a posterior portal. As the arm is brought into 90° of abduction, the Hill-Sachs lesion is demonstrated and engages in external rotation **(C). D:** Arthroscopic view through an anterosuperolateral portal of a left shoulder demonstrating an engaging Hill-Sachs lesion. Note: The lesion is oriented parallel to the anterior rim of the glenoid. **E:** Arthroscopic view of a right shoulder through a posterior portal demonstrating a nonengaging Hill-Sachs lesion. Note: The lesion is oriented at an angle to the anterior rim of the glenoid. G, glenoid; H, humeral head.

to a bony Bankart lesion or an impression (compression) lesion of the glenoid (without bony Bankart), the reverse may be true, with the inferior glenoid narrower than the superior glenoid (Fig. 4-46). This gives the impression of an inverted pear when the glenoid is viewed *en face* (Fig. 4-47).

Glenoid bone deficiency and the inverted pear configuration are best evaluated through an anterosuperolateral viewing portal. This allows an *en face* view of the glenoid and easy identification of the inverted pear configuration. Furthermore, in combined cases of an inverted pear configuration with an engaging Hill-Sachs lesion, the interplay

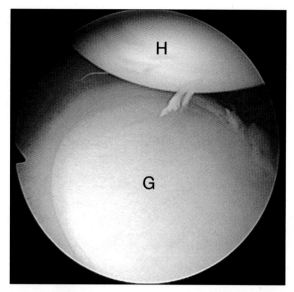

Figure 4-45 Arthroscopic view through an anterosuperolateral portal of a left shoulder demonstrating the normal pear configuration of the glenoid. Note: The inferior glenoid is wider than the superior glenoid. G, glenoid; H, humeral head.

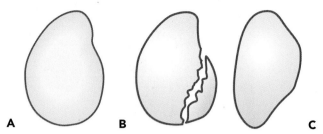

Figure 4-46 **A:** The normal shape of the glenoid is that of a pear, larger below than above. **B:** A bony Bankart lesion can create an inverted-pear configuration. **C:** A compression (impression) Bankart lesion can also create an inverted pear.

between the Hill-Sachs lesion and the residual anterior glenoid rim can be easily assessed through this portal. An inverted pear configuration signifies glenoid bone deficiency of ≥25%, as confirmed in both anatomic and clinical studies (30).

To document and accurately measure each patient individually, a different method must be used. This method relies on the position of the glenoid bare spot. When viewed *en face*, the glenoid bare spot lies roughly in the center of the inferior aspect of the glenoid. A previous study by Burkhart et al. (31) determined that the glenoid bare spot lies at the geometric center of the inferior aspect of the glenoid, equidistant from the anterior glenoid rim, the posterior glenoid rim, and the inferior glenoid rim (Table 4-1). This anatomic symmetry allows the glenoid bare spot to act as a point of reference when determining glenoid bone deficiency.

To measure accurately the amount of bone deficiency, the glenoid is viewed *en face* through the anterosuperolateral portal (Fig. 4-48). An arthroscopic probe with 3-mm laser markings is then introduced through the posterior portal and the distance from the bare spot to the posterior glenoid rim is measured (posterior length) (Fig. 4-48A). The arthroscopic probe is then advanced anteriorly and the distance from the anterior glenoid rim to the bare spot is measured (anterior length) (Fig. 4-48B). The amount of bone loss can then be calculated using the following formula.

$$\text{Glenoid bone loss} = \frac{\text{Posterior length} - \text{Anterior length}}{\text{Posterior length} \times 2} \times 100\%$$

In a series of 53 consecutive patients having instability repair, it was noted that 42 patients had a noninverted pear configuration and 11 patients had an inverted pear configuration (30). It was demonstrated that patients with an inverted pear configuration had a mean glenoid bone loss of 8.6-mm (range: 6–12-mm) representing 36% (range: 25% to 45%) of the inferior glenoid width. Interestingly, even in patients without an inverted pear configuration there was a mean glenoid bone loss of 1.5-mm (range: 0–3 mm) representing 6.2% (range: 0% to 12.5%) of the inferior

TABLE 4-1
MEAN DISTANCE FROM THE CENTER OF THE BARE SPOT TO VARIOUS POSITIONS OF THE INFERIOR GLENOID

Distance from the center of the bare spot	Living subjects (N, 56; age, 15–56 yr)			Cadavers (N, 10; age, 62–85 yr)	
	Mean	SD	Range	Mean	Range
To the posterior glenoid rim	11.4	0.85	9.0–12.0	12.3	11–15
To the anterior glenoid rim	11.1	0.91	9.0–12.0	12.1	11–15
To the inferior glenoid rim	10.7	0.98	7.5–13.5	12.1	11–15

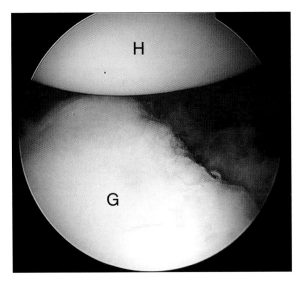

Figure 4-47 Arthroscopic view through an anterosuperolateral portal of a left shoulder demonstrating an inverted pear *cavitas* glenoid. Note: The inferior glenoid narrows to a point inferiorly. G, glenoid; H, humeral head.

glenoid width. In our clinical experience with arthroscopic Bankart repair, these more subtle degrees of bone loss have not predisposed toward recurrent instability.

BICEPS TENDON

The diagnosis and treatment of disorders of the long head of the biceps tendon remains controversial. Much of this

controversy is secondary to the uncertain role the long head of the biceps tendon plays in normal shoulder function and in pathologic conditions (e.g., massive rotator cuff tear with proximal migration). In addition, because of the extensive overlap between conditions of the long head of the biceps tendon and other disorders (e.g., biceps tendinopathy and rotator cuff tears, biceps subluxation, and subscapularis tears), it can be difficult to determine the primary cause of a patient's symptoms. Once pathology is diagnosed and treatment is required, the appropriate treatment remains controversial (i.e., débridement, tenotomy, tenodesis).

Careful evaluation of the long head of the biceps tendon involves evaluation of the biceps root, the intra-articular portion of the long head of the biceps tendon, and the portion of the biceps tendon within the intertubercular groove (Fig. 4-49). (For a complete evaluation of the biceps root, please see SLAP lesion section above.)

When evaluating the intra-articular and intertubercular portions of the long head of the biceps tendon, consider both tendinopathy and stability. Evaluate tendinopathy along the entire length of the tendon. To evaluate the intertubercular portion of the long head of the biceps tendon, use a switching stick or probe to pull the intertubercular portion of the long head of the biceps tendon intra-articularly (Fig. 4-49). The spectrum of tendinopathy can include inflammation, longitudinal splitting, partial tearing, and widening or thickening of the tendon (Fig. 4-50). Following débridement of any degenerative tissue, estimate the amount of tendinopathy as a percentage of the normal thickness of the tendon (Fig. 4-51).

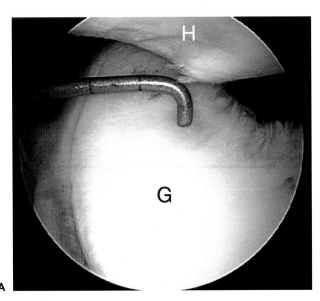 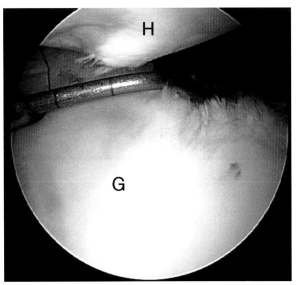

Figure 4-48 Arthroscopic view through an anterosuperolateral portal of a left shoulder demonstrating measurement of glenoid bone loss. **A:** A probe is introduced through the posterior portal to measure the distance from the bare spot to the posterior glenoid rim (12.5-mm, in this example). **B:** The probe is then advanced anteriorly to measure the distance from the anterior glenoid rim to the bare spot (5-mm, in this example). This indicates 7.5-mm of bone loss or 30% bone loss. G, glenoid; H, humeral head.

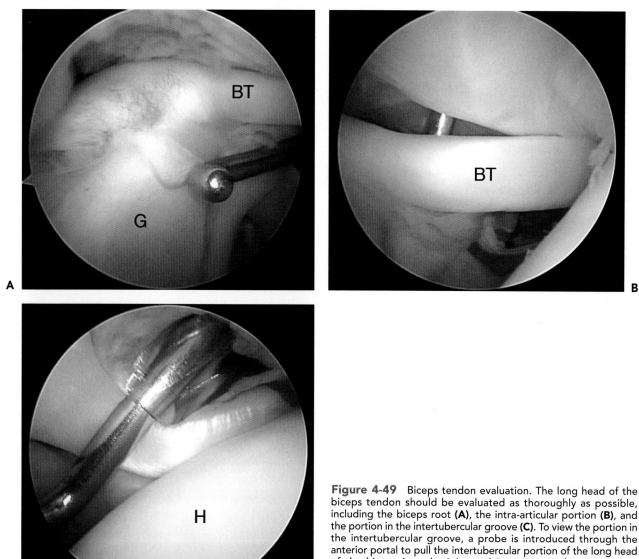

Figure 4-49 Biceps tendon evaluation. The long head of the biceps tendon should be evaluated as thoroughly as possible, including the biceps root (**A**), the intra-articular portion (**B**), and the portion in the intertubercular groove (**C**). To view the portion in the intertubercular groove, a probe is introduced through the anterior portal to pull the intertubercular portion of the long head of the biceps into the joint and into view. Arthroscopic view through a posterior glenohumeral portal of a right shoulder. G, glenoid; H, humeral head, BT, biceps tendon.

Evaluating biceps tendon stability is done in concert with evaluating the subscapularis tendon (see below for complete evaluation of the subscapularis tendon). While viewing through a posterior glenohumeral portal, evaluate the stability of the long head of the biceps tendon, both statically and dynamically, with internal and external rotation of the shoulder (Fig. 4-52). Overt biceps dislocation can be easily demonstrated statically with the long head of the biceps lying posterior to the plane of the anterior border of the subscapularis tendon, which is essentially almost always torn (Fig. 4-53), or resting within a longitudinal split of the subscapularis tendon (Fig. 4-54).

For subtle biceps subluxation or dynamic instability the arm is rotated into various positions of internal and external rotation (Fig. 4-55). Pay particular attention to encroachment of the long head of the biceps tendon against the medial sling of the biceps tendon and the subscapularis tendon. If the biceps tendon is positioned posterior to the plane of the subscapularis tendon or medial sling, this is highly suggestive of a combined upper subscapularis tear with biceps subluxation.

Once significant biceps pathology is diagnosed, surgical treatment is then carried out. In most patients with biceps dislocation, biceps tendinopathy >25% of the thickness of the tendon, or with biceps instability associated with a subscapularis tear, we prefer to perform an arthroscopic biceps tenodesis using the BioTenodesis screw system (Arthrex, Inc.; Naples, FL). In patients >70 years of age who do not require strength for activities, a tenotomy can be performed. Patients with degeneration of <25% of the tendon thickness are treated with débridement. In addition

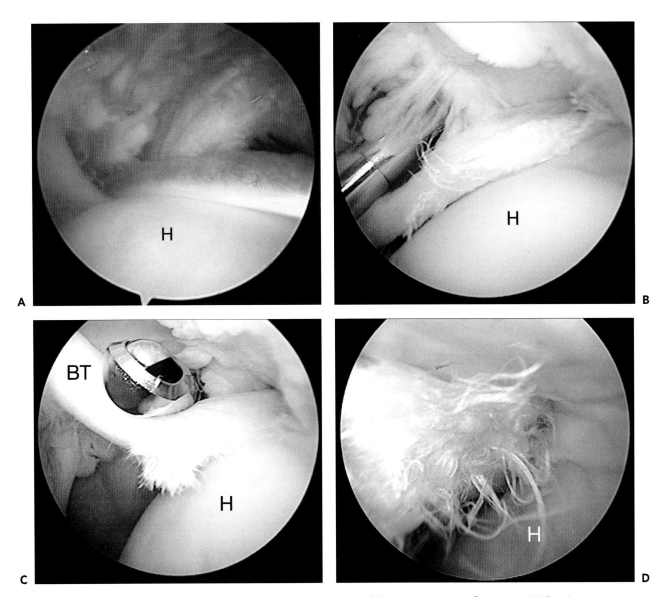

Figure 4-50   Arthroscopic view through a posterior portal demonstrating **(A)** inflammation, **(B)** longitudinal splitting, **(C)** partial tearing, and **(D)** widening or thickening of the long head of the biceps tendon. H, humeral head; BT, biceps tendon.

to treatment of biceps pathology, all concomitant shoulder pathology is arthroscopically addressed.

ROTATOR CUFF

Over the last 10 years, no reconstructive procedure of the shoulder has evolved more than rotator cuff repair. Much of the impetus for this evolution has been the result of a better understanding of the anatomy and pathoanatomy of rotator cuff pathology provided in part by the arthroscope. For decades, the goal of rotator cuff repair was to "cover the hole," and ill-advised Herculean attempts (e.g., tendon transfer, freeze-dried allograft) were made to achieve this

goal. These procedures, however, were not based on a clear understanding of the biomechanical role of the rotator cuff in shoulder function.

Force Couples

The primary function of the rotator cuff is to balance the force couples about the glenohumeral joint (32–37). A force couple is a pair of forces that act on an object and cause it to rotate. For any object to be in equilibrium, the forces must create moments (i.e., force × distance from center of rotation) about a center of rotation that are equal in magnitude and opposite in direction. In the situation where the center of rotation is equidistant from the point

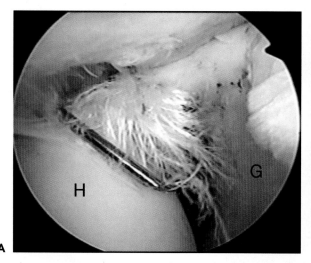
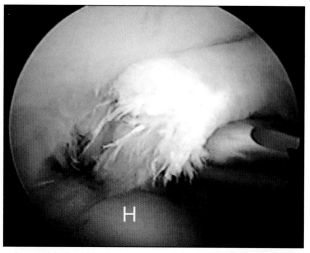

Figure 4-51 Arthroscopic view through a posterior portal of the long head of the biceps tendon in a left shoulder. **A:** Before débridement, a significant amount of partial tearing and degeneration is seen along the intra-articular portion of the long head of the biceps tendon. **B:** Following débridement, <50% of the tendon is left intact. H, humeral head; G, glenoid.

of application of each force, the forces must be equal and opposite in direction for equilibrium to exist (Fig. 4-56A). If the forces (Fig. 4-56B) are acting at different radii from the center of rotation, however, for the object to be in equilibrium, the forces will be unequal (Fig. 4-56B) but will create equal moments (force × distance).

In the shoulder, the coronal plane force couple was described by Inman et al. (38) (Fig. 4-57). This force couple is a result of the balance of moments created by the deltoid versus those created by the intact portions of the inferior rotator cuff (i.e., infraspinatus, teres minor, subscapularis).

During abduction, the coronal plane force couple will only be balanced if the line of action (centroid) of the rotator cuff force is below the center of rotation of the humeral head, so that it can oppose the moment created by the deltoid. Balancing the coronal plane force couple is essential because this maintains a stable fulcrum for glenohumeral joint motion.

An equally important force couple is the transverse plane force couple (32–37). This force couple consists of the subscapularis, anteriorly, balanced against the posterior rotator cuff (i.e., infraspinatus, teres minor) (Fig. 4-58).

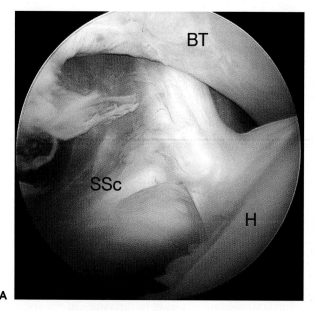
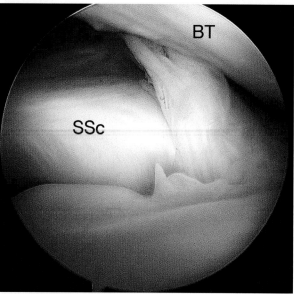

Figure 4-52 Arthroscopic views through a posterior portal of a right shoulder demonstrating the normal relationship between the long head of the biceps tendon, the medial biceps sling, and the subscapularis tendon. **A:** Internal rotation. **B:** External rotation. SSc, subscapularis; BT, biceps tendon; H, humeral head.

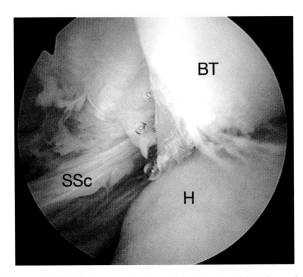

Figure 4-53 Arthroscopic view of a right shoulder through a posterior portal with a 70° arthroscope demonstrating a complete subscapularis tear with dislocation of the biceps tendon medially between the humeral head and subscapularis tendon. BT, biceps tendon; SSc, subscapularis tendon; H, humeral head.

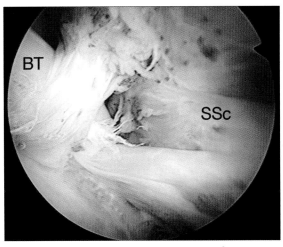

Figure 4-54 Arthroscopic view through a posterior portal of a left shoulder demonstrating a partial tear of the subscapularis tendon with the biceps tendon subluxed between the two laminae of a longitudinal split of the subscapularis. BT, biceps tendon, SSc, subscapularis.

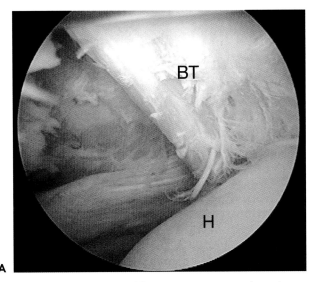

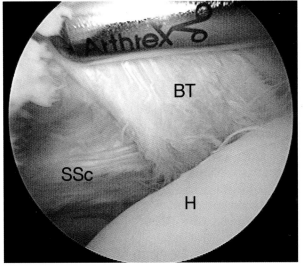

Figure 4-55 Arthroscopic views through a posterior portal showing the relationship between the long head of the biceps tendon and the subscapularis tendon. **A:** Internal rotation. **B:** External rotation. Note: With external rotation, the dislocation of the biceps tendon is accentuated medial and posterior to the subscapularis tendon. BT, biceps tendon, H, humeral head; SSc, subscapularis.

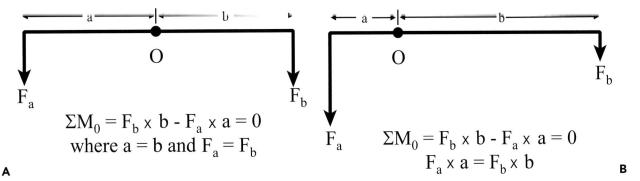

Figure 4-56   A: Force couple in which the forces are equal and are applied at equal distances from the center of rotation, creating moments (force × distance) that are equal and opposite. **B:** Force couple with unequal forces acting at different radii from the center of rotation such that the moments created by the forces (force × distance) are equal and opposite.

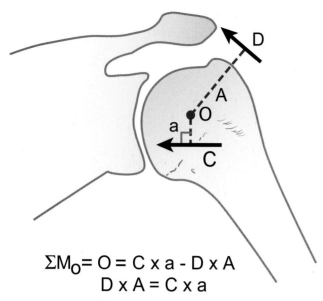

$$\Sigma M_O = O = C \times a - D \times A$$
$$D \times A = C \times a$$

Figure 4-57 *Coronal plane force couple. The inferior portion of the rotator cuff (below the center of rotation) creates a moment that must balance the deltoid moment. C, resultant of rotator cuff forces; D, deltoid force; O, center of rotation; a, moment arm of the inferior portion of the rotator cuff; A, moment arm of the deltoid.*

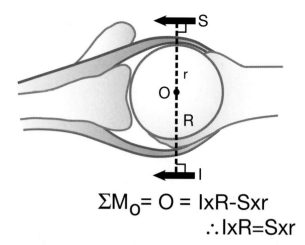

$$\Sigma M_O = O = I \times R - S \times r$$
$$\therefore I \times R = S \times r$$

Figure 4-58 *Transverse plane force couple (axillary view). The subscapularis anteriorly is balanced against the infraspinatus and teres minor posteriorly. I, infraspinatus; S, subscapularis; O, center of rotation; r, moment arm of the subscapularis; R, moment arm of the infraspinatus and teres minor.*

This force couple is particularly relevant in massive rotator cuff tears, which may extend more posteriorly, leaving only a remnant of intact posterior cuff. In many cases, the posterior rotator cuff is so weak that it cannot balance the anterior moment created by the subscapularis tendon. Furthermore, a large posterior rotator cuff tear can result in such a deficiency that the moment created by the inferior rotator cuff is also insufficient to maintain equilibrium in the coronal plane (Fig. 4-59). This, then, can result in anterior and superior translation of the humeral head and the inability to maintain a stable fulcrum of motion (Fig. 4-60). Therefore, when faced with a rotator cuff tear, the primary goal of surgery is to balance the force couples in

the transverse and coronal planes and not necessarily to "cover the hole."

Suspension Bridge Analogy

When arthroscopically viewed from the glenohumeral joint, the articular surface of the intact rotator cuff demonstrates an arching, cablelike thickening of the capsule surrounding a thinner crescent of tissue that inserts into the greater tuberosity of the humerus (39,40) (Fig. 4-61). This cablelike structure, which represents a thickening of the coracohumeral ligament, is consistently located at the avascular zone margin of the rotator cuff, extending from its anterior attachment into the greater tuberosity of the humerus just posterior to the biceps tendon, to its posterior attachment near the inferior border of the infraspinatus tendon (39,40) (Fig. 4-62). The rotator cable potentially

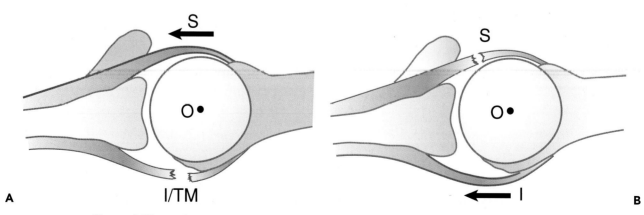

Figure 4-59 **A:** *The transverse plane force couple is disrupted because of a massive rotator cuff tear involving the posterior rotator cuff, infraspinatus, and teres minor.* **B:** *An alternative pattern of disruption of the transverse plane force couple. The transverse plane force couple is disrupted by a massive tear involving the anterior rotator cuff (i.e., subscapularis). I, infraspinatus; TM, teres minor; O, center of rotation; S, subscapularis.*

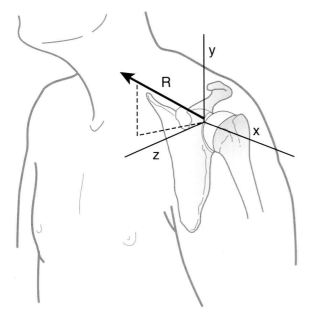

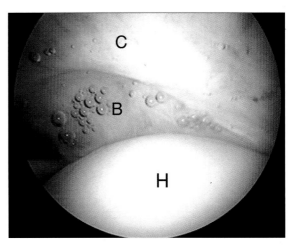

Figure 4-61 Arthroscopic view of a right shoulder demonstrating a cablelike thickening of the capsule surrounding a thinner crescent of tissue that inserts into the greater tuberosity of the humerus. C, rotator cable; B, rotator crescent; H, humeral head.

Figure 4-60 Uncoupling of the essential force couples results in anterior-superior translation of the humeral head with attempted elevation of the shoulder. R, resultant of uncoupled shoulder muscle forces.

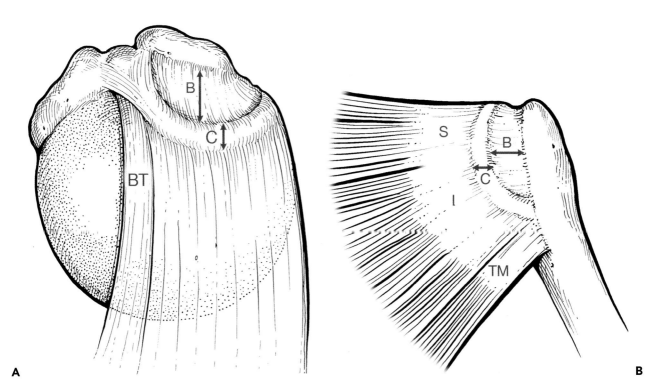

Figure 4-62 Superior **(A)** and posterior **(B)** projections of the rotator cable and crescent. The rotator cable extends from the biceps to the inferior margin of the infraspinatus, spanning the supraspinatus and infraspinatus insertions. C, rotator cable width; B, mediolateral diameter of rotator crescent; S, supraspinatus; I, infraspinatus; TM, teres minor; BT, biceps tendon.

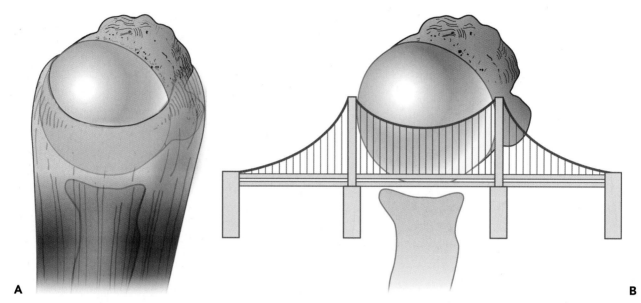

A   B

Figure 4-63 A rotator cuff tear **(A)** can be modeled after a suspension bridge **(B)**. The free margin corresponds to the cable, and the anterior and posterior attachments of the tear correspond to the supports at each end of the cable's span.

serves a protective role, transferring stress along the rotator cable, thereby stress-shielding the thinner, avascular crescent tissue, analogous to a load-bearing suspension bridge.

Similar to the intact rotator cuff, a rotator cuff tear can also be modeled after a suspension bridge where the free margin of the tear corresponds to the cable and the anterior and posterior attachments of the tear correspond to the supports at each end of the cable's span (32–34,36,40) (Fig. 4-63). This model would predict that, despite a tear in the avascular zone of the supraspinatus tendon, the supraspinatus muscle could still exert a compressive effect on the glenohumeral joint by means of its distributed load along the span of the suspension bridge configuration (32–34,36,40).

An *in vitro* biomechanical study by Halder et al. (41) has confirmed the concept of a suspension bridge model for the rotator cable-crescent complex and of rotator cuff tearing. In this study, the rotator cuff tendons of 10 cadaveric shoulders were proportionally loaded according to their cross-sectional areas, and the force transmitted by the rotator cuff to the humerus was measured using a three-component load cell. These investigators determined that detachment of one third or two thirds of the supraspinatus tendon had only a minor effect on force transmission (1% and 2%; $p > 0.05$) and that not until the entire supraspinatus tendon was detached did a significant decrease occur in force transmission (11% decrease in force transmission with complete supraspinatus detachment; $p < 0.05$). These findings support the concept that in small- and medium-sized rotator cuff tears, the rotator cuff muscle forces are effectively transmitted along the rotator cuff cable, bypassing the torn supraspinatus tendon. These observations, combined with our knowledge of the importance of balancing the force couples of the glenohumeral joint, explain why certain rotator cuff tears (termed *functional* rotator cuff tears), even massive tears, can demonstrate "normal" kinematic patterns (36) and why, after rotator cuff repair, good results can be achieved even when a water-tight closure is not obtained (42–45).

Furthermore, the implication of the cable-crescent concept contradicts the historical principle of covering the hole, particularly when using techniques such as tendon transfer to obtain closure of massive, "irreparable" rotator cuff tears. Other authors have advocated the use of tendon transfers, including the infraspinatus and subscapularis, to cover rotator cuff defects in massive tears (46–49). Transferring these muscles superiorly, however, significantly alters the normal mechanics of the rotator cuff (Fig. 4-64).

Partial Rotator Cuff Repair: Balancing the Force Couples

In situations where a massive, dysfunctional contracted immobile rotator cuff tear is not completely repairable, partial rotator cuff repair is a valid option. Partial repair respects and restores the biomechanical function of the rotator cuff. The goal of partial repair is to achieve sufficient tendon healing to regain overhead function. To accomplish this, the rotator cuff repair must satisfy the following five biomechanical criteria (33,42,43).

1. Force couples must be balanced in the coronal and transverse planes (see Figs. 4-57 and 4-58).
2. A stable fulcrum kinematic pattern must be reestablished.
3. The shoulder's "suspension bridge" must be reestablished (see Fig. 4-63).

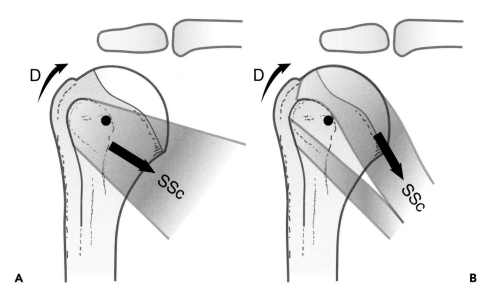

Figure 4-64 A: The centroid (line of action) of the subscapularis muscle lies inferior to the center of rotation, forming a force couple with the deltoid muscle. These two muscles have moments that are opposite in direction. **B:** The subscapularis in its transferred position now has its centroid above the center of rotation, and its moment is in the same direction as the deltoid moment. This muscle transfer destroys the important coronal plane force couple. D, deltoid moment; SSc, subscapularis.

4. The residual defect must occupy a minimal surface area.
5. The residual defect must possess edge stability.

These five criteria are primarily achieved by balancing the force couple between the anterior and posterior portions of the shoulder. This balance requires an intact subscapularis tendon anteriorly, and an intact inferior half of the infraspinatus tendon posteriorly. Anatomically, this requisite configuration corresponds to the anterior and posterior attachments of the rotator cable (see Fig. 4-62). Thus, during arthroscopic surgery, the major goal of partial rotator cuff repair is to mobilize and repair the rotator cuff to reestablish these cable attachments (Fig. 4-65). It should

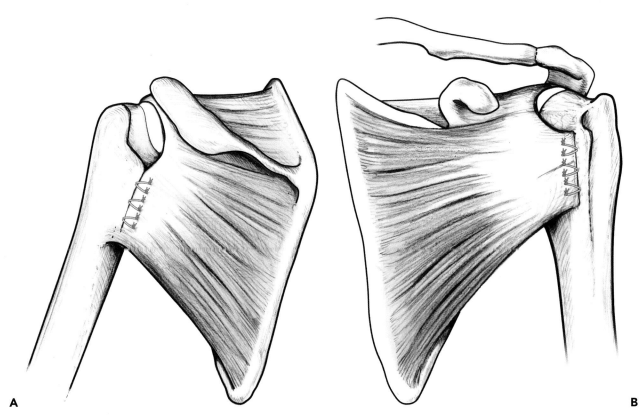

Figure 4-65 A: Partial repair of a massive posterior rotator cuff tear should include at least the lower half of the infraspinatus to repair the rotator cable and restore the force couples. **B:** Massive anterior rotator cuff tears demand as complete a repair of the subscapularis tendon as possible.

be emphasized, however, that complete anatomic closure and complete healing of the rotator cuff still achieves superior and more predictable functional results when compared with partial closure or partial healing of the rotator cuff with a persistent defect.

Four Basic Tear Patterns

Arthroscopy has greatly enhanced our understanding of rotator cuff tears. Unlike traditional open surgery, which is limited by an anterolateral exposure, arthroscopy is not restricted by spatial constraints. Using arthroscopic techniques, rotator cuff tears can now be assessed and treated from several different angles with minimal disruption to the overlying deltoid. This new perspective on evaluating and treating rotator cuff tears has led to the recognition of four major types of rotator cuff tears.

1. Crescent-shaped tears
2. U-shaped tears
3. L-shaped and reverse-L-shaped tears
4. Massive contracted immobile tears

Crescent-shaped tears are the simplest of all tears and, although they can be massive, these tears do not typically retract medially to a significant degree (Fig. 4-66A). These tears demonstrate excellent mobility from a medial-to-lateral direction and can be repaired directly to bone with minimal tension (Fig. 4-66B).

In contrast, U-shaped rotator cuff tears extend much farther medially than crescent-shaped tears, with the apex of the tear adjacent to or medial to the glenoid rim (Fig. 4-67A). Recognizing this tear pattern is critical, because attempting to medially mobilize and repair the apex of the tear to a lateral bone bed will result in overwhelming tensile stresses in the middle of the repaired rotator cuff margin (i.e., tensile overload) and subsequent failure. These tears demonstrate significant mobility from an anterior-to-posterior direction and should be initially repaired in a side-to-side fashion using the biomechanical principle of *margin convergence* (see below).

In such cases, sequential side-to-side suturing, from medial to lateral, of the anterior and posterior leaves of the tear causes the free margin of the rotator cuff to converge toward the bone bed on the humerus (Fig. 4-67B). The free margin of the rotator cuff can then be easily repaired to the bone bed in a tension-free manner (Fig. 4-67C). The technique of *margin convergence* both allows repair of seemingly irreparable tears and minimizes strain at the repair site (50). Theoretically, this decreases the risk of rupture and subsequent failure of the rotator cuff repair.

The L-shaped and reverse-L-shaped tears are similar to U-shaped tears. One of the leaves (usually the posterior leaf), however, is more mobile than the other leaf and can be easily brought to the bone bed and to the other leaf (Fig. 4-68A). In these cases, side-to-side suturing is first performed along the longitudinal split (Fig. 4-68B) and then the converged margin is repaired to bone (Fig. 4-68C). In more chronic cases, the physiologic pull of the rotator cuff muscles posteriorly will cause an L-shaped tear to assume a more U-shaped configuration (Fig. 4-69A). In chronic L-shaped tears, it is imperative to determine which leaf is more mobile and where the "corner" of the L-shaped tear needs to be restored. In these cases, side-to-side suturing is first performed along the longitudinal split (Fig. 4-69B) and then the converged margin is repaired to bone (Fig. 4-69C).

These first three tear patterns represent >90% of posterosuperior rotator cuff tears and can be repaired using the principles outlined here. Thus, most rotator cuff tears,

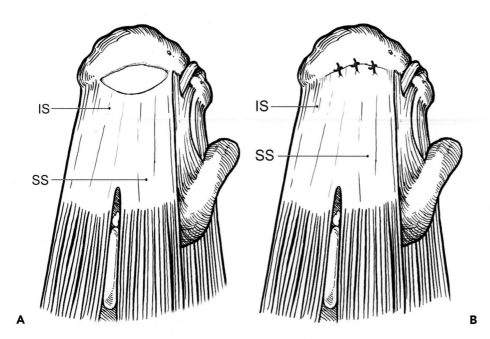

A

B

Figure 4-66 Crescent-shaped rotator cuff tear. **A:** Superior view of a crescent-shaped rotator cuff tear involving the supraspinatus and infraspinatus tendons. **B:** Crescent-shaped tears demonstrate excellent mobility from a medial to lateral direction and can be repaired directly to bone. SS, supraspinatus; IS, infraspinatus.

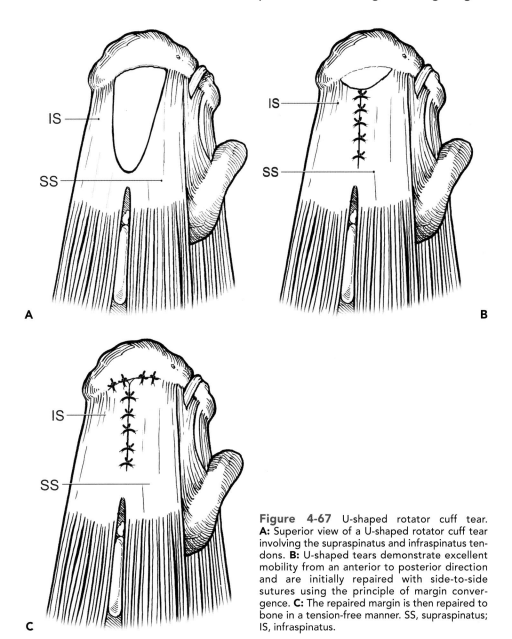

Figure 4-67 U-shaped rotator cuff tear. **A:** Superior view of a U-shaped rotator cuff tear involving the supraspinatus and infraspinatus tendons. **B:** U-shaped tears demonstrate excellent mobility from an anterior to posterior direction and are initially repaired with side-to-side sutures using the principle of margin convergence. **C:** The repaired margin is then repaired to bone in a tension-free manner. SS, supraspinatus; IS, infraspinatus.

even massive tears, can be repaired without extensive mobilization with an understanding and recognition of these tear patterns. Repairing tears according to their tear pattern can lead to excellent results (51,52). In the fourth tear pattern, the massive, contracted, immobile rotator cuff tear, other techniques must be used (see Chapter 5, *The Tough Stuff*).

Margin Convergence: Optimizing Mechanics through Understanding Anatomy

Although some massive rotator cuff tears are crescent shaped and can be repaired directly to bone, U-shaped and L-shaped tears are amenable to repair using the principle of margin convergence. These tears demonstrate significant mobility from an anterior to posterior direction and should initially be repaired in a side-to-side fashion, using the biomechanical principle of *margin convergence* (50–52).

When addressing U-shaped or L-shaped tears, the tears are initially repaired with sequential side-to-side suturing, from medial to lateral, of the anterior and posterior leaves of the tear. This causes the free margin of the rotator cuff to converge toward the bone bed on the humerus (see Fig. 4-67B), and the free margin of the rotator cuff can then easily be repaired to the bone bed in a tension-free manner (see Fig. 4-67C). The technique of margin convergence both allows repair of seemingly irreparable tears and minimizes strain at the repair site (50).

To estimate the amount of strain reduction following margin convergence, consider the case of a U-shaped

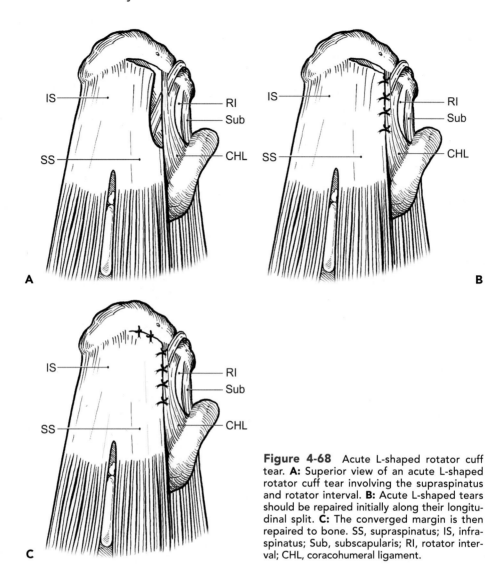

Figure 4-68 Acute L-shaped rotator cuff tear. **A:** Superior view of an acute L-shaped rotator cuff tear involving the supraspinatus and rotator interval. **B:** Acute L-shaped tears should be repaired initially along their longitudinal split. **C:** The converged margin is then repaired to bone. SS, supraspinatus; IS, infraspinatus; Sub, subscapularis; RI, rotator interval; CHL, coracohumeral ligament.

tear that is closed side-to-side for two thirds of its length. Assume that (a) the rotator cuff consists of an elastic, isotropic, homogeneous material; (b) the cross-sectional area remains constant along the tear length; and (c) the load is the resultant force caused by contraction of the rotator cuff musculature across the tear. Strain in the rotator cuff tear (Fig. 4-70) is defined as the change in the medial-to-lateral dimension of the tear (ΔL) divided by the initial (L) medial-to-lateral dimension of the tear ($\Delta L / L$) and is related to the cross-sectional area of the intact tissue according to the formula (53):

$$\varepsilon \text{ (strain)} = \frac{\Delta L}{L} = \frac{F}{AE}$$

Where

L = medial-to-lateral dimension of the cuff tear
A = cross-sectional area of intact cuff at level of strain measurement
F = resultant longitudinal rotator cuff force
E = modulus of elasticity (Young's modulus)

In our case, where a U-shaped tear is closed side-to-side along two thirds of its length, then $L_1 = 3L_2$, where L_1 is the initial length and L_2 is the length after side-to-side suturing (Fig. 4-71). Also assume that the cross-sectional area (A_2) after side-to-side repair is twice the original area (A_1). In this example, the resultant rotator cuff force (F) acting on the areas does not change and thus $F = F_1 = F_2$. Therefore,

$$\Delta L_1 = \frac{F_1 L_1}{A_1 E} \text{ and } \Delta L_2 = \frac{F_2 L_2}{A_2 E}$$

And, thus,

$$\frac{\Delta L_1}{\Delta L_2} = \frac{L_1 A_2}{L_2 A_1} = \frac{(3L_2)(2A_1)}{L_2 A_1} = 6$$

In other words, $\Delta L_1 = 6\Delta L_2$. Clinically this means that under the same force, the fiber elongation of our side-to-side repaired U-shaped rotator cuff tear would only be one sixth the elongation of the original configuration, clearly an advantageous clinical scenario. This strain reduction would be protective against a rupture of a rotator cuff

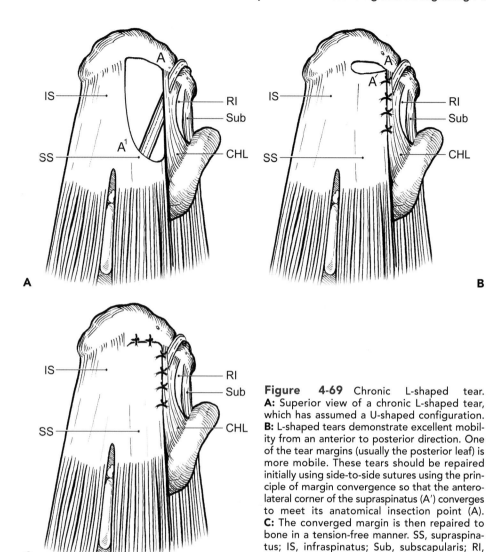

Figure 4-69 Chronic L-shaped tear. **A:** Superior view of a chronic L-shaped tear, which has assumed a U-shaped configuration. **B:** L-shaped tears demonstrate excellent mobility from an anterior to posterior direction. One of the tear margins (usually the posterior leaf) is more mobile. These tears should be repaired initially using side-to-side sutures using the principle of margin convergence so that the antero-lateral corner of the supraspinatus (A') converges to meet its anatomical insection point (A). **C:** The converged margin is then repaired to bone in a tension-free manner. SS, supraspinatus; IS, infraspinatus; Sub, subscapularis; RI, rotator interval; CHL, coracohumeral ligament.

repair construct to bone and would also be protective against propagation of the tear if it were left in a crescent-shaped configuration and not repaired to bone.

An *in vitro* mechanical study performed by Halder et al. (41) also confirmed the utility of the cable-crescent concept where, following complete removal of the supraspinatus tendon, side-to-side repair of the residual rotator cuff tear (i.e., repair of infraspinatus to rotator interval) restored the normal force transmission of the rotator cuff to 90% of the intact cuff, even if the tear was not repaired to bone. This improvement in force transmission is likely explained by the restoration of the rotator cable integrity.

In cases where there is a deficient rotator interval, a margin convergence type repair can still be performed. In these situations, the posterior rotator cuff is converged to the bone bed by suturing it to the long head of the biceps tendon (Fig. 4-72) (54). A partial closure of the rotator cuff defect is obtained by advancing the posterior rotator cuff

anteriorly and laterally along the biceps tendon by means of sequential side-to-side sutures and then securing it to the bone bed (Fig. 4-73). A similar strain reduction is obtained at the interface between the bone and the rotator cuff tendon. The goal is not to have the rotator cuff tendon heal to the biceps tendon, but to optimize the conditions for healing of the rotator cuff tendon to bone.

PARTIAL THICKNESS ROTATOR CUFF TEARS

Partial thickness rotator cuff tears are roughly twice as common as full-thickness rotator cuff tears in both clinical and cadaveric studies. Partial thickness tears can be divided anatomically into articular surface tears, bursal surface tears, and insubstance (interstitial) tears (Fig. 4-74). Codman (55) was likely the first to describe partial thickness tears, which he called rim rents, on the articular surface

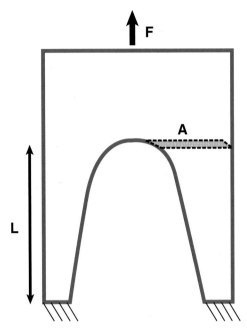

Figure 4-70 Diagrammatic representation of linear strain and elongation. A force *(F)* applied to a rotator cuff tear of length *(L)* will cause an elongation of the tear (ΔL). Elongation is related to strain according to the formula

$$\varepsilon(\text{strain}) = \frac{\Delta L}{L} = \frac{F}{AE}$$

where A, cross-sectional area of intact cuff at level of strain measurement and E, modulus of elasticity (Young's modulus).

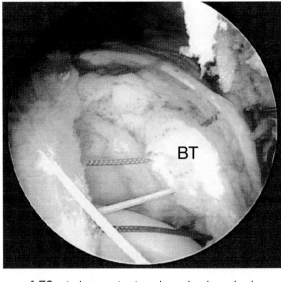

Figure 4-72 Arthroscopic view through a lateral subacromial portal of a right shoulder demonstrating margin convergence sutures passed through the rotator cuff posteriorly and the biceps tendon anteriorly. BT, biceps tendon.

of the rotator cuff and stated: "I am confident that these rim rents account for the great majority of sore shoulders." It was not until the development of arthroscopy, which allowed an inside-out view of the rotator cuff, that the diagnosis of partial thickness tears (in particular articular surface tears) became commonplace (56–58).

It has been a long-held belief that the amount of partial thickness damage to the tendon correlates with the severity of symptoms (55,56). Assessment of partial thickness rotator

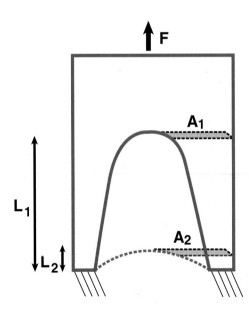

Figure 4-71 Free body diagram showing the mechanical conditions before and after partial side-to-side repair. The length of the tear has been reduced from L_1 to L_2, and the cross-sectional area of the cuff tissue at the apex of the margin of the tear has been increased from A_1 to A_2. These changes decrease the elongation of the tear and decrease the strain at the tear margin.

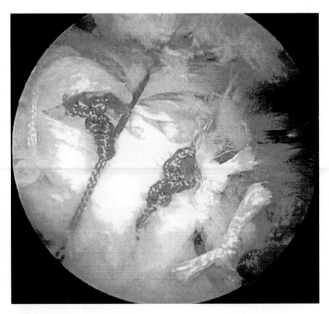

Figure 4-73 Arthroscopic view through a posterior subacromial portal of a right shoulder demonstrating a repaired massive rotator cuff tear with the margin convergence sutures from the posterior cuff to the biceps tendon and the posterior rotator cuff anchored firmly to bone.

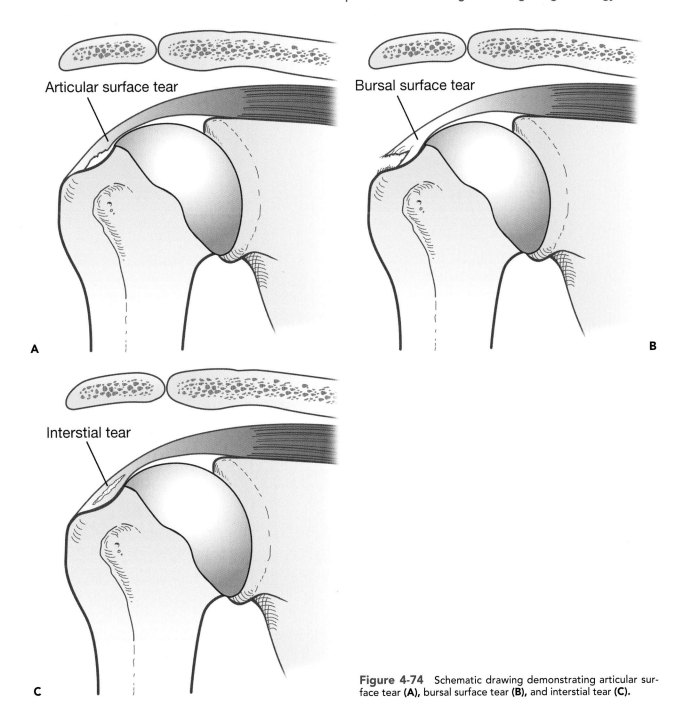

Figure 4-74 Schematic drawing demonstrating articular surface tear **(A)**, bursal surface tear **(B)**, and interstial tear **(C)**.

cuff tear size and thickness, however, is difficult and imprecise. Despite this, several authors have recommended different treatment regimens for partial thickness rotator cuff tears based on the thickness of tendon involvement. For example, Weber (59,60) has recommended that partial thickness rotator cuff tears involving >50% of the tendon thickness should be repaired.

Despite his recommendations, which have become a standard of treatment (56–58), measuring tear thickness remains difficult. In fact, in his study, Weber (59) noted that "objective means of assessing the depth of tear have

proved elusive," and further Ruotolo and Nottage (61), in 2004, stated that ". . . to date, no technique to accurately measure the thickness of a supraspinatus partial thickness rotator cuff tear has been described."

The current measurement method arbitrarily compares the amount of exposed bone in the rotator cuff footprint with historical anatomic data to determine the percentage of tendon involvement. Recently, Ruotolo and Nottage (61) demonstrated that the mean medial to lateral thickness of the supraspinatus tendon insertion was ~12 mm and recommended that all tears with >7 mm of exposed bone lateral to the articular surface (representing >50% of the tendon substance) should be repaired.

Although this method may work "on average," in fact, the medial to lateral thickness of the tendon can be remarkably diverse and has a range from 9 to 15-mm (61). Thus, 6 to 7-mm of exposed bone can represent anywhere from 37% to 69% of the tendon thickness. Current treatment algorithms based on thickness involvement must, therefore, be interpreted in light of this variability. Because partial thickness tears are so common, however, we use a simple and accurate method of measuring tendon thickness and tear involvement with an intra-articular depth gauge.

Intra-articular Depth Gauge

The intra-articular depth gauge is a simple two-piece tool that functions similarly to a depth gauge used in a trauma situation. It can be used to measure thickness involvement for both bursal surface and articular surface tears. It consists of an inner needle-tipped metallic probe that is used to penetrate the rotator cuff in a minimally traumatic fashion. This tip is marked distally (near the tip) by 3-mm lines [Fig. 4-75; (A)]. These 3-mm lines allow direct measurement of the exposed portion of the footprint by counting the number of lines exposed. Proximally (near the surgeon), the inner metallic tube is also marked with numbers [see Fig. 4-75; (B)]. The outer metallic sleeve slides freely over the inner metallic probe [see Fig. 4-75; (C)].

To measure the thickness of the entire rotator cuff, the instrument is used similarly to that of a standard depth gauge. With the tip of the inner metallic tube placed adjacent to the articular cartilage edge [Fig. 4-76; (A)], the outer metallic sleeve is slid to the edge of the rotator cuff [see Fig. 4-76; (C)]. The thickness of the entire rotator cuff is then read off the numbers on the distal portion of the inner metallic tube [see Fig. 4-76; (B)].

Partial Articular Surface Tear: Measuring Tendon Involvement

Following identification and débridement of the partial articular surface tear, the subacromial bursa is débrided to ensure that no obstruction remains to the depth gauge

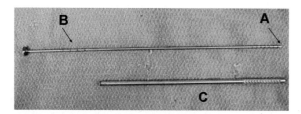

Figure 4-75 The intra-articular depth gauge. Needle tip with 3-mm markings (A); depth markings to measure total tendon thickness (B); and sliding outer metallic sleeve (C).

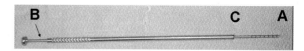

Figure 4-76 The intra-articular depth gauge. The needle tip (A), which is used to penetrate the residual intact rotator cuff and measure the exposed footprint, is marked with 3-mm markings. The outer metallic sleeve (C) is then slid down to contact the bursal surface of the rotator cuff. Total tendon thickness can then be measured by the number of exposed markings on (B).

from exuberant or thickened subacromial bursa. While viewing through a posterior glenohumeral portal, an 18-gauge spinal needle is used initially to localize the correct angle of approach from the lateral aspect of the shoulder to the partial thickness tear.

A small (2-mm) stab incision is made in the lateral skin (localized using the spinal needle), and the rotator cuff is penetrated by the needle-tipped inner probe, tangential to the footprint of the rotator cuff and adjacent to the articular surface of the humeral head (Fig. 4-77). The thickness of footprint exposed is then measured by counting the number of exposed 3-mm markers. To measure the entire thickness of the rotator cuff footprint, the outer metallic sleeve is then slid down the shaft of the inner probe through the deltoid to engage the rotator cuff. This can be confirmed by viewing through a subacromial portal (Fig. 4-78). The tendon thickness can then be read off the numbers on the shaft extracorporeally (Fig. 4-79).

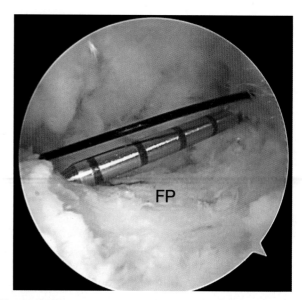

Figure 4-77 Arthroscopic view from a posterior glenohumeral portal of a right shoulder demonstrating a partial articular surface tear of the supraspinatus tendon. The needle-tipped inner probe is used to penetrate the rotator cuff tangential to the footprint and adjacent to the articular surface of the humeral head. The five marks exposed allow exposure of 15 mm of the footprint. FP, footprint.

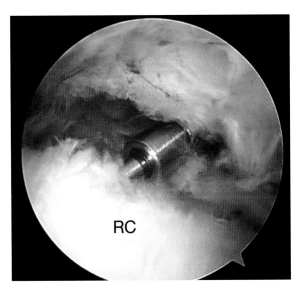

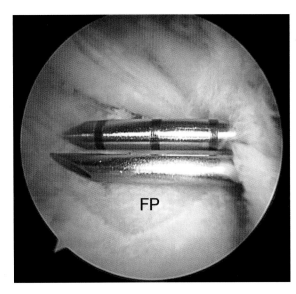

Figure 4-78 Arthroscopic view from a posterior subacromial portal of a right shoulder demonstrating the outer metallic sleeve contacting the bursal surface of the rotator cuff. RC, rotator cuff.

Figure 4-80 Arthroscopic view through a subacromial portal of a right shoulder demonstrating the exposed bursal footprint measurement using the inner metallic probe and counting the number of markings; in this case, 9-mm. FP, footprint.

Bursal Surface Rotator Cuff Tear: Measuring Tendon Involvement

Bursal surface rotator cuff tears can be similarly measured. The tear is initially débrided and the subacromial bursa removed. A spinal needle is again used to determine the correct angle of approach and a small (2 mm) stab incision is used to introduce the inner metallic probe. The probe is used initially to measure the thickness of the footprint exposed by counting the number of markings (Fig. 4-80). The inner metallic probe, which is then used to penetrate the residual rotator cuff, is placed against the medial aspect of the footprint. The outer sleeve is then slid down the shaft of the inner probe to lie adjacent to the "shoulder" of the greater tuberosity

(Fig. 4-81). To determine the thickness of the entire rotator cuff footprint, the numbers off the shaft are read. To confirm that the inner metallic probe has been placed adjacent to the articular surface against the medial footprint, we prefer to do so by viewing directly through a posterior glenohumeral portal before reading the numbers off the shaft (Fig. 4-82).

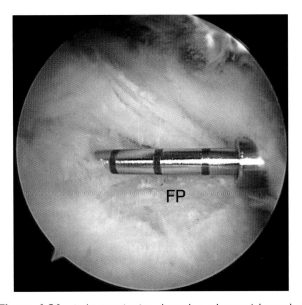

Figure 4-81 Arthroscopic view through a subacromial portal of a right shoulder. To measure the entire thickness of the footprint, the inner metallic probe is advanced through the residual rotator cuff and into the medial aspect of the footprint. The outer sleeve is then advanced to the shoulder of the greater tuberosity and the entire thickness of the footprint can be measured by reading the numbers on the shaft; in this case, 12-mm, or 75% thickness is involved. FP, footprint.

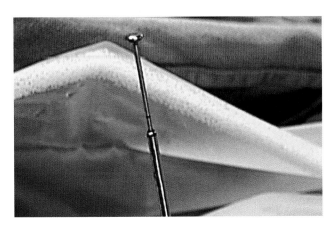

Figure 4-79 Clinical photo demonstrating the numbers on the shaft of the depth gauge, in this case 21-mm. In this case, the thickness of the footprint exposed is 15-mm/21-mm, 71%.

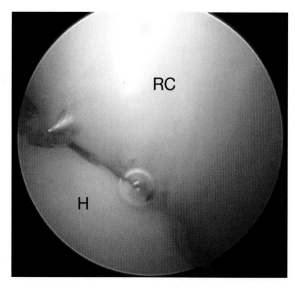

Figure 4-82 Arthroscopic view through a posterior gleno-humeral portal of a right shoulder. To ensure that the inner metallic probe has been placed adjacent to the articular surface and along the medial aspect of the footprint, the probe and cuff are viewed through a posterior glenohumeral portal. H, humeral head; RC, rotator cuff.

Figure 4-83 T2-weighted magnetic resonance image shows a possible intratendinous rotator cuff tear (*arrow*).

Interstitial Tears: Identifying the Tear Location—The Bubble Sign

Treatment of interstitial rotator cuff tears remains controversial. These tears are usually identified by preoperative MRI (Fig. 4-83) and, although they do not extend to the bursal or articular surface, they can be extensive and symptomatic. Because these tears do not extend to the bursal or articular surface, they can be very difficult to localize arthroscopically. We have used the "bubble sign" as a method of localizing the insubstance tear (62).

Following subacromial bursectomy and decompression, the rotator cuff is evaluated. Usually, minimal overt evidence is seen of the location of the insubstance tear. An initial impression can be gained of the tear location by close evaluation of the MRI. A probe is then used to palpate the rotator cuff. In patients with significant insubstance tearing, the two laminae of the rotator cuff are commonly unstable and can be felt "rolling" or "sliding" over one another (Fig. 4-84).

Once this area is localized, an 18-gauge spinal needle is used to penetrate the superficial lamina of the insubstance tear and then attempt to inject saline. In cases of an intact rotator cuff, significant resistance to injection will be noted and no significant amount of saline can be injected. In patients with significant insubstance tearing, however, the saline will flow freely until the contained cuff defect is filled, and a localized dome-shaped bubble of the rotator cuff will appear as saline is injected between the two laminae of the rotator cuff (Fig. 4-85). This bubble sign confirms the location and the unstable nature of the two laminae.

We next débride the outer lamina and repair it to the bone bed (Fig. 4-86). When performing a bubble test, take

care not to inadvertently place the spinal needle through the entire rotator cuff and into the glenohumeral joint. In addition, if the needle is not correctly placed, the depth of the needle position may have to be altered to ensure that the tip is between the two laminae.

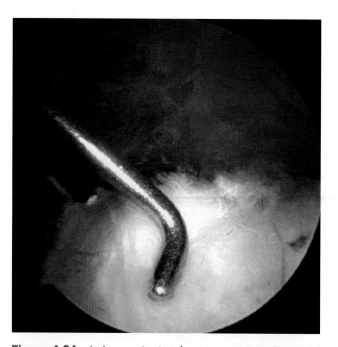

Figure 4-84 Arthroscopic view from a posterior subacromial portal of a left shoulder shows "sliding" of the rotator cuff tendon insertion under a hooked probe. The relative motion between the superficial and deep tendon layers that has been created by the intratendinous defect cause this sliding sensation.

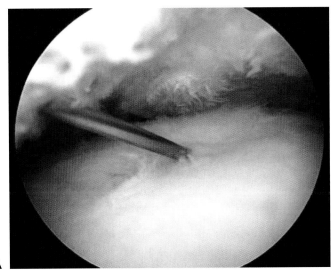
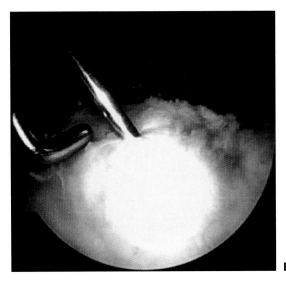

Figure 4-85 The bubble sign seen via arthroscopic views from a posterior subacromial portal of a left shoulder. **A:** An 18-gauge spinal needle is inserted into the suspected lesion, and saline is injected. **B:** The saline flows into the contained cuff defect and the rotator cuff expands locally, forming a bubble.

To Fix or Not to Fix?

Once the thickness and the tear involvement have been measured and calculated, the arthroscopist must make the surgical decision on whether to débride or repair the interstitial rotator cuff tear. We generally repair all insubstance tears that we believe are symptomatic, because the unstable nature of the two laminae will likely continue to progress without repair. For bursal and articular surface

Figure 4-86 Rotator cuff débridement. Arthroscopic view from a posterior subacromial portal of a left shoulder shows a shaver introduced through the lateral portal, which easily falls into a localized area of degeneration.

tears, we base our decision on tendon involvement, the patient's symptoms, and the patient's age. Tendon involvement of >50% is repaired. In young patients who have significant weakness or who require strength for vocational or sports activities, however, we repair tears with >33% tendon thickness involvement. In older patients who do not require strength and who do not wish to undergo a longer rehabilitation process, we either débride or repair the tear and institute a standard "decompression" rehabilitation protocol without immobilization.

Footprint Reconstruction

The rotator cuff insertion is not a simple linear structure. Several studies have documented that the footprint of the rotator cuff is a complex three-dimensional structure overlying a large surface of the proximal humerus. One potential shortcoming of suture anchor repair of the rotator cuff (either arthroscopically or in a mini-open fashion) is that suture anchors provide point fixation only (Fig. 4-87). Therefore, when performing an arthroscopic rotator cuff repair with a single row of lateral anchors, the normal footprint of the rotator cuff is not restored and the medial aspect of the rotator cuff tendon insertion can lift away from the bone bed during abduction of the shoulder. This is particularly relevant when repairing partial articular surface rotator cuff tears, because if we complete the partial tear and fix the tendon only laterally, we merely recreate the partial articular surface tear (Fig. 4-88).

In an elegant study by Apreleva et al. (63), the post-repair three-dimensional rotator cuff footprint was evaluated after using several different methods of rotator cuff repair. These authors determined that suture anchor repair

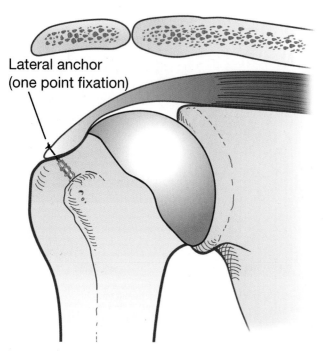

Figure 4-87 Schematic drawing of a single row suture anchor repair demonstrating point fixation. With abduction of the shoulder, the rotator cuff tendon will lift from the medial footprint.

constructs using a single row of anchors restored only 67% of the original footprint of the rotator cuff.

A double row repair using a row of medial anchors and a row of lateral anchors, however, more adequately restores the footprint of the rotator cuff and increases the area of contact for healing. Furthermore, by providing a second row of fixation, the number of points of fixation is increased (usually doubled), thereby (a) increasing the strength of the initial repair construct; (b) decreasing the load each suture loop and knot must resist; (c) decreasing the load each anchor must resist; and (d) decreasing the stress at each suture-cuff contact point. All these factors can potentially improve the mechanical strength and function of the repaired rotator cuff by providing more complete healing across the anatomic footprint.

When performing a double row rotator cuff repair, we generally insert anchors and perform suture passage for the medial row first. The medial row of suture anchors is placed on the medial aspect of the footprint just lateral to the articular margin. Sutures are passed in a mattress fashion. We then insert anchors and pass sutures for the lateral row. The lateral row of suture anchors is placed in the lateral aspect of the footprint at the "shoulder" of the greater tuberosity. The lateral row sutures are passed in a simple suture fashion and tied, which lateralizes the rotator cuff to the lateral aspect of the footprint. The arm is then brought down into adduction and the medial mattress sutures are tied. These sutures are meant to compress the rotator cuff against the bone bed. As can be seen arthroscopically before tying the medial row of anchors, the medial aspect

of the rotator cuff is elevated off the bone bed in a partial articular surface tear fashion (Fig. 4-89A). Tying the medial sutures, however, reduces the cuff fully to the articular margin and compresses the rotator cuff against the medial aspect of the footprint (Fig. 4-89B).

In our hands, most arthroscopic rotator cuff repairs are secured in a double row fashion. Even with large or massive tears, if sufficient mobility is present, then a double row repair is possible. It should be stressed, however, that to obtain a double row repair, the rotator cuff must not be repaired under tension. It is important to avoid the temptation of routinely pulling the rotator cuff laterally and placing the repair under tension to obtain a double row repair. This will undoubtedly fail from tension overload. Instead, the mobility (in the medial to lateral and anterior to posterior directions) and tear configuration should be closely evaluated and the tear should be repaired accordingly.

The clinical and anatomic results of double row rotator cuff repair appear promising. Recently, DeBeer et al. (64) reviewed their results of 58 arthroscopic rotator cuff repairs using a modified double row technique and an interlocking suture method for rotator cuff footprint reconstruction. At a mean of 15 months follow-up, 90% of their patients had good or excellent results and, more importantly, 89% of patients at follow-up demonstrated an intact rotator cuff on postoperative ultrasound. These results are particularly exciting considering the results of Galatz et al. (45), who demonstrated excellent clinical results following arthro-

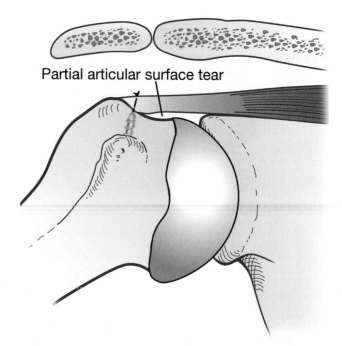

Figure 4-88 Schematic drawing demonstrating a partial thickness articular surface rotator cuff tear. The tear is completed and repaired with a single row of suture anchors laterally. When the shoulder is abducted, a similar lesion, with lifting of the medial footprint, is created, despite lateral repair.

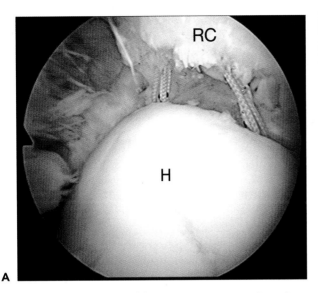
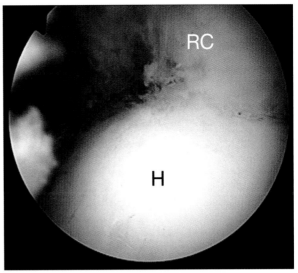

Figure 4-89   Arthroscopic views through a posterior glenohumeral portal of a right shoulder demonstrating a double row rotator cuff repair, following tying of the lateral row of sutures (**A**) and following tying of the lateral and medial row of sutures (**B**). Note: Tying only the lateral row of sutures leaves the rotator cuff elevated off the medial footprint. With tying of the medial sutures, the rotator cuff is compressed against the medial footprint. H, humeral head; RC, rotator cuff.

scopic rotator cuff repair using a single row technique but had a retear rate of 94% on follow-up ultrasound.

SUBSCAPULARIS TENDON

Anatomy and Function

Despite the subscapularis tendon being the largest rotator cuff tendon of the shoulder, the function and clinical relevance of subscapularis pathology has been largely ignored in the literature. The subscapularis muscle originates from the medial two thirds of the anterior scapula, courses laterally beneath the coracoid process, and becomes tendinous near the level of the glenoid rim. As it travels laterally, its tendinous portion intermingles with the fibers of the joint capsule and inserts onto the lesser tuberosity. In many shoulders there is a second, more muscular attachment distal to the lesser tuberosity and ~2 to 3 cm in length.

The footprint of the subscapularis tendon insertion on the lesser tuberosity is roughly trapezoidal in shape, with its widest portion located superiorly. It has a mean superior to inferior length of ~2.5 cm (range 1.5–3.0 cm) (Tehrany AM, Burkhart SS, Wirth MA; unpublished data).

Classically, the subscapularis has been described as an internal rotator of the glenohumeral joint (65), and its contribution to anterior shoulder stability has also been investigated (66,67). As described above in the section, *Rotator Cuff*, the subscapularis tendon is an essential component of the transverse plane force couple. Thus, any

major disruption of the subscapularis tendon leads to a relative deficiency of the anterior cuff and the anterior moment. Fluoroscopic triplane imaging on patients with massive cuff tears involving most of the anterior cuff has demonstrated that these tears display unbalanced force couples, resulting in an unstable fulcrum and potential superior migration of the humeral head (36). Restoration of the subscapularis and its moment as a means of balancing the force couple, therefore, is essential in providing a stable fulcrum for glenohumeral motion.

Etiology of Subscapularis Tears: Subcoracoid Impingement, The Roller Wringer Effect, and Tensile Undersurface Fiber Failure (TUFF) Lesions of the Subscapularis Tendon

Whereas the pathology associated with rotator cuff disease is well documented, the etiology and pathogenesis of rotator cuff disease remains controversial. In particular, the various etiologic factors associated with subscapularis tears remain unclear (68). Although it seems intuitively obvious that intrinsic degeneration of the subscapularis tendon and, collectively, the rotator cuff contributes to tendon tearing, this phenomenon has only recently been investigated in the subscapularis tendon.

In 1998, Sakurai et al. (69) reported on the gross morphologic and histologic findings in 46 cadaveric shoulders. A total of 20 shoulders had supraspinatus tears and an almost equal number (17) of cadavers had subscapularis tears. All of these tears were partial thickness, articular-sided tears. All of the subscapularis tears appeared to begin at the most superior portion of its insertion, which was where most of the tendon degeneration was identified. In 1999, Sano et al. (70) histologically evaluated the supraspinatus, infraspinatus, and subscapularis tendons in 76 cadaveric shoulders. They demonstrated that a similar amount of degeneration (i.e., fiber thinning, granulation tissue, incomplete tearing) was present in all three tendons and that this degeneration was most prominent on the articular (as opposed to bursal) surface of the tendon. These findings collectively suggest that intrinsic tendon degeneration can be an important etiologic factor in subscapularis tendon tears.

Although it is clear that intrinsic degeneration likely contributes to subscapularis tendon tearing, we have also observed that subcoracoid stenosis and subcoracoid impingement can contribute to and exacerbate subscapularis tendon degeneration and tearing (68). In patients with subcoracoid stenosis and subcoracoid impingement, the upper subscapularis tendon appears to "bowstring" tightly across the prominent coracoid tip. With rotation of the shoulder during a dynamic arthroscopic examination, the coracoid can be seen "rolling" along and anterior to the subscapularis tendon. As the arm is rotated into slight internal rotation, the subscapularis tendon is forced to travel between a prominent coracoid tip and the "relatively" prominent humerus (Fig. 4-90). This situation is analogous to an old-fashioned clothes wringer, where an article of clothing (representing the subscapularis tendon) is squeezed between two rollers (the coracoid and lesser tuberosity) to wring the water from the clothes (Fig. 4-91).

In contrast to the hypothetical role of extrinsic subacromial impingement in contributing to supraspinatus tears, whereby the acromion abrasively compresses and erodes the supraspinatus tendon, we believe the coracoid has a different effect on the subscapularis tendon. We propose that the mechanical forces across the convex surface of the subscapularis tendon, as it is bowstrung across the coracoid tip, would primarily be tensile and would be located at the articular surface. Thus, the tensile load would be greatest at the articular surface, or the undersurface, of the subscapularis tendon.

This scenario can be modeled after a simply supported beam, where the subscapularis tendon is represented by the beam, and the lesser tuberosity of the humerus and the scapula represent the supports on either end of the beam (Fig. 4-92). Coracoid impingement would be represented by a load directed perpendicular to the top (surface) of the beam. Thus, the stress distribution would be compressive on the top half of the beam and tensile on the bottom half of the beam. In addition, the tensile fiber stress would increase with progression from the neutral axis of the beam toward the bottom of the beam, reaching a maximum at the undersurface of the beam, corresponding to the articular surface of the subscapularis tendon (71).

Our model predicts that the highest amount of tensile stress would occur on the deep articular surface of the subscapularis tendon, exactly where Sano et al. (70) have demonstrated histologically that the tendon degeneration is most prominent. Previous studies by Sano et al. (72) and Uhthoff and Sano (73) have demonstrated an inverse correlation between the tensile strength of a tendon insertion and the degree of degeneration. That is, as the degree of degeneration of the tendon insertion increases, the tendon insertion becomes weaker. Therefore, whereas the tensile loads on the deep articular surface of the subscapularis tendon (created by subcoracoid impingement and the roller-wringer effect) may, in part, contribute to degeneration, they may also lead to mechanical failure by tensile overload of the weakened degenerative articular surface fibers of the subscapularis tendon. Subcoracoid impingement,

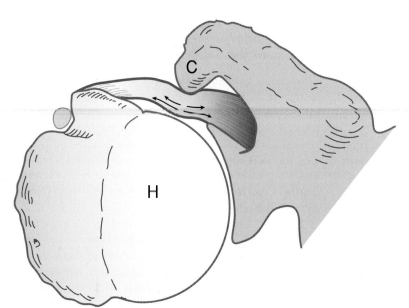

Figure 4-90 Schematic drawing of the roller-wringer effect. In patients with subcoracoid impingement, the prominent coracoid tip indents the superficial surface of the subscapularis tendon. This creates tensile forces on the convex, articular surface of the subscapularis tendon and can lead to failure of the subscapularis fibers (i.e., *tensile undersurface fiber failure* [TUFF] lesion). C, coracoid; H, humerus.

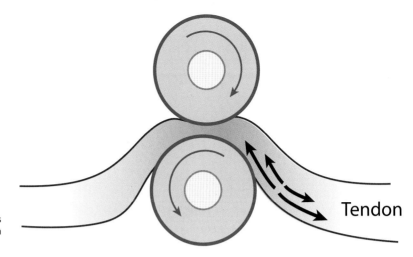

Figure 4-91 Schematic drawing of a clothes wringer demonstrating increased tensile forces on the convex surface of the clothes.

therefore, can be both an etiologic and an exacerbating factor.

This sets the scenario for a tensile undersurface fiber failure (TUFF) lesion, where the tensile undersurface loads are focused on the weakened degenerative tissue, leading to fiber failure. This situation correlates with the cadaveric study of Sakurai et al. (69) who reported that the most common pattern of subscapularis tearing was the partial thickness, articular-surface tear. This scenario of subscapularis failure can be further compounded by an eccentric tensile load on the subscapularis tendon (i.e., forced external rotation), a common cause of subscapularis tendon tear.

Making a Diagnosis of Subcoracoid Impingement

It is important to remember, however, that not all patients with subscapularis tendon tears have subcoracoid stenosis or impingement nor do all patients with subcoracoid steno-

sis or impingement have subscapularis tendon tears. We make a diagnosis of subcoracoid stenosis and subcoracoid impingement based on clinical, imaging, and arthroscopic findings (74). All patients with subcoracoid stenosis or impingement must have:

1. Pain and tenderness anteriorly in the region of the coracoid
2. Pain with combined forward flexion, internal rotation, and adduction (Fig. 4-93)
3. A subcoracoid space (coracohumeral interval) of <6 mm on MRI (Fig. 4-94)
4. A subcoracoid space of <6 mm at arthroscopy (Fig. 4-95)
5. Direct contact of the coracoid against the lesser tuberosity or subscapularis tendon at arthroscopy (Fig. 4-96).

In addition to isolated subscapularis tendon tears, we commonly also diagnose subcoracoid impingement in patients with combined subscapularis, supraspinatus, and infraspinatus tears (74). In our experience, approximately 20% of patients with combined subscapularis, supraspinatus, and infraspinatus tears have subcoracoid impingement. It is important to remember that in patients with these massive tears, proximal migration can give the false impression of subcoracoid impingement with anterosuperior migration of the humeral head with a corresponding decrease in the subcoracoid space. In these patients, it is important that the arm be placed in traction (either through a traction boom or manually through an assistant) to reduce the proximal migration and limit this effect when measuring the subcoracoid space arthroscopically.

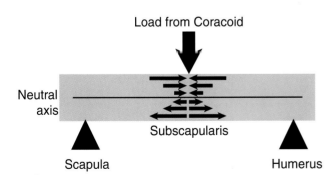

Figure 4-92 Schematic diagram of a simply supported beam. In this scenario, the beam is supported at each end by the scapula and the humerus, respectively. Subcoracoid impingement is represented by a load perpendicular to the beam, which results in compressive forces on the superficial side of the beam and tensile forces on the deep convex side of the beam.

Arthroscopic Evaluation of the Subscapularis Tendon and the Subcoracoid Space

Because arthroscopy of the subscapularis tendon and the subcoracoid space can be a challenging undertaking in

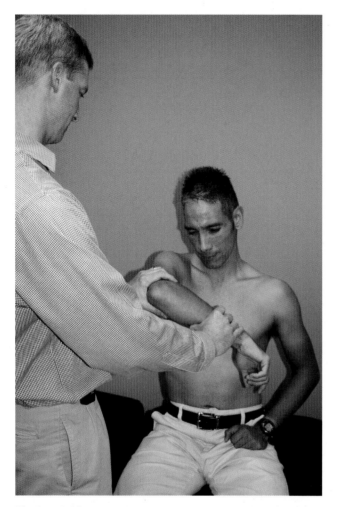

Figure 4-93 Clinical photo demonstrating the subcoracoid impingement position of combined flexion, adduction, and internal rotation.

unfamiliar territory, we highlight the procedure here. For a complete discussion of shoulder arthroscopic procedures, please refer to Part II.

Subscapularis Evaluation

Diagnostic glenohumeral arthroscopy is performed through a standard posterior portal with an arthroscopic pump maintaining pressure at 60 mm Hg. Visualization of the subscapularis and its tendinous insertion into the lesser tuberosity is first done through a posterior viewing portal with the arm in abduction and internal rotation. These maneuvers lift the fibers of the intact portion of the subscapularis away from the footprint, allowing excellent visualization of its insertion (Fig. 4-97).

Usually, a 70° arthroscope is necessary for complete assessment of the subscapularis insertion (Fig. 4-98). Because degeneration of the subscapularis begins on the articular side of the upper portion of the subscapularis, partial ruptures are also easily diagnosed by observing a bare footprint or bare bone bed on the lesser tuberosity in association with tearing of the subcapularis tendon fibers

(Fig. 4-99). The extent of tearing can be estimated by relating the size of the observed bare area to the known mean dimensions of the subscapularis footprint.

Biceps Tendon Evaluation

The long head of the biceps tendon is evaluated next. Subluxation of the biceps tendon, a common finding associated with subscapularis tears, can be dynamically evaluated by moving the arm into internal and external rotation. The long head of the biceps is also assessed for degeneration, and the amount of partial tearing is estimated. The biceps tendon can be completely assessed by pulling the intertubecular portion of the biceps tendon intra-articularly using a switching stick through an anterior portal. Pay particular attention to the junction of the medial sling, the subscapularis tendon, and the posterior rotator cuff, an area of confluent structures that is commonly abnormal in biceps disorders. A proximal biceps tendon situated posterior to the projected fibers of the subscapularis tendon is diagnostic for medial subluxation of the biceps tendon. Furthermore, abrasive injury to the medial biceps where it contacts the medial sling suggests an incompetent sling with biceps subluxation (Fig. 4-100).

Our indications for biceps tenodesis include degeneration involving >50% of the thickness of the tendon, or biceps tendon instability. If any evidence is seen of biceps tendon instability, particularly if associated with a subscapularis tear, we perform an arthroscopic biceps tenodesis (75).

Subcoracoid Space Evaluation

After inspecting the subscapularis tendon insertion and the biceps tendon, we turn our attention to the coracoid and

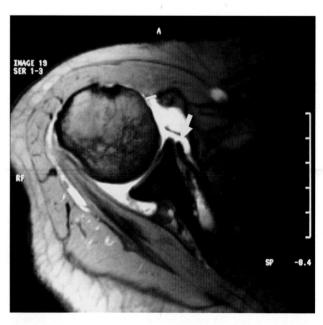

Figure 4-94 T-2 weighted axial magnetic resonance imaging (MRI) view demonstrating a decreased coracohumeral space (*yellow line*) and complete tear of the subscapularis tendon. *Yellow arrow*, edge of the retracted subscapularis tendon.

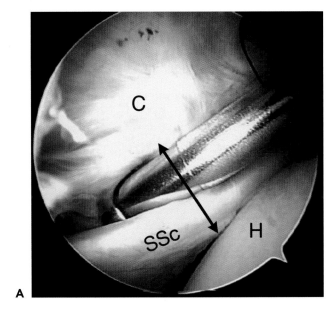
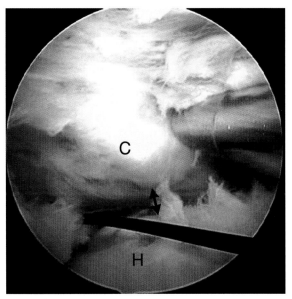

Figure 4-95 Palpation of the prominent coracoid tip. Posterior arthroscopic view of right shoulders using a 70° arthroscope. A shaver is introduced through an anterolateral portal and the prominent coracoid is palpated. An initial assessment of the coracohumeral space is made. Note the minimal space available (↔) for the subscapularis tendon signifying coracohumeral stenosis. **A:** Intact subscapularis tendon. **B:** Torn subscapularis tendon with a severely stenotic subcoracoid space. H, humerus; SSc, subscapularis tendon C, coracoid.

the subcoracoid space. The subcoracoid space is defined as the interval between the tip of the coracoid and the humeral head (i.e., the coracohumeral interval) (76,77). This space must be large enough to accommodate the articular cartilage of the humerus, the subscapularis tendon, the subscapularis bursa and the rotator interval tissue, and portions of the insertions of the coracoacromial ligament and the conjoint tendon. The normal coracohumeral interval has been demonstrated in anatomic and imaging studies to be between 8.4 and 11.0 mm (74,77,78). We define

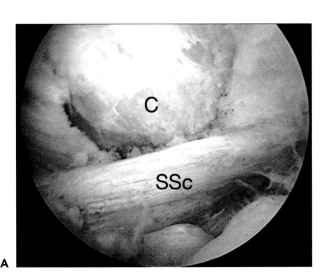
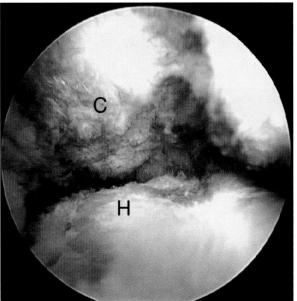

Figure 4-96 Confirming subcoracoid impingement. Posterior arthroscopic view of right shoulders using a 70° arthroscope. Manipulation of the arm into flexion, adduction, and internal rotation demonstrates subcoracoid impingement with contact between the coracoid and the subscapularis tendon or lesser tuberosity of the humerus. **A:** Intact subscapularis tendon. **B:** Torn subscapularis tendon. C, coracoid; H, humerus; SSc, subscapularis.

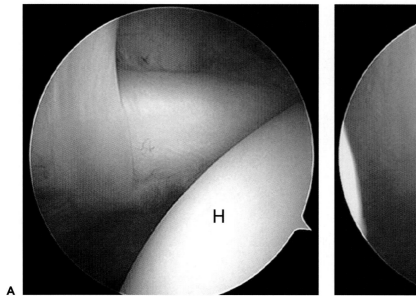
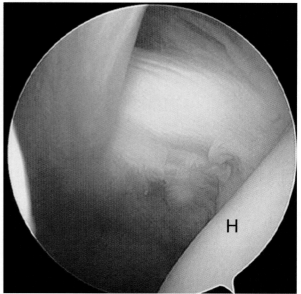

Figure 4-97 Arthroscopic view of the subscapularis insertion of a right shoulder from the posterior portal using a 30° arthroscope with the arm in 30° of abduction and neutral rotation **(A)**; internal rotation **(B)**. Note: The internal rotation slackens the overlying subscapularis fibers and reveals the intact subscapularis insertion. H, humeral head.

subcoracoid stenosis as a coracohumeral interval of <6 mm (i.e., narrowing of the subcoracoid space) (74,79,80). Although an initial appreciation of the size of the coracohumeral interval can be gained on MRI (see Fig. 4-94), it is most accurate to directly measure the coracohumeral space intraoperatively.

In patients with complete subscapularis tears, the coracoid can be felt as a bony prominence in the soft tissues anterior to the subscapularis tendon (see Fig. 4-95B). The size of the coracohumeral interval is estimated by introducing an instrument of known size through an anterosuperolateral portal and placing it between the

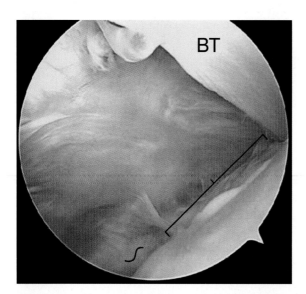

Figure 4-98 Arthroscopic "aerial" view of a right shoulder from a posterior portal using a 70° arthroscope demonstrating a full-thickness tear of the upper portion of the subscapularis tendon. Note: The bare area of the subscapularis footprint (demonstrated by the bracket) has only the most inferior portion of the tendon intact (~) and the biceps tendon is subluxed posterior to the upper subscapularis tendon. BT, biceps tendon.

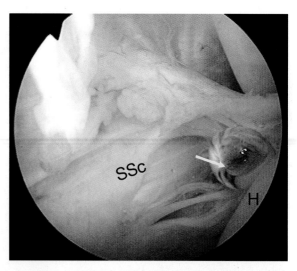

Figure 4-99 Arthroscopic view of the subscapularis insertion of a right shoulder from a posterior portal with the arm in 30° of abduction and internal rotation demonstrating a partial tear of the articular surface of the subscapularis tendon. Note: The tearing of the fibers exposes the underlying footprint of the subscapularis insertion (*arrow*). SSc, subscapularis. H, humeral head.

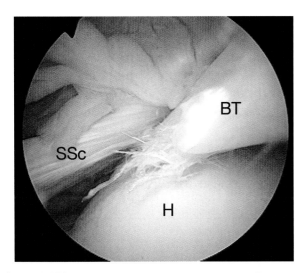

Figure 4-100 Arthroscopic view of a right shoulder from a posterior portal using a 70° arthroscope demonstrating a degenerative and subluxed biceps tendon *(BT)*, and a torn subscapularis tendon *(SSc)*. Note: The proximal biceps tendon appears to be situated posterior to the projected fibers of the subscapularis tendon, implying medial subluxation or dislocation. H, humeral head.

coracoid and humerus. In many cases, particularly those involving combined subscapularis, supraspinatus, and infraspinatus tears, the coracoid will be so prominent and the subcoracoid space so tight that even a 5-mm shaver will not fit between the coracoid and humerus. When evaluating the subcoracoid space and measuring the coracohumeral interval (particularly when associated with massive rotator cuff tears), it is important that traction be applied to the arm manually or by a traction boom to

minimize any potential effect of proximal humeral migration.

If the coracohumeral interval is <6 mm, a diagnosis is made of subcoracoid stenosis (i.e., narrowing of the subcoracoid space). In and of itself, subcoracoid stenosis may not be pathologic or symptomatic. To diagnose subcoracoid impingement (defined as impingement of the coracoid against the humerus [usually the lesser tuberosity]), it is important to demonstrate direct contact of the coracoid against the lesser tuberosity in a coracoid impingement position. To demonstrate this, the arm is brought into a combination of flexion, adduction, and internal rotation (see Fig. 4-96B), a position that generally corresponds to the position of discomfort determined during preoperative physical examination. If subcoracoid stenosis and subcoracoid impingement are diagnosed intraoperatively with correlative signs and symptoms clinically, we proceed with subcoracoid decompression and coracoplasty (for a complete discussion of arthroscopic coracoplasty, see Part II) (74,80) (Fig. 4-101).

In many cases, the subcoracoid space will be so tight and the coracohumeral interval so small that the coracoid will impinge against the subscapularis tendon and the humerus in adduction and internal rotation and not in the classic position of flexion, adduction, and internal rotation. In contrast to the situation above, these cases are frequently associated with full-thickness, partial tears of the upper subscapularis tendon or partial articular-surface tears of the subscapularis tendon (i.e., TUFF lesions of the subscapularis tendon).

At arthroscopy, the coracoid typically will appear as a prominent bulge anterior to the upper subscapularis tendon,

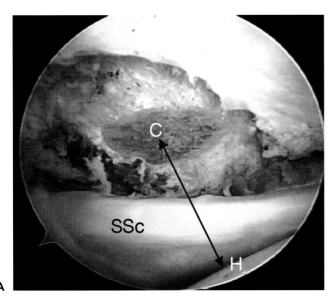

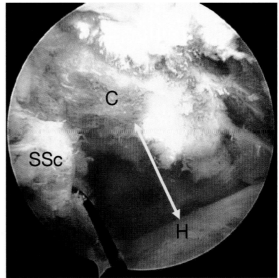

A   B

Figure 4-101 Posterior arthroscopic view of right shoulder demonstrating an increased coracohumeral space *(double-headed arrows)* following subcoracoid decompression and coracoplasty allowing room for the subscapularis repair. **A:** Intact subscapularis tendon. **B:** Torn subscapularis tendon. C, coracoid; SSc, subscapularis; H, humeral head.

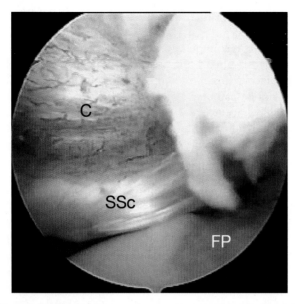

Figure 4-102 Posterior arthroscopic view of a right shoulder using a 70° arthroscope demonstrating a tear of the upper subscapularis tendon and a corresponding bare subscapularis footprint. Note: The prominent coracoid tip appears as a bulge anterior to the upper subscapularis tendon, "bowstringing" the subscapularis fibers. C, coracoid; SSc, subscapularis tendon; FP, bare footprint of the subscapularis tendon.

"bowstringing" the subscapularis fibers across the prominent coracoid process (Fig. 4-102). Furthermore, by rotating the arm in internal and external rotation with the shoulder in adduction, the coracoid can be seen rolling anterior to the subscapularis tendon, indenting the superficial surface of the

subscapularis while stretching (i.e., tensile loading) the deep surface of the subscapularis (Figs. 4-103 and 4-104).

Identifying the Margin of the Torn Subscapularis Tendon: The Comma Sign

In chronic subscapularis tears, the lesser tuberosity will appear bare (see Figs. 4-98 and 4-101B) and the subscapularis tendon can be difficult to identify. This difficulty occurs because the tendon is commonly retracted medially and can be found at, or medial to, the glenoid. The situation is further compounded if the tendon is scarred to the inner deltoid fascia or to the coracoid, because this further obscures the tendon edges.

We use a systematic method in delineating the retracted tendon edge. It is important to recognize that, in retracted subscapularis tears, because of the close proximity and interdigitation between the subscapularis tendon and the medial sling of the biceps (composed of portions of the superior glenohumeral ligament and the coracohumeral ligament), the entire complex is torn off the humerus collectively and remains together. This forms a "comma-shaped" arc (called the "comma sign") just above the superolateral corner of the subscapularis and provides a marker for the subscapularis tendon (Fig. 4-105) (81). Identifying and following the comma sign will lead to the superolateral border of the subscapularis tendon. After identifying the superolateral corner of the subscapularis tendon, we find it useful to use a tendon grasper to pull the medially retracted tissues laterally until we can definitively identify the upper border of subscapularis (Fig. 4-106).

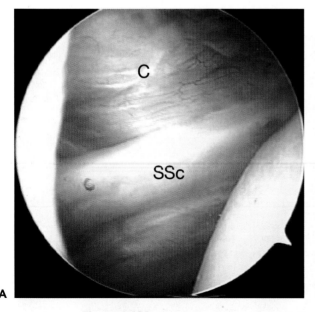

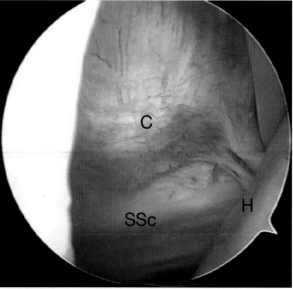

A   B

Figure 4-103 The "roller-wringer effect." Arthroscopic views of a right shoulder from a posterior portal. **A:** The coracoid tip can be seen as a prominent bulge anterior to the upper border of the subscapularis tendon. **B:** With rotation of the arm, the coracoid "rolls" toward the subscapularis tendon insertion, bulging the insertional fibers and creating a tensile load on the undersurface fibers of the subscapularis. C, coracoid; SSc, subscapularis tendon; H, humeral head.

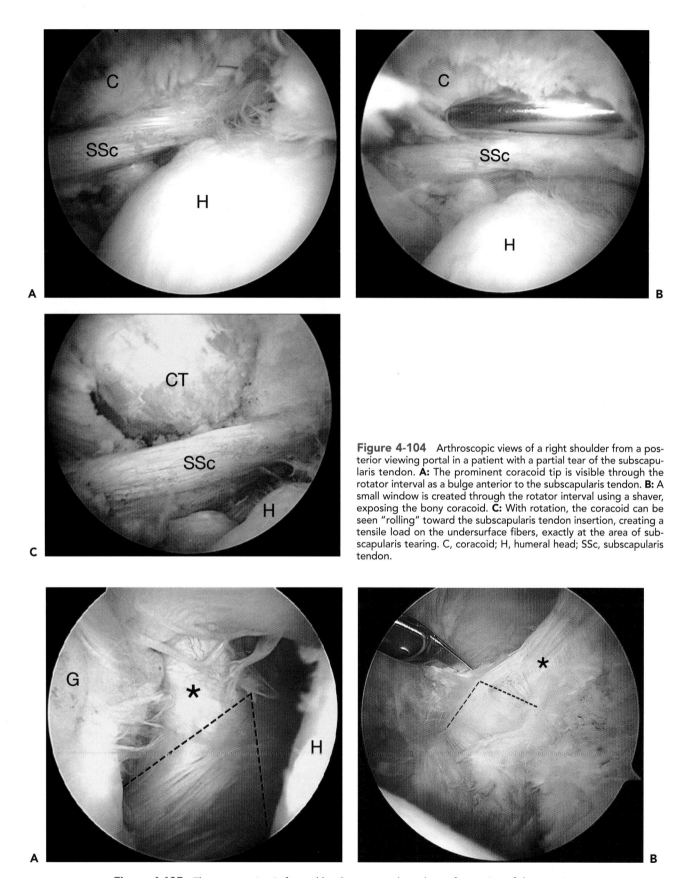

Figure 4-104 Arthroscopic views of a right shoulder from a posterior viewing portal in a patient with a partial tear of the subscapularis tendon. **A:** The prominent coracoid tip is visible through the rotator interval as a bulge anterior to the subscapularis tendon. **B:** A small window is created through the rotator interval using a shaver, exposing the bony coracoid. **C:** With rotation, the coracoid can be seen "rolling" toward the subscapularis tendon insertion, creating a tensile load on the undersurface fibers, exactly at the area of subscapularis tearing. C, coracoid; H, humeral head; SSc, subscapularis tendon.

Figure 4-105 The comma sign is formed by the comma-shaped arc of a portion of the superior glenohumeral ligament–coracohumeral ligament complex (*) (the medial sling of the biceps), which has torn off the humerus. The comma-shaped arc (*) extends to the superolateral corner of the subscapularis tendon (-------). **A:** Arthroscopic view of a right shoulder through a posterior viewing portal demonstrating a retracted subscapularis tear with its associated comma sign. **B:** Posterior viewing portal of a left shoulder shows the subscapularis adhesed to the overlying fascia. The comma sign (*) leads the surgeon to the superolateral corner of the subscapularis. G, glenoid, H, humeral head.

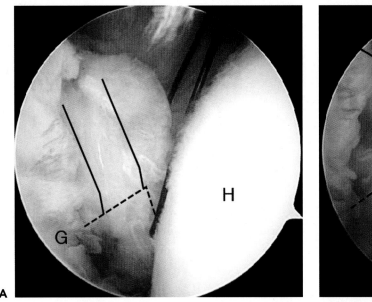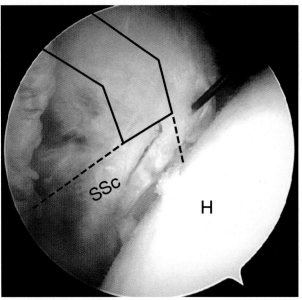

Figure 4-106   Arthroscopic views from a posterior portal of a right shoulder demonstrating a complete subscapularis (SSc) tendon tear retracted to the glenoid margin. **A:** A traction stitch has been placed in the superolateral corner of the subscapularis tendon. Do not confuse the soft tissues superior to the superolateral corner of the subscapularis tendon as the edge of the subscapularis tendon. This area represents the "comma sign." **B:** Traction on the subscapularis tendon reveals the true borders of the subscapularis demonstrating that the subscapularis tendon had been significantly retracted medially and inferiorly. G, glenoid; H, humeral head; dashed line (------), upper border of the subscapularis tendon; solid line (——), outlines the comma sign.

(For a complete step-by-step discussion of subscapularis tendon repair, see Part II. For a more complete discussion of the comma sign see Chapter 5, section entitled, "Finding the Subcapularis.")

REFERENCES

1. Williams MM, Snyder SJ, Buford D Jr. The Buford complex—the cord-like middle glenohumeral ligament and absent anterosuperior labrum complex: a normal anatomic capsulolabral variant. *Arthroscopy.* 1994;10(3): 241–247.
2. Andrews JR, Carson W Jr, McLeod W. Glenoid labrum tears related to the long head of the biceps. *Am J Sports Med.* 1985;13:337–341.
3. Snyder SJ, Karzel RP, Delpizzo W, et al. SLAP lesions of the shoulder. *Arthroscopy.* 1990;6:274–279.
4. Walch G, Boileau J, Noel E, et al. Impingement of the deep surface of the supraspinatus tendon on the posterior superior glenoid rim: an arthroscopic study. *J Shoulder Elbow Surg.* 1992;1:238–243.
5. Jobe CM. Posterior superior glenoid impingement: expanded spectrum. *Arthroscopy.* 1995;11:530–537.
6. Halbrecht JL, Tirman P, Atkin D. Internal impingement of the shoulder: comparison of findings between the throwing and nonthrowing shoulders of college baseball players. *Arthroscopy.* 1999;15:253–258.
7. Burkhart SS, Morgan CD, Kibler WB. The disabled throwing shoulder: spectrum of pathology. Part I: Pathoanatomy and biomechanics. *Arthroscopy.* 2003;19(4):404–420.
8. Burkhart SS, Morgan CD, Kibler WB. The disabled throwing shoulder: spectrum of pathology. Part II: Evaluation and treatment of SLAP lesions in throwers. *Arthroscopy.* 2003;19(5):531–539.
9. Burkhart SS, Morgan CD, Kibler WB. The disabled throwing shoulder: spectrum of pathology. Part III: The SICK scapula, scapular dyskinesis, the kinetic chain and rehabilitation. *Arthroscopy.* 2003;19(60):641–661.
10. Jobe FW, Giangarra CE, Kvitne RS, et al. Anterior capsulolabral reconstruction of the shoulder in athletes in overhead sports. *Am J Sports Med.* 1991;19:428–434.
11. Garth WP, Allman FL, Armstrong NS. Occult anterior subluxation of the shoulder. *Am J Sports Med.* 1987;15:579–585.
12. Kvitne RS, Jobe FW. The diagnosis and treatment of anterior instability in the throwing athlete. *Clin Orthop.* 1993;291:107–123.
13. Jobe CM, Pink MM, Jobe FW, et al. Anterior shoulder instability, impingement, and rotator cuff tear: theories and concepts. In: Jobe FW, ed. *Operative Techniques in Upper Extremity Sports Injuries.* St. Louis: Mosby; 1996:164–176.
14. Glousman RE, Jobe FW. Anterior shoulder instability: impingement and rotator cuff tear. Anterior and multidirectional instability. In: Jobe FW, ed. *Operative Techniques in Upper Extremity Sports Injuries.* St. Louis: Mosby; 1996:191–209.
15. Verna C. Shoulder flexibility to reduce impingement. Presented at the 3rd annual PBATS (Professional Baseball Athletic Trainer Society) Meeting, Mesa, Arizona, March 1991.
16. Kibler WB. The relationship of glenohumeral internal rotation deficit to shoulder and elbow injuries in tennis players: a prospective evaluation of posterior capsular stretching. Presented at the annual closed meeting of the American Shoulder and Elbow Surgeons, New York, October 1998.
17. Koffler KM, Bader D, Eager M, et al. The effect of posterior capsule tightness on glenohumeral translation in the late cocking phase of pitching: a cadaveric study. Presented at the 21st Annual Meeting of the Arthroscopy. Association of North America, Washington, DC, April 25, 2004.
18. Tibone J, Lee T. Biomechanical derangements caused by tightening the posterior capsule of the shoulder. Presented at the annual closed meeting of the American Shoulder and Elbow Surgeons, Dana Point, CA, October 20, 2003.
19. Morgan CD, Burkhart SS, Palmeri M, et al. Type II SLAP lesions: three subtypes and their relationship to superior instability and rotator cuff tears. *Arthroscopy.* 1998;14:553–565.
20. Curl LA, Warren RF. Glenohumeral joint stability. Selective cutting studies on the static capsular restraints. *Clin Orthop.* 1996;330:54–65.
21. Pagnani MJ, Warren RF. Stabilizers of the glenohumeral joint. *J Shoulder Elbow Surg.* 1994;3:173–190.
22. Warren RF, Kornblatt IB, Marchand R. Static factors affecting shoulder stability. *Orthop Trans.* 1984;8:89.
23. O'Brien SJ, Warren RF. Anterior shoulder instability. *Orthop Clin North Am.* 1987;18:395–408.
24. Pagnani MJ, Deng XH, Warren RF, et al. Effect of lesions of the superior portion of the glenoid labrum on glenohumeral translation. *J Bone Joint Surg Am.* 1995;77:1003–1010.
25. Speer KP, Deng X, Borrero S, et al. Biomechanical evaluation of a simulated Bankart lesion. *J Bone Joint Surg Am.* 1994;76:1819–1826.
26. Bui-Mansfield LT, Taylor DC, Uhorchak JM, et al. Humeral avulsion of the glenohumeral ligament: Imaging features and a review of the literature. *AJR Am J Roentgenol.* 2002;179:649–655.
27. Wolf EM, Cheng JC, Dickson K. Humeral avulsion of the glenohumeral ligaments as a cause of anterior shoulder instability. *Arthroscopy.* 1995; 11:600–607.
28. Bokor DJ, Conboy VB, Olson C. Anterior instability of the glenohumeral joint with humeral avulsion of the glenohumeral ligament. A review of 41 cases. *J Bone Joint Surg Br.* 1999;81:93–96.

29. Burkhart SS, DeBeer JF. Traumatic glenohumeral bone defects and their relationship to failure of arthroscopic Bankart repairs: significance of the inverted-pear glenoid and the humeral engaging Hill-Sachs lesion. *Arthroscopy.* 2000;16(7):677–694.

30. Lo IK, Parten PM, Burkhart SS. The inverted pear glenoid: an indicator of significant glenoid bone loss. *Arthroscopy.* 2004;20(2):169–174.

31. Burkhart SS, DeBeer JF, Tehrany AM, et al. Quantifying glenoid bone loss arthroscopically in shoulder instability. *Arthroscopy.* 2002;18(5):488–491.

32. Burkhart SS. Current concepts. Reconciling the paradox of rotator cuff repair versus debridement: a unified biomechanical rationale for the treatment of rotator cuff tears. *Arthroscopy.* 1994;10:4–19.

33. Burkhart SS. Shoulder arthroscopy. New concepts. *Clin Sports Med.* 1996;15:635–653.

34. Burkhart SS. Arthroscopic debridement and decompression for selected rotator cuff tears. Clinical results, pathomechanics, and patient selection based on biomechanical parameters. *Orthop Clin North Am.* 1993;24:111–123.

35. Burkhart SS. Arthroscopic treatment of massive rotator cuff tears. *Clin Orthop.* 2001;390:107–118.

36. Burkhart SS. Fluoroscopic comparison of kinematic patterns in massive rotator cuff tears. A suspension bridge model. *Clin Orthop.* 1992;284:144–152.

37. Burkhart SS. Arthroscopic treatment of massive rotator cuff tears. Clinical results and biomechanical rationale. *Clin Orthop.* 1991;267:45–56.

38. Inman VT, Saunders JB, Abbott LC. Observations on the function of the shoulder. *J Bone Joint Surg Am.* 1944;26:1–30.

39. Clark JM, Harryman DT II. Tendons, ligaments, and capsule of the rotator cuff. *J Bone Joint Surg Am.* 1992;74:713–725.

40. Burkhart SS, Esch JC, Jolson RC. The rotator crescent and rotator cable: an anatomic description of the shoulder's "suspension bridge". *Arthroscopy.* 1993;9:611–616.

41. Halder AM, O'Driscoll SW, Heer G, et al. Biomechanical comparison of effects of supraspinatus tendon detachments, tendon defects and muscle retractions. *J Bone Joint Surg Am.* 2002;84:780–785.

42. Burkhart SS. Partial repair of massive rotator cuff tears: the evolution of a concept. *Orthop Clin North Am.* 1997;28:125–132.

43. Burkhart SS, Wesley MN, Ogilvie-Harris DJ, et al. Partial repair of irreparable rotator cuff tears. *Arthroscopy.* 1994;10:363–370.

44. Harryman DT II, Mach LA, Wang KY, et al. Repairs of the rotator cuff: correlation of functional results with integrity of the cuff. *J Bone Joint Surg Am.* 1991;73:982–989.

45. Galatz LM, Ball CM, Teefey SA, et al. The outcome and repair integrity of completely arthroscopically repaired large and massive rotator cuff tears. *J Bone Joint Surg Am.* 2004;86A(2):219–224.

46. Cofield RH. Subscapular muscle transposition for repair of chronic rotator cuff tears. *Surg Gynecol Obstet.* 1982;154:667–672.

47. Cofield RH. Tears of the rotator cuff. *Instr Course Lect.* 1981;30:258–273.

48. Neer CS II. Impingement lesions. *Clin Orthop.* 1983;173:70–77.

49. Neviaser RJ, Neviaser TJ. Transfer of subscapularis and teres minor for massive defects of rotator cuff. In: Bayley I, Kessel L, eds. *Shoulder Surgery.* Berlin: Springer-Verlag; 1982:60–63.

50. Burkhart SS, Athanasiou KA, Wirth MA. Margin convergence: a method of reducing strain in massive rotator cuff tears. *Arthroscopy.* 1996;12:335–338.

51. Burkhart SS, Danaceau SM, Pearce CE Jr. Arthroscopic rotator cuff repair: analysis of results by tear size and by repair technique- margin convergence versus direct tendon-to-bone repair. *Arthroscopy.* 2001;17:905–912.

52. Burkhart SS. Arthroscopic repair of massive rotator cuff tears: concept of margin convergence. *Techniques in Shoulder and Elbow Surgery.* 2000;1:232–239.

53. Riley WF, Zachary LW. Axial loading: applications and pressure vessels. In *Introduction to Mechanics.* New York: John Wiley; 1989:87–89.

54. Richards DP, Burkhart SS. Margin convergence of the posterior rotator cuff to the biceps tendon. *Arthroscopy.* 2004;20(7):771–775.

55. Codman E. *The Shoulder.* Boston: Thomas Todd; 1934.

56. McConfille OR, Iannotti JP. Partial-thickness tears of the rotator cuff: evaluation and management. *J Am Acad Orthop Surg.* 1999;7:32–43.

57. Fukuda H. Partial thickness rotator cuff tears: a modern view on Codman's classic. *J Shoulder Elbow Surg.* 2000;9:163–168.

58. Breazeale NM, Craig EV. Partial thickness rotator cuff tears. *Orthop Clin North Am.* 1997;28:145–155.

59. Weber SC. Arthroscopic debridement and acromioplasty versus mini-open repair in the treatment of significant partial-thickness rotator cuff tears. *Arthroscopy.* 1999;15:126–131.

60. Weber SC. Arthroscopic debridement and acromioplasty versus mini-open repair in the management of significant partial-thickness tears of the rotator cuff. *Orthop Clin North Am.* 1997;28:79–82.

61. Ruotolo C, Fow JE, Nottage WM. The supraspinatus footprint: an anatomic study of the supraspinatus tendon insertion. *Arthroscopy.* 2004;20:246–249.

62. Lo IK, Gonzalez DM, Burkhart SS. The bubble sign: an arthroscopic indicator of an intratendinous rotator cuff tear. *Arthroscopy.* 2002;18(9):1029–1033.

63. Apreleva M, Ozbaydar M, Fitzgibbons PG, et al. Rotator cuff tears: the effect of the reconstruction method on three-dimensional repair site area. *Arthroscopy.* 2001;18:519–526.

64. De Beer J, Berghs B, van Rooyen K. Arthroscopic rotator cuff repair by footprint reconstruction. *19th Annual San Diego Meeting Syllabus* 2002:425–431.

65. Dick TP, Howden R. *Gray's Anatomy: The Classic Collectors Edition.* London: Crown Publishers; 1977.

66. Bowen MK, Warren RF. Ligamentous control of shoulder stability based on selective cutting and static translation experiments. *Clin Sports Med.* 1994;10:757–782.

67. Turkel SJ, Panio MW, Marshall JL, et al. Stabilizing mechanism preventing anterior dislocation of the gleno-humeral joint. *J Bone Joint Surg Am.* 1981;63:1208–1217.

68. Lo IK, Burkhart SS. The etiology and assessment of subscapularis tendon tears: a case for subcoracoid impingement, the roller-wringer effect, and TUFF lesions of the subscapularis. *Arthroscopy.* 2003;19(1):1142–1150.

69. Sakurai G, Ozaki J, Tomita Y, et al. Incomplete tears of the subscapularis tendon associated with tears of the supraspinatus tendon: cadaveric and clinical studies. *J Shoulder Elbow Surg.* 1998;7:510–515.

70. Sano H, Ishii H, Trudel G, et al. Histologic evidence of degeneration at the insertion of 3 rotator cuff tendons: a comparative study with human cadaveric shoulders. *J Shoulder Elbow Surg.* 1999;8:574–579.

71. Leet KL. *Fundamentals of Structural Analysis.* New York: Macmillan Publishing Co.; 1988;9.

72. Sano H, Ishii H, Yeadon A, et al. Degeneration at the insertion weakens the tensile strength of the supraspinatus tendon. A comparative mechanical and histologic study of bone-tendon complex. *J Orthop Res.* 1997;15:719–726.

73. Uhthoff HK, Sano H. Pathology of failure of the rotator cuff tendon. *Orthop Clin North Am.* 1997;28:31–41.

74. Lo IK, Parten PM, Burkhart SS. Combined subcoracoid and subacromial impingement in association with anterosuperior rotator cuff tears: an arthroscopic approach. *Arthroscopy.* 2003;19(10):1068–1078.

75. Lo IK, Burkhart SS. Arthroscopic biceps tenodesis using a bioabsorbable interference screw. *Arthroscopy.* 2004;20(1):85–95.

76. Gerber C, Terrier F, Ganz R. The role of the coracoid process in the chronic impingement syndrome. *J Bone Joint Surg Br.* 1985;67:703–708.

77. Gerber C, Terrier F, Zehnder R, et al. The subcoracoid space. An anatomic study. *Clin Orthop.* 1987;215:132–138.

78. Friedman RJ, Bonutti PM, Genez B. Cine magnetic resonance imaging of the subcoracoid region. *Orthopedics.* 1998;21:545–548.

79. Nove-Josserand L, Boulahia A, Levigne C, et al. Coraco-humeral space and rotator cuff tears. *Rev Chir Orthop. Reparatrice Appar Mot.* 1999;85:677–683.

80. Lo IK, Burkhart SS. Arthroscopic coracoplasty through the rotator interval. *Arthroscopy.* 2003;19(6):667–671.

81. Lo IK, Burkhart SS. The comma sign: an arthroscopic guide to the torn subscapularis tendon. *Arthroscopy.* 2003;19(3):334–337.

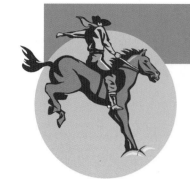

The Tough Stuff

Massive Contracted Adhesed Rotator Cuff Tears, Subscapularis Tears, and Biceps Pathology

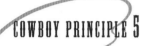

COWBOY PRINCIPLE 5

On a gentle horse, every man is a rider.

This cowboy principle speaks for itself. Sometimes silence can be a speech.

-Interval Slide in Continuity

MASSIVE CONTRACTED IMMOBILE ROTATOR CUFF TEARS

Rarely, massive rotator cuff tears are immobile and severely contracted, with poor mobility from both a medial to lateral direction and an anterior to posterior direction. This lack of mobility precludes either a repair directly to bone (as in crescent-shaped tears) or a repair to bone following margin convergence (as in U-shaped tears or L-shaped tears). We refer to these tears as massive contracted immobile rotator cuff tears (1). A simple capsular release deep to the retracted tendons will not restore sufficient lateral excursion for tendon repair to bone. These tears, however, can be repaired using the techniques of single and double interval slides.

Massive, contracted, immobile rotator cuff tears, which represent <10% of massive rotator cuff tears, can be classified into two common patterns: (a) massive contracted

longitudinal tears (Fig. 5-1A) and (b.) massive contracted crescent tears (Fig. 5-1B). In general, massive contracted crescent tears are wider (in an anterior to posterior direction) than massive contracted longitudinal tears and, thus, more difficult to repair. Furthermore, massive contracted longitudinal tears have an intact rotator interval as well as a "tongue" of supraspinatus tendon at the anterior margin of the tear. This tongue of tissue is useful during subsequent repair of these tears.

For repair of massive contracted longitudinal tears, a single anterior interval slide is used. In these patients, the tissue between the rotator interval and supraspinatus tendon is released, essentially incising the posterior portion of the coracohumeral ligament (Fig. 5-2A). In most massive contracted longitudinal tears, the improved lateral mobility of ~2 cm following a single anterior interval slide is sufficient to allow repair of the supraspinatus tendon to bone (Fig. 5-2B). The infraspinatus and teres minor are then advanced superiorly and laterally and the posterior defect is closed with side-to-side sutures (Fig. 5-2C).

For repair of massive contracted crescent tears, a double interval slide is necessary. In these patients, even with an anterior interval release, the 2-cm gain in lateral excursion is insufficient to allow a tension-free repair of the supraspinatus tendon to bone. An additional posterior interval slide is performed, releasing the interval between the supraspinatus and infraspinatus tendons all the way to the base of the scapular spine (Fig. 5-3A). Following a double interval slide, the supraspinatus tendon's lateral mobility is significantly improved, usually by 4 to 5 cm, allowing a tension-free repair to bone (Fig. 5-3B). The double interval slide also

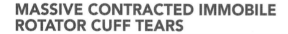

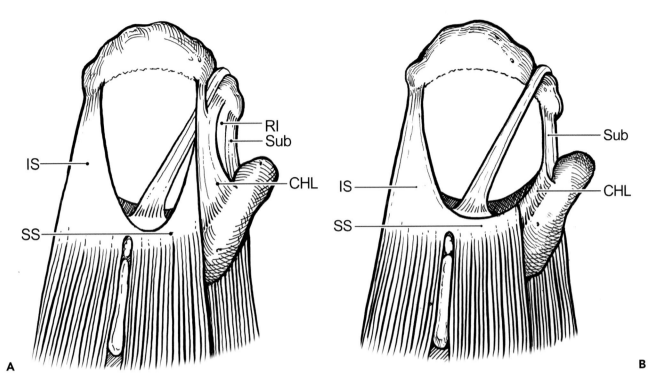

Figure 5-1 Massive contracted immobile rotator cuff tears. **A:** Superior view of a massive contracted immobile longitudinal rotator cuff tear. **B:** Superior view of massive contracted immobile crescent rotator cuff tear. SS, supraspinatus; IS, infraspinatus; Sub, subscapularis; RI, rotator interval; CHL, coracohumeral ligament. (From Lo IK, Burkhart SS. Arthroscopic repair of massive, contracted, immobile rotator cuff tears using single and double interval slides: technique and preliminary results. *Arthroscopy.* 2004;20(1):22–33, Fig. 1; with permission.)

significantly increases the lateral excursion of the posterior leaf, permitting the infraspinatus and teres minor to be similarly advanced superiorly and laterally (Fig. 5-3C). The posterior defect is then closed with side-to-side sutures (Fig. 5-3D).

Technique

Following complete removal of the overlying bursa, the tear is identified and assessed for mobility. With the arthroscope posterior, the medial to lateral mobility of the tear is assessed using a soft tissue grasper introduced through the lateral portal. Noncontracted crescent-shaped tears have excellent medial to lateral mobility and reduce easily to the bone bed. Such tears are repaired directly to bone. Those tears with poor medial to lateral mobility are then further assessed for anterior and posterior mobility.

With the arthroscope lateral, the mobility of the anterior and posterior leaves of the rotator cuff tear is similarly assessed using a soft tissue grasper. The posterior leaf mobility is assessed by pulling the posterior leaf anteriorly with the grasper placed through the anterior portal, whereas the anterior leaf is assessed by pulling the anterior leaf posteriorly with the grasper placed through the posterior portal. If the anterior and posterior leaves are sufficiently mobile to allow side-to-side closure, then the tear is classified as a U-shaped massive tear and the technique of margin conver-

gence is used. The converged rotator cuff margin is then repaired to bone as previously described in Chapter 4. In contracted cases with immobile tendon margins, we first try to improve tendon mobility by releasing the capsule deep to the tendon. We have found, however, that this technique does not usually produce much improvement in tendon excursion—only 2 to 3 mm at most.

If the anterior and posterior leaves are not amenable to margin convergence and the tendons are not mobile from medial to lateral even after releasing the tendon–capsule interface, then the tear is classified as a massive contracted immobile rotator cuff tear (Fig. 5-4). In these cases, a single or double interval slide technique can be used for repair. In most cases, massive contracted longitudinal tears can be repaired using a single anterior interval slide because these tears are not as wide (in an anterior to posterior dimension) as massive contracted crescent tears. They also have an additional "tongue" of supraspinatus tissue, which is important during repair of the supraspinatus tendon to bone. Massive contracted crescent tears are usually amenable to repair using a double interval slide.

To perform an anterior interval slide, the supraspinatus tendon is initially identified and a traction stitch is placed near the anterolateral corner of the tendon and pulled out through a separate accessory lateral portal. The

Text continues on page 114.

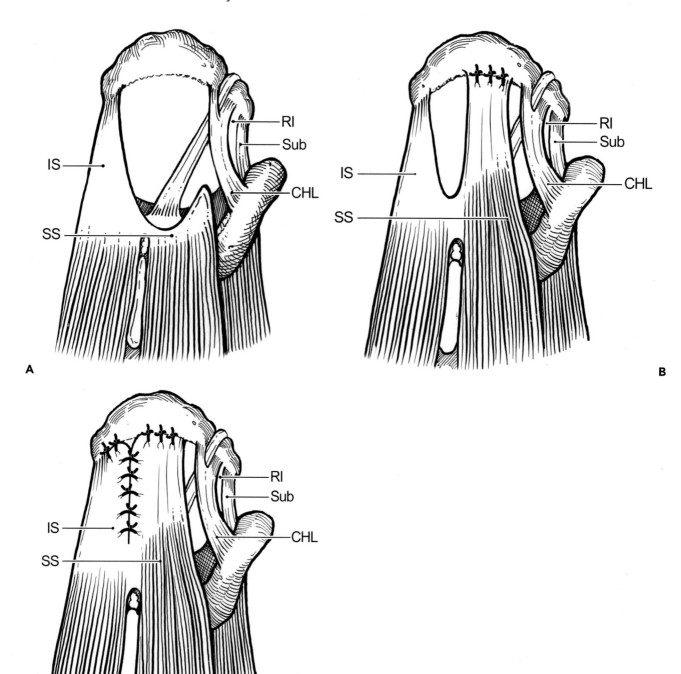

Figure 5-2 Repair of a massive contracted immobile longitudinal rotator cuff tear. **A:** An anterior interval slide is performed by incising the interval between the supraspinatus tendon and rotator interval. This incision releases the posterior portion of the coracohumeral ligament. **B:** The improved mobility from the release allows repair of the supraspinatus tendon to a lateral bone bed. **C:** The posterior leaf of the tear, consisting of the infraspinatus and teres minor tendons is then advanced superiorly and laterally and the residual longitudinal defect is closed by side-to-side sutures. SS, supraspinatus; IS, infraspinatus; Sub, subscapularis; RI, rotator interval; CHL, coracohumeral ligament. (From Lo IK, Burkhart SS. Arthroscopic repair of massive, contracted, immobile rotator cuff tears using single and double interval slides: technique and preliminary results. *Arthroscopy.* 2004;20(1):22–33, Fig. 2; with permission.)

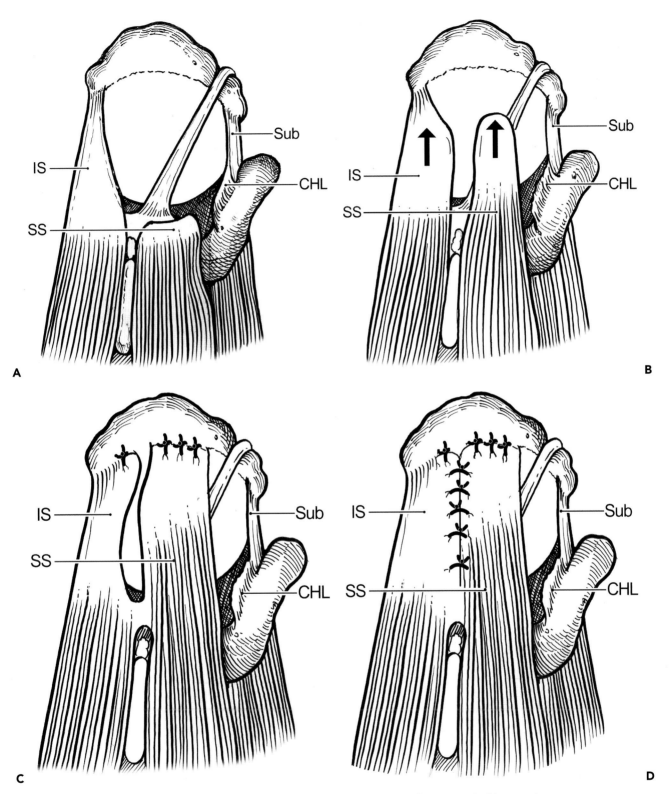

Figure 5-3 Repair of a massive contracted immobile crescent rotator cuff tear. **A:** A double interval slide is performed by first completing an anterior interval slide and then performing a posterior interval slide by releasing the interval between the supraspinatus and infraspinatus tendons. **B:** Following release, improved mobility is found in the supraspinatus tendon and the infraspinatus and teres minor tendons posteriorly. **C:** The supraspinatus can then be repaired to a lateral bone bed in a tension-free manner and the infraspinatus and teres minor tendons are advanced laterally and superiorly. **D:** The residual defect is then closed with side-to-side sutures. SS, supraspinatus; IS, infraspinatus; Sub, subscapularis; CHL, coracohumeral ligament. (From Lo IK, Burkhart SS. Arthroscopic repair of massive, contracted, immobile rotator cuff tears using single and double interval slides: technique and preliminary results. *Arthroscopy*. 2004;20(1):22–33, Fig. 3; with permission.)

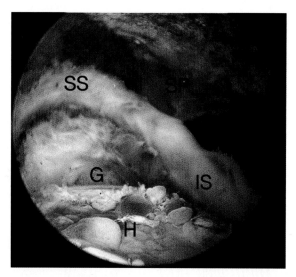

Figure 5-4 Arthroscopic view of a left shoulder from a lateral viewing portal demonstrating a typical massive severely contracted rotator cuff tear not amenable to direct tendon-to-bone repair or margin convergence and requiring an interval slide technique. G, glenoid; H, humeral head; SS, supraspinatus; IS, infraspinatus; SP, scapular spine.

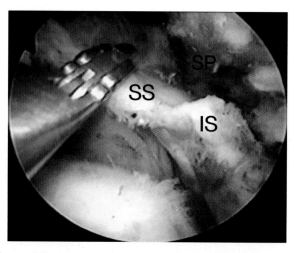

Figure 5-6 Arthroscopic view of a left shoulder from a lateral portal demonstrating the arching column of the scapular spine (SP), which serves as a marker between the supraspinatus (SS) and infraspinatus tendons (IS). A Viper suture passer (Arthrex Inc; Naples, FL) is used to pass traction sutures into each tendon.

anterior margin of the supraspinatus tendon is located just above the root of the biceps tendon. The tissue anterior to that point is the rotator interval. The posterior margin of the supraspinatus is delineated by the scapular spine.

When performing an anterior interval slide, it is easiest to view from the lateral, posterolateral, or posterior subacromial portal. These viewing portals allow the correct orientation and visualization of the release. A basket punch or arthroscopic scissor (Arthrex, Inc.; Naples, FL) is introduced through the accessory lateral portal, and the

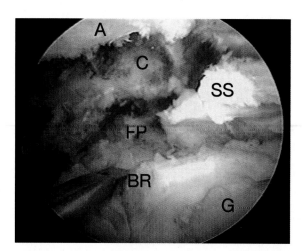

Figure 5-5 Arthroscopic view of a left shoulder from a posterolateral viewing portal demonstrating an anterior interval slide with release of the anterior margin of the supraspinatus (SS) tendon. The release is stopped when the fat pad that overlies the coracoid base comes into view. BR, biceps root (after tenotomy); G, glenoid; A, acromion; C, clavicle; FP, fat pad above coracoid base.

supraspinatus tendon is then released from lateral to medial, starting at the free margin of the cuff tear just above the root of the biceps tendon, and progressing to the base of the coracoid. The release is stopped when the surgeon sees at the apex of the cut the fat pad that overlies the coracoid base (Fig. 5-5). This release incises the coracohumeral ligament. A single anterior interval slide usually provides ~1 to 2 cm of supraspinatus tendon excursion from medial to lateral.

If more mobility is required than an anterior interval slide will produce, a double interval slide can be performed (e.g., during repair of massive, contracted, crescent tears). This procedure combines the standard anterior interval slide, as just described, with a posterior interval slide, which releases the interval between supraspinatus and infraspinatus tendons. It is critical to expose arthroscopically the lateral border of the scapular spine, which marks the interval between the supraspinatus and infraspinatus, by resecting the medial fibrofatty tissue until the arching column of the scapular spine is visible (Fig. 5-6). Traction sutures are placed at the anterolateral corner of the infraspinatus tendon and at the posterolateral corner of the supraspinatus tendon. The posterior interval slide is performed while viewing through the lateral portal and using a basket punch or arthroscopic scissor through a posterolateral portal (Fig. 5-7A). As traction is placed on the two sutures, the posterior edge of the supraspinatus tendon is released from the anterior margin of the infraspinatus tendon by incising the interval between supraspinatus and infraspinatus tendons (i.e., the interval between the two traction sutures) and progressing toward the scapular spine (Fig. 5-7B). Care is taken to avoid injury to the suprascapular nerve by lifting the arthroscopic

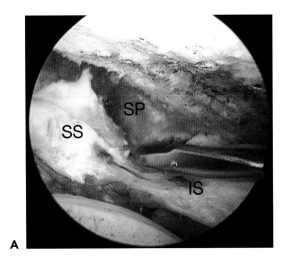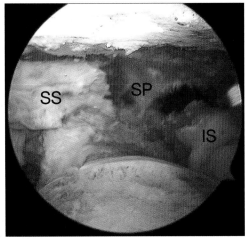

A   B

Figure 5-7   Arthroscopic views of a left shoulder from a lateral portal demonstrating a posterior interval slide. **A:** Release of the posterior margin of the supraspinatus tendon *(SS)* from the infraspinatus *(IS)* tendon using an arthroscopic scissor. **B:** Completed posterior interval slide demonstrating complete release of the *IS* from the *SS* tendon, revealing the scapular spine *(SP)*. Care is taken to avoid injury to the underlying suprascapular nerve.

punch or scissors away from the bone as the posterior interval slide is performed. Furthermore, pulling on the traction sutures as the posterial interval slide is done helps protect the suprascapular nerve by pulling the tendon margin away from the nerve.

With a combined anterior and posterior interval slide, ~3 to 5 cm of additional medial to lateral mobility of the supraspinatus tendon is obtained. Thus, tendon mobility after release may be sufficient to allow a tension-free repair of the supraspinatus tendon to the lateral bone bed (Fig. 5-8A,B). In addition, the posterior interval slide improves mobility of the infraspinatus tendon and the remaining posterior rotator cuff. This usually allows superior and

lateral mobilization of the infraspinatus tendon and repair in a tension-free manner (Fig. 5-9).

We commonly use suture anchors [BioCorkscrew, or BioCorkscrew-FT (Arthrex, Inc.; Naples, FL)] double-loaded with #2 FiberWire (Arthrex) for tendon-to-bone fixation. In addition, if the released tendon does not reach well onto the prepared bone bed, the rotator cuff footprint can be medialized 0.5 cm to maximize tendon-to-bone contact and ensure a tension-free repair. The residual defect between the supraspinatus and infraspinatus tendons is then closed (Fig. 5-10). This side-to-side repair is essential to reduce strain at the tendon–bone interface by the principle of margin convergence.

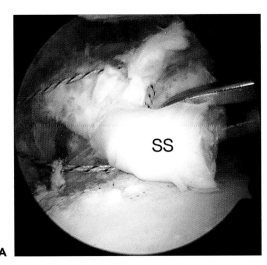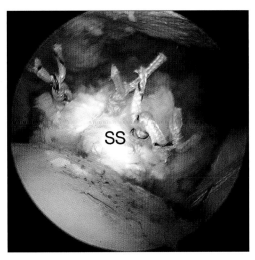

A   B

Figure 5-8   Arthroscopic views of a left shoulder from a lateral portal following anterior and posterior interval slides. **A:** Improved mobility of the supraspinatus *(SS)* tendon is obtained following release. This allows a tension-free repair of the *SS* tendon to the lateral bone bed. **B:** Completed *SS* tendon repair using BioCorkscrew (Arthrex, Inc.; Naples, FL.) suture anchors double loaded with #2 FiberWire (Arthrex) suture.

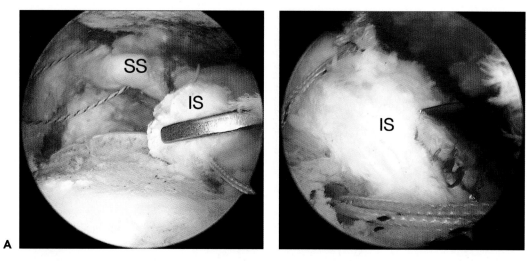

Figure 5-9   Arthroscopic views of a left shoulder from a lateral portal demonstrating improved mobility of the infraspinatus tendon following posterior interval slide. **A:** The infraspinatus *(IS)* tendon demonstrates improved medial to lateral mobility following posterior interval slide, allowing a tension-free repair to the lateral bone bed. Note: Compare the position of the Tigerwire suture in Figure 5-8A with that in Figure 5-9A, indicating how much lateral excursion of the supraspinatus *(SS)* has been gained by the release. **B:** Tendon-to-bone fixation of the *IS* tendon using BioCorkscrew (Arthrex, Inc.; Naples, FL) suture anchors double loaded with #2 FiberWire (Arthrex) suture and retrograde suture passage with a Penetrator (Arthrex) suture passer. G, glenoid; H, humerus.

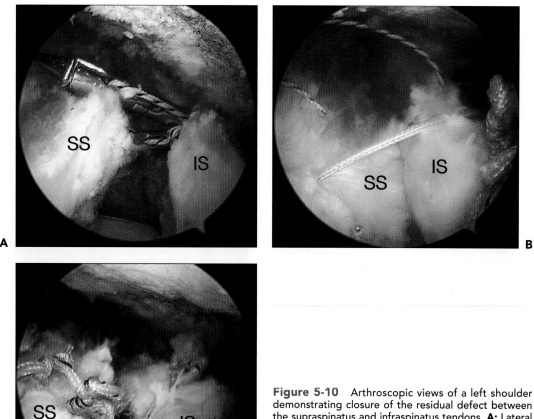

Figure 5-10   Arthroscopic views of a left shoulder demonstrating closure of the residual defect between the supraspinatus and infraspinatus tendons. **A:** Lateral arthroscopic view demonstrating side-to-side suturing of the supraspinatus *(SS)* and infraspinatus *(IS)* tendons using a hand-off technique with two Penetrator (Arthrex, Inc.; Naples, FL) suture passers. **B:** Completed side-to-side suture passage between the *SS* and *IS* tendons. **C:** Completed repair of the *SS* tendon to the *IS* tendon following repair of each tendon to bone.

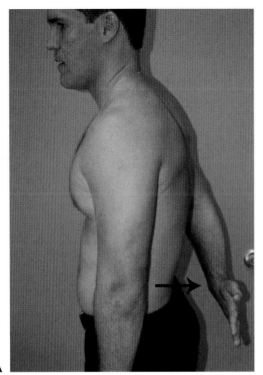 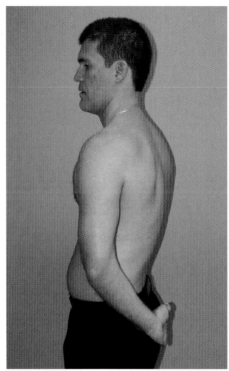

Figure 5-11 Clinical photo demonstrating the lift-off test. The back of the hand is placed on the lower back with the shoulder in maximal internal rotation, and the patient is asked to lift the hand off the back. **A:** Right hand can be lifted off the back demonstrating an intact subscapularis tendon function. **B:** Left hand cannot be lifted off the back—a positive test consistent with a subscapularis tear.

SUBSCAPULARIS TENDON TEARS

Arthroscopic subscapularis tendon repair has been the last component of arthroscopic rotator cuff repair to be perfected (2–4). Three unique aspects of the subscapularis can make it particularly difficult to repair. First, the chronic subscapularis tear tends to retract much more than the rest of the rotator cuff, causing great difficulty in mobilizing that tendon. Second, mobilizing the retracted subscapularis can be daunting because it tends to scar against the coracoid, in close proximity to important neurovascular structures. Third, visualization and manipulation of arthroscopic instruments in the tightly constricted subcoracoid space can be challenging. It is essential to address the torn subscapularis as the first step during arthroscopic shoulder surgery before fluid extravasation and swelling cause further constriction and compromise of the subcoracoid space. The goal of this section is to provide some technical hints and pearls for safely performing arthroscopic subscapularis repair (5).

Safety of the Approach

The key to success in this procedure is to know the arthroscopic anatomy around the coracoid. The anatomy at risk includes the axillary nerve, the axillary artery, the musculocutaneous nerve, and the lateral cord of the brachial plexus. All of these are >25 mm from the coracoid on anatomic cadaver dissections (5).

The safety of mobilizing the subscapularis tendon has been called into question because of the potential for neurovascular injury with subscapularis release, a complication that has only been reported at open surgery (6). It is important to recognize that the arthroscopic approach should be safer than the open approach simply because of the topographic differences between them. In the open approach, the surgeon must cross above the neurovascular structures as the release is done, putting these structures at risk for injury as the lower part of the tendon is released. In contrast, with the arthroscopic approach, the surgeon does an inside-out approach that does not cross the neurovascular structures.

Step-by-Step Procedure

Before You Begin (Preoperative Planning)
The clinician should be suspicious of a torn subscapularis based on preoperative physical examination. Recently, the senior author examined the sensitivity and specificity of several physical examination techniques in terms of identifying a torn subscapularis. The lift-off test (Fig. 5-11) is not positive until at least three fourths of the subscapularis tendon is detached and, therefore, is not a good test for upper subscapularis tears. The

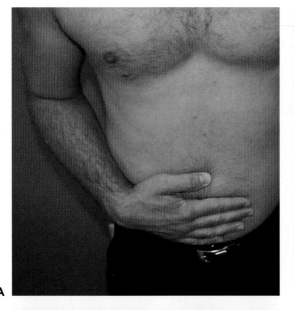
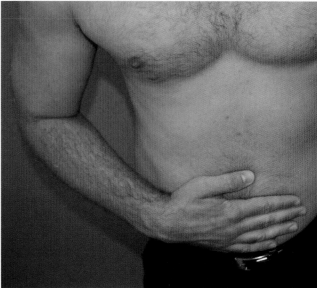
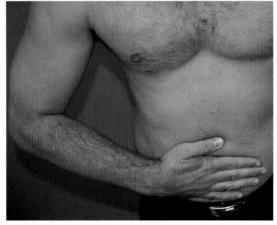

Figure 5-12 Napoleon test. **A:** Positive Napoleon sign indicates a nonfunctional subscapularis tendon. The patient can press on the belly only by flexing the wrist 90°, using the posterior deltoid rather than the subscapularis for this function. **B:** Intermediate Napoleon sign indicates partial function of the subscapularis tendon. As patient presses on the belly, the wrist flexes 30° to 60° because of partial function of the subscapularis tendon. **C:** Negative Napoleon sign indicates normal subscapularis tendon function. Patient is able to maintain the wrist extended while pressing on the belly.

Napoleon test can be useful to gain a preoperative estimation of how much of the subscapularis has been torn (Fig. 5-12). After tearing of the upper 50% to 60% of the subscapularis, the patient will develop an intermediate Napoleon sign (Fig. 5-12B). When the subscapularis is completely torn, the patient can push against the belly only by activating the posterior deltoid while the wrist is flexed 90°. This is a positive Napoleon test (Fig. 5-12A). The most sensitive test for a torn subscapularis (particularly a partial tear involving only the upper subscapularis) is the "bear hug" test (7). In this test, the patient places the hand of the affected side on the opposite shoulder with the fingers extended and the elbow elevated into a forward position. The examiner then tries to pull the patient's hand off the shoulder perpendicular to the plane of the forearm as the patient resists (Fig. 5-13). If the examiner is able to lift the patient's hand off the shoulder, this is a positive finding and is suggestive of at least a partially torn subscapularis. Another useful procedure is to check each patient's external rotation while

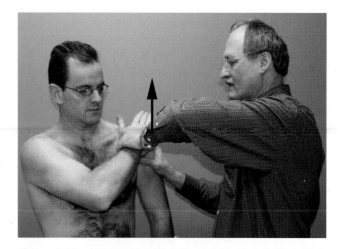

Figure 5-13 The bear hug test. The hand on the affected side is placed on the opposite shoulder with the fingers extended and the elbow elevated forward. The patient resists as the examiner tries to pull the hand off the shoulder in a direction that is perpendicular to the plane of the forearm (*arrow*). If the examiner is able to lift the hand off the shoulder, the patient likely has a torn (either partial or complete) upper subscapularis tendon.

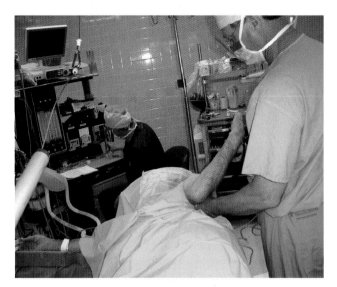

Figure 5-14 Passive external rotation >90° is suggestive of a complete subscapularis tendon tear.

under anesthesia. Significantly increased external rotation suggests a complete subscapularis tear (Fig. 5-14).

Portal Placement ("Portal Positioning Can be Your Best Friend or Your Worst Enemy")

Proper placement of an anterior portal and an anterosuperolateral portal is essential. Once subscapularis pathology is recognized, the next step is to place these two portals. First the anterosuperolateral portal is established (Fig. 5-15). An 18-gauge spinal needle is inserted off the anterolateral tip of the acromion. It is directed into the glenohumeral joint in a direction that is appropriate for preparation of the lesser tuberosity. This is accomplished if the spinal needle

makes a 5° to 10° angle of approach toward the lesser tuberosity. An additional benefit of this angle is that it ends up being relatively parallel to the direction of the subscapularis so that it can be used for working on that tendon (lysis of adhesions; antegrade suture passage) in addition to working on the lesser tuberosity (Fig. 5-16). This is the primary working portal during subscapularis repair. We place an 8.25-mm threaded, clear cannula (Arthrex) in this portal.

The anterior portal used for subscapularis repair is positioned somewhat more medially on the skin in comparison to the standard anterior portal. An 18-gauge spinal needle is inserted such that it enters the glenohumeral space just lateral to the coracoid tip and approaches the lesser tuberosity at a 30° to 45° angle. This portal will be used primarily for anchor placement. Because of humeral retroversion, the surgeon's hand must be placed quite medial during anchor placement, often in close proximity to the patient's jaw (see *Anchor Insertion* section below).

Address the Biceps Tendon ("To Fix the Subscap, You Must First SEE the Subscap")

Before addressing the subscapularis pathology, the biceps tendon should be thoroughly examined. The insertional footprint of the medial sling of the biceps is directly adjacent to the footprint of the upper subscapularis. A tear of the upper subscapularis is usually accompanied by disruption of the adjacent insertion of the medial sling, causing medial subluxation of the biceps. If biceps instability is noted, the biceps tendon must be addressed via tenodesis or tenotomy because a persistently subluxed biceps will stress the subscapularis repair and cause it to fail. If the biceps is intact but subluxed and the subscapularis is not retracted, visualization will be much easier if a biceps tenotomy (in

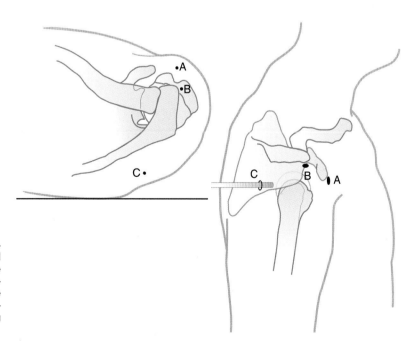

Figure 5-15 Portals for arthroscopic subscapularis tendon repair. The anterior portal (A) is used for anchor placement and suture passage. The anterosuperolateral portal (B) is used for subscapularis tendon mobilization and preparation of the bone bed, as well as for traction sutures. The posterior portal (C) is used as an arthroscopic viewing portal.

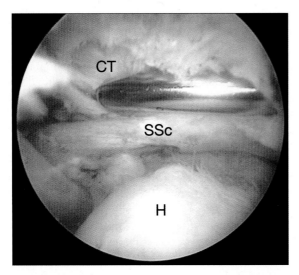

Figure 5-16 A shaver placed through the anterosuperolateral portal has an approach angle that is essentially parallel to the subscapularis *(SSc)* tendon (posterior viewing portal with 70° arthroscope). CT, coracoid tip; H, humerus.

preparation for tenodesis) is done before repairing the subscapularis. We generally prefer to do a biceps tenodesis except in elderly patients who have low demands and, in these elderly patients, we do a simple biceps tenotomy. For those patients in whom we plan to do a tenodesis, we ini-

tially place two half-racking sutures in the intra-articular portion of the biceps tendon to hold it securely (Fig. 5-17). Then, the tendon is tenotomized at its root, adjacent to the anterosuperior labrum. Next, we exteriorize the biceps through the anterosuperior portal to place a secure interlocking whipstitch (three or four passes on each side of the biceps tendon) (Fig. 5-18). By flexing the elbow and the shoulder, a greater length of tendon can be pulled out through the portal. Then, we bring the sutures from the whipstitch through an anterior portal that serves as a holding area before doing a tenodesis with a BioTenodesis (Arthrex) interference screw after the subscapularis repair. Once the tenotomy of the biceps has been done (in preparation for the tenodesis), the visualization for subscapularis repair is greatly improved (Fig. 5-19). It is important to recognize that biceps tenotomy or tenodesis is essential in the case of biceps subluxation or dislocation because, if the biceps is not transferred out of the way of the subscapularis to a tenodesis site, the persistent force of the subluxed biceps over the top of the subscapularis repair will cause the repair to fail.

Identify the Coracoid

The coracoid tip can be found routinely anterior to the upper border of the subscapularis (Fig. 5-20). It is important to use the 30° arthroscope when searching for the coracoid

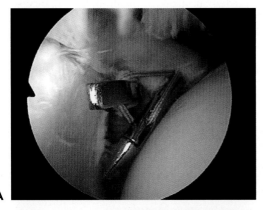

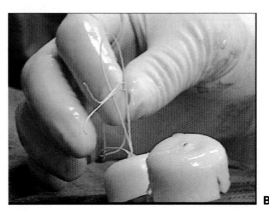

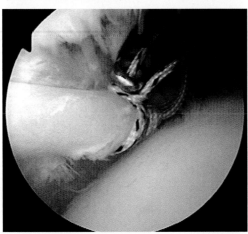

Figure 5-17 Two half-racking sutures are placed to secure the biceps tendon before tenotomy. **A:** A Penetrator (Arthrex, Inc.; Naples, FL) hands off a FiberWire suture (Arthrex) to a suture retriever. **B:** The FiberWire loop is then exteriorized and the free ends of the suture are passed through the loop. **C:** The free ends of the suture are tensioned to bring the suture loop down to the tendon. This causes the suture to "lock" down on the tendon, having a "strangulation" effect and preventing cut-out of the suture through the tendon. Sometimes, using a single diameter knot pusher to push the loop down (as seen here) assists in securing the loop.

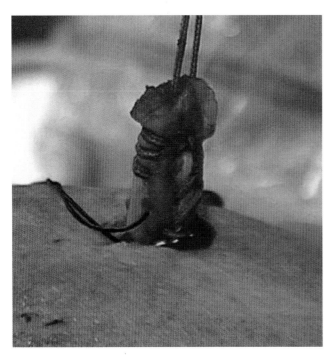

Figure 5-18 The cut end of the biceps tendon is pulled out through the anterosuperolateral portal by means of the two half-racking sutures. Then, a locking whipstitch is placed in the biceps, four throws on each side of the tendon.

because this allows the surgeon to maintain proper orientation. Use of a 70° arthroscope increases the potential to become disoriented and stray inferior to the coracoid tip. If inadvertent dissection proceeds inferior to the coracoid, danger of neurovascular injury increases substantially.

Two situations occur in which the surgeon must locate the coracoid: (a) the subscapularis is not retracted (e.g., partial tear) and (b) the subscapularis is retracted (complete full-thickness tear). The technique for locating the coracoid is different for these two situations.

If the subscapularis is not retracted, the surgeon should make a window in the rotator interval just above the upper border of the subscapularis tendon to identify the coracoid. In making this window, both the medial sling of the biceps and the superior glenohumeral ligament should be preserved (Fig. 5-21). If the subscapularis tendon is retracted, the surgeon should identify the coracoacromial (CA) ligament as it goes from the anterolateral aspect of the acromion and heads in an inferomedial direction toward the coracoid tip. These diagonal fibers of the CA ligament can always be identified and then followed directly to the coracoid tip where they insert (Fig. 5-22). The conjoined tendon can be identified just inferior to the bony tip of the coracoid, which can be palpated easily with an instrument. Be careful not to confuse these structures with a scarred subscapularis (Fig. 5-23).

Once the coracoid tip is located, its posterolateral aspect can then be easily skeletonized with electrocautery, arthroscopic elevators, and motorized shaver. This is all performed through the anterosuperolateral portal while visualizing through the posterior portal (usually with a 70° arthroscope) (Fig. 5-24). In exposing the coracoid, it is important to preserve the attachments to the conjoined tendon. The attachments from the CA ligament into the coracoid can be sacrificed, if necessary, so that an adequate coracoplasty can be done.

Perform the Coracoplasty

The plane of the coracoplasty is parallel to the plane of the subscapularis tendon. This is easily accomplished through the anterosuperolateral portal. The goal of the coracoplasty is to create a 7- to 10-mm space between the reconfigured coracoid tip and the anterior plane of the subscapularis. This subcoracoid decompression protects the repaired subscapularis from any abrasive effect from the coracoid during tendon healing. Typically, the burr is placed into the anterosuperolateral portal and directed anterior to the medial sling (comma sign) tissue into the subcoracoid space (Fig. 5-25).

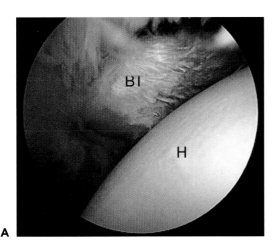 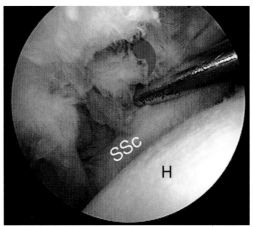

Figure 5-19 A: Subluxed biceps tendon *(BT)* obscures the upper subscapularis tendon (which cannot be seen) and comma sign (,) in this right shoulder. **B:** After biceps tenotomy (in preparation for tenodesis), the subscapularis tendon *(SSc)* and the comma sign (,) are easily visualized. H, humerus.

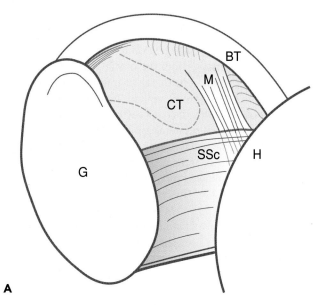

A

Figure 5-20 This drawing represents the arthroscopic view from the posterior portal of a right shoulder. The shadow of the coracoid tip *(CT)* is typically found at the superior border of the subscapularis tendon *(SSc)*. G, glenoid; H, humerus; M, medial biceps sling; BT, biceps tendon.

Improving Anterior Exposure (Creating More Anterior Subcoracoid Space)

Although a 70° arthroscope allows better overall visualization of the subscapularis and its footprint on the lesser tuberosity, some patients have such a tight subcoracoid space that visualization is very difficult. In such cases, we have found the "posterior lever push" to be helpful in enlarging the subcoracoid space (Fig. 5-26). This maneuver requires a second assistant positioned anterior to the

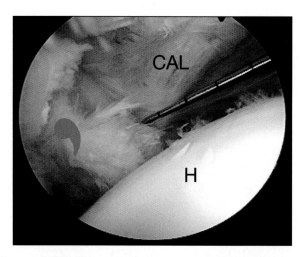

Figure 5-22 The comma sign (‚) is visible adjacent to a retracted subscapularis tendon. The coracoacromial ligament *(CAL)* inserts onto the tip of the *processus coracoideus scapulae* (coracoid), which is being palpated by a metal probe. H, humerus.

patient, who is in a lateral decubitus position. This assistant levers the humeral head posteriorly by simultaneously pushing the proximal humerus posteriorly and pulling the distal humerus anteriorly. This maneuver typically expands the field of view in the anterior aspect of the shoulder by 5 to 10 mm (Fig. 5-27).

Finding the Subscapularis ("The Key Is in the Comma")

In the case of a complete subscapularis tear, the tendon will dramatically retract. In fact, it frequently retracts almost to the level of the anterior labrum medially. The key to finding the subscapularis and differentiating it from the conjoined tendon and the coracoacromial ligament is to

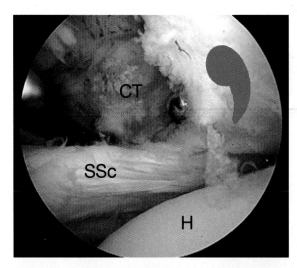

Figure 5-21 A window has been made in the rotator interval with care taken to preserve the comma (‚). The coracoid tip *(CT)* is located just anterior to the upper border of the subscapularis tendon *(SSc)*. H, humerus.

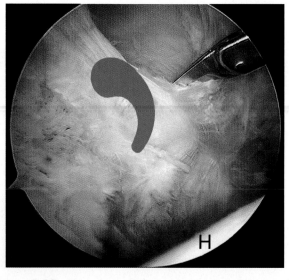

Figure 5-23 The subscapularis tendon is scarred against the coracoid. The comma sign (‚) leads to the lateral border of the subscapularis, which is being dissected from the coracoid. H, humerus.

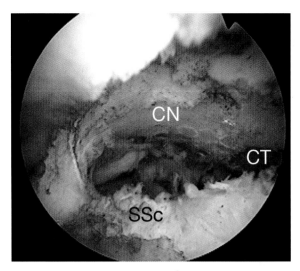

Figure 5-24 Posterior viewing portal. A 70° arthroscopic view of a right shoulder. The coracoid has been skeletonized to reveal the coracoid neck (CN) and the coracoid tip (CT), which has undergone coracoplasty. The subscapularis (SSc) is still encased by the scar tissue that has been dissected from the coracoid.

locate the "comma sign." The comma sign is a comma-shaped arc of tissue located at the superolateral border of the subscapularis, which will always lead to the superolateral border of the subscapularis (Fig. 5-28).

The comma is actually the remnant of the medial sling of the biceps, whose footprint before tearing from the bone had been directly adjacent to the superior portion of the footprint of the subscapularis on the lesser tuberosity of the humerus (Fig. 5-29). Typically, when the subscapularis fails completely, the medial sling of the biceps pulls away from the lesser tuberosity as well so that these struc-

tures remain together (Figs. 5-30 and 5-31). This is convenient because the comma then allows the surgeon to be able to fully delineate the superolateral aspect of the subscapularis. The comma is composed of fibers of the medial head of the coracohumeral ligament as well as a portion of the superior glenohumeral ligament. Progression from the intact situation to a completely torn and retracted subscapularis is best understood by means of sequential schematic drawings (Fig. 5-32).

Subscapularis Tendon Mobilization
For the retracted subscapularis tendon, a three-sided release must be done. The release is done anteriorly, superiorly, and posteriorly on the subscapularis. This technique is facilitated by placing a traction suture at the junction of the comma with the subscapularis (Fig. 5-33). The traction suture is placed using a free FiberWire suture (Arthrex) on a Viper suture passer (Arthrex). The traction suture is then positioned outside the cannula through the anterosuperolateral portal so that the sutures will not obstruct instruments while working through this portal. Next, the three-sided release is performed in stages.

Anterior Subscapularis Tendon Release
The first stage is the anterior release. A retracted subscapularis tendon tends to adhere to the posterolateral aspect of the coracoid. The anterior release is achieved by using a combination of shaver and electrocautery to dissect the subscapularis from the coracoid. Starting at the previously identified coracoid tip, dissection is continued medially along the posterolateral aspect of the coracoid until this structure is essentially skeletonized to the level of the coracoid neck and base (Fig. 5-34). Once the coracoid has been skeletonized all the way around to the coracoid neck, it is

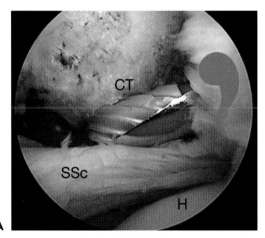 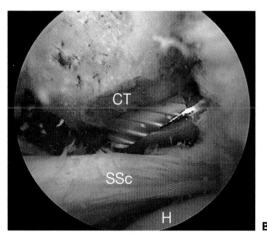

Figure 5-25 A: Posterior viewing portal, 70° "aerial" view. The power burr has a diameter of 5.5 mm and does not fit into the space between the coracoid tip (CT) and the subscapularis tendon (SSc). The comma (ɔ) is visible at the superolateral border of the subscapularis (SSc). **B:** After the coracoplasty has been completed, the space between the coracoid tip (CT) and subscapularis tendon (SSc) should be ~7 to 10 mm, which can be estimated from the diameter of the power burr. CT, coracoid tip; SSc, subscapularis; H, humerus.

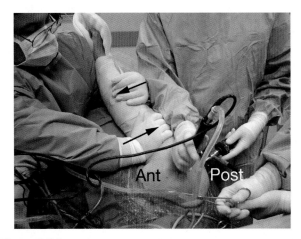

Figure 5-26 Posterior lever push. The second assistant simultaneously pushes the proximal humerus posteriorly and pulls the distal humerus anteriorly.

virtually impossible to see all the way to the coracoid base. At that point, it is important to use the traction suture to pull the subscapularis as far laterally as possible and then make a window through the rotator interval tissue, preserving the comma tissue. By preserving the comma, this tissue can later be used to aid in the repair of the residual portion of the cuff tear (infraspinatus and supraspinatus). While pulling laterally on the subscapularis, the electrocautery probe is used to make a window in the rotator interval (Fig. 5-35). Then the 70° arthroscope is "parked" in that rotator interval window so that the neck of the coracoid can be visualized. Now, the remaining portion of the coracoid is skeletonized down to the base. In doing this, the attachment of the coracohumeral ligament to the coracoid is completely released, allowing maximal lateral excursion of the subscapularis. Incidentally,

by releasing the coracohumeral ligament, an anterior interval slide has also been performed, thereby improving lateral excursion of the supraspinatus (if it is torn). This type of anterior interval slide, in which the coracohumeral ligament is released while preserving the comma tissue, is termed as interval slide in continuity.

Superior Subscapularis Tendon Release
Next, we progress to the superior release. This is essentially an extension of the anterior release. Using 15° and 30° arthroscopic elevators (Arthrex), adhesions between the lateral arch of the coracoid and the upper border of the subscapularis are broken up (Fig. 5-36). We never dissect medial to the midpoint of the base of the coracoid because this is an area where neurovascular structures are potentially at risk. We have not found it necessary to dissect further medial than this because the dense adhesions are always at the inferolateral aspect of the coracoid neck and coracoid base. As long as the surgeon stays just underneath or lateral to the coracoid, neurovascular structures are not at risk (5).

Posterior Subscapularis Tendon Release
Finally, the posterior release is performed. While pulling on the traction suture, an arthroscopic elevator is used to break adhesions between the posterior surface of the subscapularis and the anterior surface of the glenoid neck (Fig. 5-37). This is actually the safest area to release because the substance of the subscapularis muscle protects the neurovascular structures.

Prepare the Bone Bed
Next, using electrocautery, ring curettes, arthroscopic shaver, and an arthroscopic burr, the lesser tuberosity bone bed is

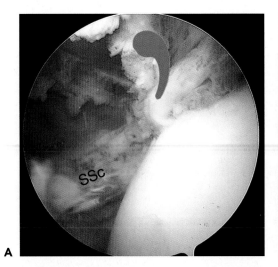

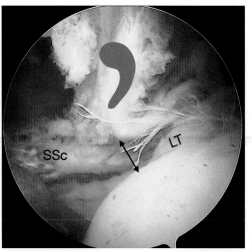

A   B

Figure 5-27 **A:** Right shoulder. Posterior viewing portal with 70° arthroscope. This is the "exposure" of the upper subscapularis tendon footprint with the patient in a standard lateral decubitus position without a posterior lever push. The upper tendon of the subscapularis is tightly draped across the lesser tuberosity, and the footprint is not visible. SSc, subscapularis; (ʾ), comma. **B:** Same shoulder with a 70° arthroscope with a posterior lever push. This maneuver dramatically increases the exposure of the subscapularis footprint, providing much more room for visualization, instrumentation, and bone bed preparation. LT, lesser tuberosity footprint.

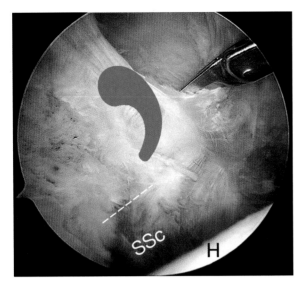

Figure 5-28   The comma sign. Right shoulder, posterior viewing portal. This comma-shaped arc of tissue always leads to the superolateral border of the subscapularis tendon *(SSc)*. This tissue is the remnant of the medial sling of the biceps, superior border of subscapularis; H, humerus.

prepared down to a bleeding base without decorticating the bone. In some cases of chronic tears, the aforementioned mobilization techniques may not bring the subscapularis tendon as far laterally as would be preferred to obtain a good footprint on the lesser tuberosity. In such cases, consider medialization of the bone bed up to 5 mm to create a larger footprint (Fig. 5-38). This degree of medialization of the footprint has not caused any loss of function in the senior author's experience. It is better to medialize the footprint than to risk disruption of the repair by overtensioning it.

Anchor Insertion

In general, we use one doubly loaded suture anchor for each linear centimeter of subscapularis tear. In anatomic dissections, we have found that the superior-to-inferior length of the footprint of the normal subscapularis is 2.45 cm (Burkhart SS and Tehrany AM, unpublished data). Therefore, for a 50% tear, we will place one anchor; for a 100% tear, two anchors. Occasionally, sufficient lateral excursion of the subscapularis tendon exists to allow a double row fixation, but not as frequently as in other rotator

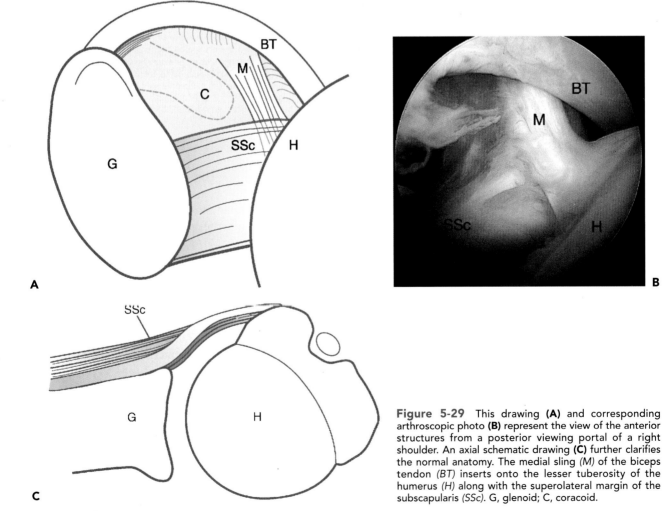

Figure 5-29   This drawing **(A)** and corresponding arthroscopic photo **(B)** represent the view of the anterior structures from a posterior viewing portal of a right shoulder. An axial schematic drawing **(C)** further clarifies the normal anatomy. The medial sling *(M)* of the biceps tendon *(BT)* inserts onto the lesser tuberosity of the humerus *(H)* along with the superolateral margin of the subscapularis *(SSc)*. G, glenoid; C, coracoid.

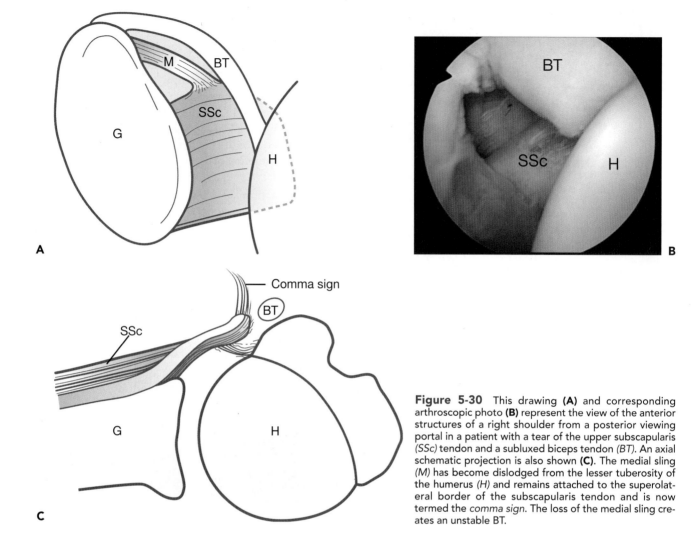

Figure 5-30 This drawing **(A)** and corresponding arthroscopic photo **(B)** represent the view of the anterior structures of a right shoulder from a posterior viewing portal in a patient with a tear of the upper subscapularis *(SSc)* tendon and a subluxed biceps tendon *(BT)*. An axial schematic projection is also shown **(C)**. The medial sling *(M)* has become dislodged from the lesser tuberosity of the humerus *(H)* and remains attached to the superolateral border of the subscapularis tendon and is now termed the *comma sign*. The loss of the medial sling creates an unstable BT.

cuff tendons. Even so, single row repair has provided generally good results. We will focus this discussion on single row repair of the subscapularis.

Because of humeral neck retroversion, the angle of approach for anchor placement in the lower half of the lesser tuberosity requires that a "hand on jaw" position be used during anchor insertion. That is, the surgeon's hand is almost up against the patient's jaw when holding the bone punch to make the hole into the lesser tuberosity (Fig. 5-39). Our anesthesiologist routinely places eye protection on the patient (e.g., disposable plastic goggles) to avoid inadvertent trauma to the eye by instruments or anchor inserter handles.

In the case of a complete subscapularis tear, the inferior anchor is placed first. Both sutures are then passed (as will be outlined below) and the sutures are sequentially tied. To simplify suture management, sutures from the lower anchor are tied before placing the superior anchor.

Subscapularis Tendon Suture Passage
The surgeon must recognize that the coracoid is in such a location that retrograde passage of sutures through the

subscapularis tendon is difficult and instruments to pass the sutures antegrade are much more useful. After the anchors are inserted through the anterior portal, one suture strand from the lower anchor is pulled out the anterosuperolateral 8.25-mm clear cannula. As noted, this anterosuperolateral portal is the primary working portal because of its parallel orientation with the subscapularis. The suture strand is then loaded onto a standard Viper (Arthrex) suture passer. While pulling tension on the traction suture (which is outside the cannula through the same portal), a "bite" of subscapularis tendon is grasped by the viper and the suture passed through the lateral aspect of the tendon in an antegrade fashion. This process is repeated with the other color suture strand.

When passing the sutures from the superior anchor, we grasp the subscapularis tendon at the junction of the tendon with the comma sign (Fig. 5-40). If coverage of the footprint is adequate, we pass the sutures from the anchor through the upper border of the tendon at a point just medial to the junction of the comma with the upper border of the subscapularis tendon. In this manner, the vertical

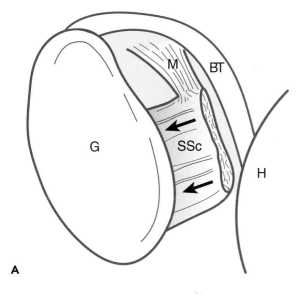

A

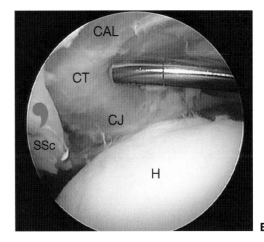

B

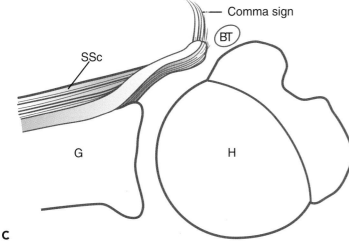

C

Comma sign

SSc

BT

G

H

Figure 5-31 This drawing **(A)** and corresponding arthroscopic photo **(B)** represent a complete subscapularis tendon tear with medial retraction almost to the level of the glenoid *(G)* in association with a medially dislocated biceps tendon. An axial projection is also shown in **(C)**. In this situation, the comma sign (ͽ) leads to the superolateral border of the subscapularis tendon *(SSc)*. CAL, coracoacromial ligament; CJ, conjoined tendon; CT, *processus coracoideus scapulae* (coracoid) tip; H, humerus; BT, biceps tendon; M, medial sling.

fibers of the comma tissue (medial sling) will prevent linear cut-through of the sutures in the subscapularis tendon. Typically, sutures are tied through the anterosuperolateral portal. We find the use of the Surgeon's Sixth Finger (Arthrex) knot pusher helpful in that it allows manipulation of the tissue while tying the knot and also maintains the tightest loop security possible (Fig. 5-41). Grasping the subscapularis tendon at the junction with the comma tissue also provides a rolled edge to the upper border of the subscapularis tendon (Fig. 5-42).

Does Fatty Degeneration of the Subscapularis Tendon Matter?

Some reports in the orthopedic literature suggest that fatty degeneration of the rotator cuff might be a contraindication to rotator cuff repair and that muscle tendon units with fatty degeneration do not have an ability to heal (8,9). In the case of the subscapularis tendon, this does not seem to hold true. It appears to be unique among the rota-

tor cuff tendons in that a significant part of its function is a tenodesis function and it is needed as an anterior restraint (10). That is, it can help provide a fulcrum of motion even if it functions only as a tenodesis with no contractile elements. We believe, therefore, that function can be enhanced by repairing all subscapularis tears regardless of the degree of fatty degeneration. In fact, we have observed dramatic improvements in overhead function after repair of subscapularis tears that had virtually complete fatty degeneration of the subscapularis muscle.

What If the Subscapularis Tendon Is Not Repairable?

The subscapularis is almost always repairable through meticulous mobilization techniques and through medialization of the bone footprint. Occasionally, the surgeon encounters a subscapularis tendon that is not repairable. In such a case, one should consider an Achilles tendon allograft or a subcoracoid pectoralis major transfer (11,12).

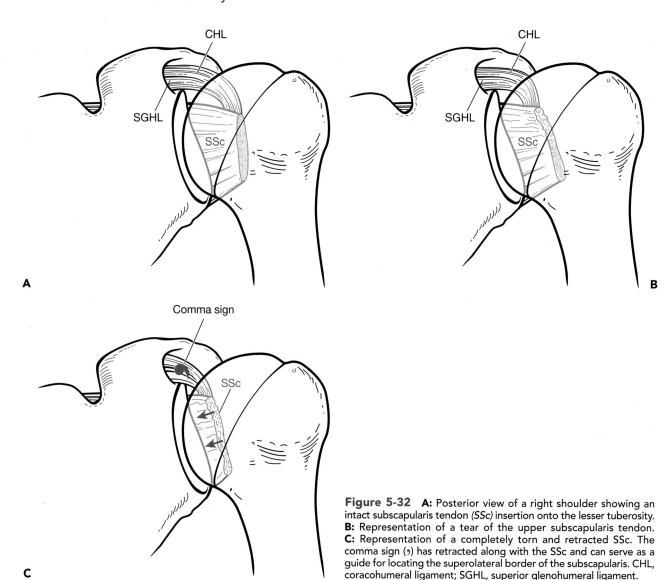

Figure 5-32 A: Posterior view of a right shoulder showing an intact subscapularis tendon *(SSc)* insertion onto the lesser tuberosity. **B:** Representation of a tear of the upper subscapularis tendon. **C:** Representation of a completely torn and retracted SSc. The comma sign (ɔ) has retracted along with the SSc and can serve as a guide for locating the superolateral border of the subscapularis. CHL, coracohumeral ligament; SGHL, superior glenohumeral ligament.

Proximal Humeral Migration

Proximal humeral migration can occur with massive anterosuperior tears (combined subscapularis, supraspinatus, and infraspinatus tendon tears). When proximal humeral migration occurs as a result of these large tears, a loss of overhead function frequently occurs. In our series of subscapularis repairs (2), 10 of the 25 were anterosuperior rotator cuff tears with proximal humeral migration. All of these had lost overhead function. With subscapularis repair and repair of the residual rotator cuff, 8 of these 10 had durable reversal of proximal humeral migration, which was radiographically confirmed. Each of these eight patients had restoration of overhead function, whereas the two patients without reversal of proximal humeral migration did not regain overhead function.

Postoperative Protocol

After repair of the subscapularis, with or without associated repair of other rotator cuff tendons, the patient is

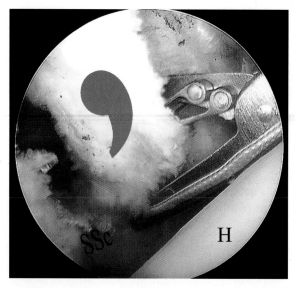

Figure 5-33 Right shoulder, posterior viewing portal. A traction suture is placed at the junction of the comma (ɔ) and the subscapularis tendon *(SSc)*. H, humerus.

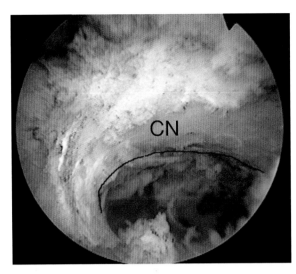

Figure 5-34 Right shoulder, posterior viewing portal through a 70° arthroscope. Anterior release. The coracoid dissection *(solid line)* has skeletonized the posterolateral coracoid to the level of the coracoid neck *(CN)*.

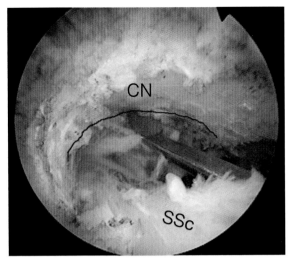

Figure 5-36 Right shoulder, posterior viewing portal through a 70° arthroscope. Superior release: A 30° arthroscopic elevator, introduced through an anterosuperolateral portal, is used to perform the superior release, lysing adhesions between the subscapularis and the *processus coracoideus scapulae* (coracoid) neck or base. CN, coracoid neck; SSc, subscapularis.

placed in a sling for 6 weeks. In the case of a complete subscapularis tear, external rotation beyond 0° is not allowed for 6 weeks. With partial subscapularis tears, we allow passive external rotation to ~30°. No overhead motion is allowed for 6 weeks. The patient, however, can use the hand in the straight-ahead position for writing or eating. The sling is removed daily for a shower.

After 6 weeks, the patient's sling is discontinued and a stretching program of passive external rotation and overhead stretching (using a rope and pulley) is begun. At 12 weeks postoperative, strengthening is initiated, first with Thera-Band elastic resistive bands followed by light weights,

as dictated by the patient's progress. Unrestricted activities are delayed until 6 to 12 months postoperative, depending on the size of the tear and the restoration of strength.

BICEPS PATHOLOGY: TENDINITIS TO CHRONIC RUPTURES

Treatment of disorders of the long head of the biceps tendon remains controversial. This is, in part, because of the unclear

Text continues on page 133.

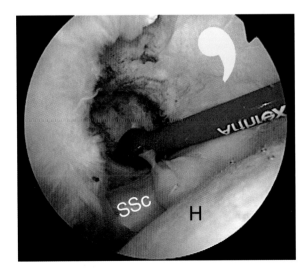

Figure 5-35 Posterior viewing portal through a 70° arthroscope. While pulling the subscapularis *(SSc)* laterally with traction sutures, the surgeon uses the electrocautery probe to make a window in the rotator interval, which provides access to the base of the coracoid.

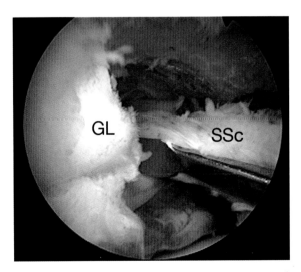

Figure 5-37 Right shoulder; posterior release. A 15° arthroscopic elevator is used to develop the plane between the posterior aspect of the subscapularis tendon *(SSc)* and the anterior glenoid neck and glenoid labrum *(GL)*, thereby releasing adhesions that may be restricting lateral excursion of the subscapularis.

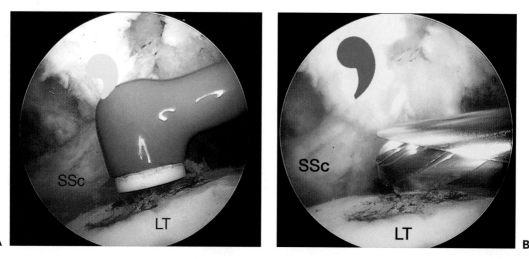

Figure 5-38   A: Right shoulder, posterior viewing portal through a 70° arthroscope. An electrocautery probe is used to delineate a medialized footprint on the lesser tuberosity. **B:** Right shoulder. Power burr prepares the medialized footprint that was first delineated by electrocautery probe by "burring off the charcoal" down to bleeding bone. SSc, subscapularis; LT, lesser tuberosity of humerus.

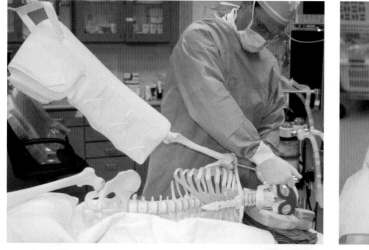

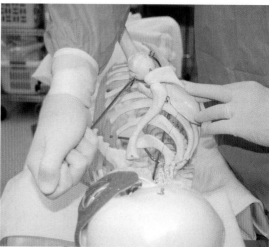

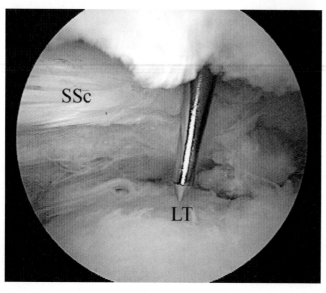

Figure 5-39   A: This skeleton demonstrates how the arm is held in 30° of abduction and 30° of forward flexion during shoulder arthroscopy in the lateral decubitus position. **B:** Photograph from the head looking downward demonstrates how the combination of abduction, forward flexion, and normal humeral retroversion necessitates a "hand on face" position during anchor insertion into the lesser tuberosity. This highlights the need for protective goggles on the patient. **C:** This "hand on face" position allows the surgeon to achieve an appropriate "deadman" angle to insert suture anchors into the lesser tuberosity (LT). SSc, subscapularis.

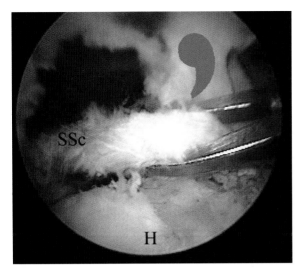

Figure 5-40 Right shoulder; posterior viewing portal. During suture passage into the upper subscapularis tendon, the tendon is grasped and the suture passed at the junction of the subscapularis (*SSc*) and the comma (*,*). H, humerus.

Figure 5-42 Right shoulder; posterior viewing portal. Sutures from the upper anchor have been placed at the junction of the vertically oriented comma tissue and the upper border of subscapularis tendon (*SSc*). This suture placement prevents suture cut-out and provides a rolled edge to the upper subscapularis tendon repair. H, humerus.

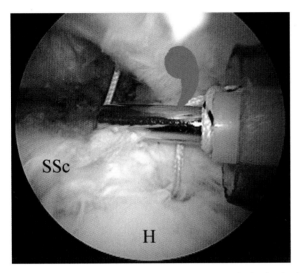

Figure 5-41 Right shoulder; posterior viewing portal. The Sixth-Finger knot pusher allows the subscapularis (*SSc*) tendon to be manipulated and held in the appropriate position while each half-hitch of the knot is tied. This provides maximal loop security. H, humerus.

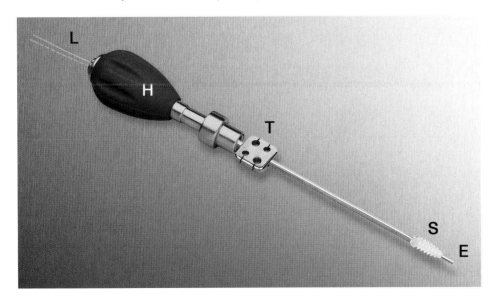

Figure 5-43 Clinical photo of the Bio-Tenodesis (Arthrex, Inc.; Naples, FL) cannulated screwdriver with driver handle (*H*), reverse threaded sleeve and thumbpiece (*T*), bioabsorbable Bio-Tenodesis screw (*S*), and a loop of suture (*L*) loaded through the cannulated tip. Turning the handle (*H*) and holding the thumbpiece (*T*) advances the screw (*S*) by means of the reverse-threaded sleeve which advances on the driver shaft while the driver end (*E*) remains stationary at the base of the bone socket. The measuring guides on the thumbpiece (*T*) are used to size the biceps tendon.

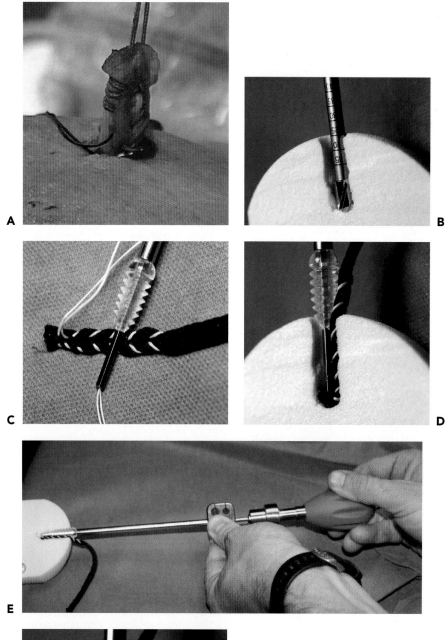

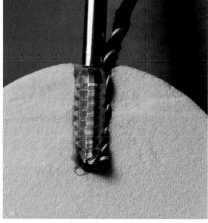

Figure 5-44 **A:** Biceps tendon has been exteriorized and a Krakow whipstitch has been placed In the bicep tendon. **B:** A bone socket is drilled over a guide pin using a cannulated headed reamer to a depth of 25-mm. **C:** Suture ends from the whipstitch are threaded through the cannulated driver tip. **D:** The screwdriver tip pushes the tendon to the base of the bone socket. **E:** The screw is advanced by turning the driver handle while holding the thumbplate that is attached to the reverse-threaded metal sleeve. **F:** The interference fit of the tendon between bone and the Bio-Tenodesis (Arthrex, Inc.; Naples, FL) screw gives excellent fixation.

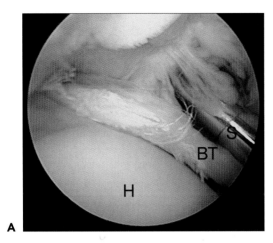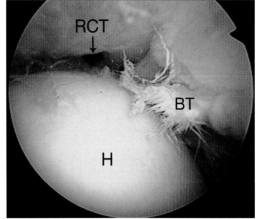

A   B

Figure 5-45 **A:** Posterior arthroscopic view of a left shoulder with a 70° scope after the shaver has been levered downward on the biceps tendon to pull additional tendon into the joint, demonstrating significant degeneration of the biceps tendon. **B:** A 30° scope view showing associated rotator cuff tear. BT, biceps tendon; H, humerus; S, shaver blade; RCT, rotator cuff tear.

role of the long head of the biceps tendon during normal glenohumeral motion and its primary or secondary function in the presence of shoulder pathology (e.g., instability versus rotator cuff tears). The spectrum of pathology demonstrated by the long head of the biceps tendon can include tendinitis, instability (subluxation or dislocation), and tears (partial or complete). The major surgical treatment modalities for disorders of the long head of the biceps tendon include débridement, tenotomy, or tenodesis (13–15).

We commonly débride tears involving <50% of the biceps tendon without instability. However, we perform an arthroscopic biceps tenodesis for (a) biceps tears involving >50% of the tendon; (b) medial subluxation of the biceps tendon; and (c) combined subscapularis tears and biceps subluxation, in which biceps tenodesis is performed to protect the arthroscopic subscapularis repair. The indications for arthroscopic biceps tenotomy are similar to the indications for arthroscopic biceps tenodesis; however, tenotomy is reserved for older patients (usually, >70 years of age) with lower physical demands.

Because the functional outcome of patients with chronic unrepaired ruptures of the long head of the biceps tendon can be normal or near normal, complete tears of the biceps tendon are rarely an indication for tenodesis. Some young active individuals, however, can have unsatisfactory outcomes from tenotomy with ongoing pain and cramping in their biceps lump. In these patients, an arthroscopic-assisted biceps tenodesis is still sometimes possible and can restore the normal contour of the biceps and function of the biceps (see Part II: Chapter 18A, *The Cobra Procedure,* also discussed later in Chapter 5) (16).

The Bio-Tenodesis Screw System

Our technique for arthroscopic biceps tenodesis incorporates the Bio-Tenodesis Screw System (Arthrex), which uses

a uniquely designed Bio-Tenodesis screwdriver. This cannulated screwdriver (Fig. 5-43) is specially designed with a reverse threaded sleeve and thumbpiece on the driver shaft. During insertion of the Bio-Tenodesis interference screw, this design allows the biceps tendon to be maintained at the bottom of the bone socket under tension as the screw is advanced in the bone socket by the hex driver and by the advancing reverse-threaded pitch of the metal sleeve. Fixation is achieved using bioabsorbable PLLA (poly-L-lactic acid) cannulated screws, which are available in four diameters (5.5, 7, 8, and 9-mm) and are 23-mm in length.

In brief, following tenotomy and whipstitching of the biceps tendon (Fig. 5-44A), a bone socket is drilled over a guide pin with a cannulated headed reamer to a depth of 25 mm (Fig. 5-44B). Next, the suture ends are passed directly through the cannulated screwdriver (Fig. 5-44C) via a nitinol suture threader. Alternatively, the suture ends can be passed through a loop of suture at the end of the cannulated screwdriver. These sutures are pulled, advancing the biceps tendon to the end of the cannulated driver and allowing the biceps tendon to be manipulated and controlled by the cannulated screwdriver tip. The screwdriver tip, along with the biceps tendon, is then inserted into the base of the previously drilled bone socket (Fig. 5-44D) and the screw is advanced by turning the driver handle while holding the thumbpiece at the top of the reverse-threaded metal sleeve. This maneuver advances the tendon in the bone socket while the leading end of the tendon is maintained in a stationary position at the base of the bone socket (Fig. 5-44E). This guarantees an adequate bone-tendon-screw interface within the bone socket (Fig. 5-44F) and eliminates the need for transosseous drilling. Note that the FiberWire whipstitch provides additional friction against the screwthreads, adding to the interference fit and helping to further resist pull-out of the screw.

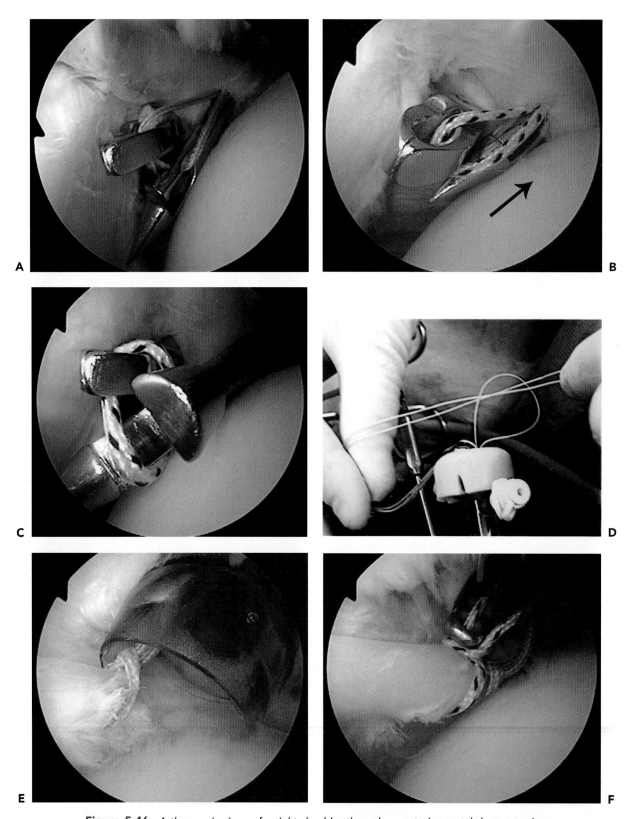

Figure 5-46 Arthroscopic views of a right shoulder through a posterior portal demonstrating placement of the half-racking stitch. **A:** A Penetrator (Arthrex, Inc.; Naples, FL) is loaded with #2 FiberWire (Arthrex) and is used to pierce the biceps tendon distal to its origin. **B:** The suture loop is temporarily held using a suture retriever through the anterior portal while the Penetrator is withdrawn from the biceps tendon and reinserted into the joint posterior to the biceps tendon. **C:** The Penetrator is then used to retrieve the suture loop out through the lateral cannula. **D:** Clinical photo. The free ends of the suture are then fed through the suture loop and pulled. **E:** The suture loop is drawn into the joint creating a grasping half-racking stitch securing the long head of the biceps tendon. **F:** A second half-racking stitch is placed for added security. A single-hole knot pusher is used to push the loop down tightly against the biceps tendon.

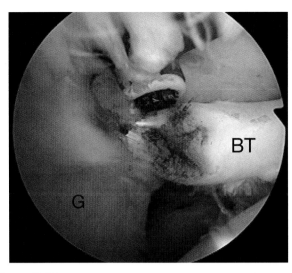

Figure 5-47 Arthroscopic views of a right shoulder from a posterior portal. The biceps tendon is released close to its insertion on the superior labrum using a 90° hooked electrocautery bovie (Arthrex, Inc.; Naples, FL). BT, biceps tendon; G, glenoid.

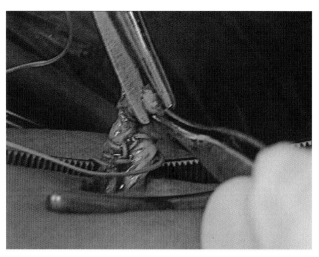

Figure 5-49 The biceps tendon is whipstitched and contoured to a uniform shape. The bulbous end of the tendon, as seen in this photo, must be trimmed to pass easily into the bone socket.

Operative Technique: Arthroscopic Biceps Tenodesis in the Presence of a Torn Rotator Cuff

Diagnostic glenohumeral arthroscopy is performed through a standard posterior portal; an anterior portal is created just superior to the lateral half of the subscapularis tendon and the biceps–labrum complex, and the long head of the biceps is assessed. A complete assessment of the biceps tendon is performed by pulling the intertubecular portion of the biceps tendon intra-articularly and assessing the amount of degeneration, partial tearing, and instability (Fig. 5-45A).

After completing diagnostic arthroscopy, we débride any tendon degeneration. If a concomitant rotator cuff tear is present (Fig. 5-45B), a lateral portal is established directly through the torn rotator cuff. A half-racking stitch traction suture is place in the posterior portion of the tendon just distal to its insertion on the superior labrum. This is performed by piercing the biceps tendon with a Penetrator (Arthrex) suture passer loaded with #2 FiberWire (Arthrex) (Fig. 5-46A). The suture loop is then held using a suture retriever through the anterior portal as the Penetrator is withdrawn from the biceps tendon (Fig. 5-46B). The Penetrator is then used to retrieve the suture loop out through the lateral cannula (Fig. 5-46C). The free ends of the suture limbs are then fed through the suture loop and pulled (Fig. 5-46D). This draws the suture loop into the joint and creates a grasping half-racking stitch that securely holds the long head of the biceps tendon, even in cases of degeneration (Figs. 5-46E and 5-46F).

The biceps tendon is then tenotomized close to its insertion on the superior labrum. A 90° OPES electrocautery probe (Arthrex) is used to perform the tenotomy while preserving as much length as possible (Fig. 5-47), and the residual stump on the superior labrum is débrided to a stable and smooth margin.

The traction sutures are then rerouted to the lateral portal and the biceps tendon is pulled out through the rotator cuff defect, the subacromial space (Fig. 5-48), the deltoid, and finally out through the skin. To solidly secure the biceps tendon, a whipstitch of #2 FiberWire (Arthrex) is sutured along the biceps tendon for ~1.5 cm (Fig. 5-49). The initial entry point and final exit point of the whipstitch should be side by side at a distance of 5 mm from the end

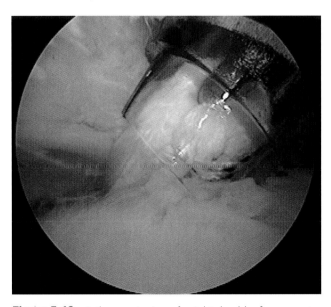

Figure 5-48 Arthroscopic view of a right shoulder from a posterior subacromial portal. Pulling on the traction sutures draws the biceps tendon through the rotator cuff tear, into the subacromial space, and out through the skin. It is useful to guide the biceps tendon into the mouth of the clear cannula and to withdraw the cannula as traction on the tendon is maintained so that the biceps will not hang up on deltoid muscle.

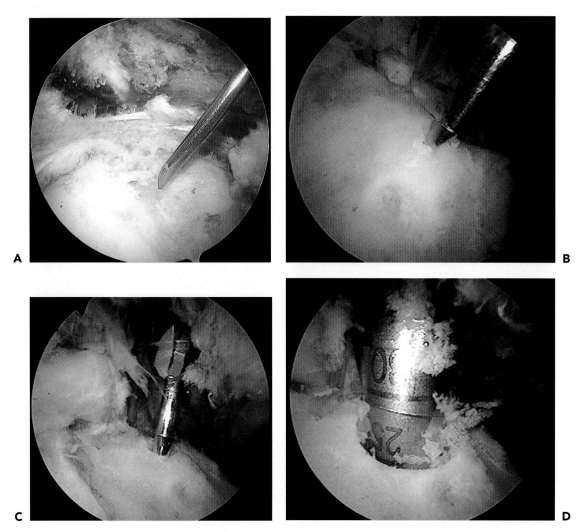

Figure 5-50 Arthroscopic views from the posterior portal of a right shoulder demonstrating drilling of the bone socket. **A:** An 18-gauge needle is used as a guide to position the drill hole. **B:** A 2.4-mm guide pin is placed in the anterolateral aspect of the greater tuberosity. **C:** A cannulated headed reamer is inserted over the guide pin and drill hole placement is assessed. **D:** A bone socket is then drilled to ~25 mm in depth to accommodate a 23-mm screw.

of the tendon so that the tip of the Bio-Tenodesis screwdriver, when brought down to the base of the whipstitch, can effectively manipulate the tendon and push it to the bottom of the bone socket. To increase the length of excursion of the biceps tendon through the skin during suturing, the shoulder and elbow are positioned in flexion to decrease the tension in the biceps tendon and maximize the length of tendon that can be exteriorized. The biceps tendon is then contoured to a uniform shape (removing the bulbous tip) and is sized using the measuring guide on the thumbpiece of the Bio-Tenodesis screwdriver.

Subacromial bursoscopy is then performed using a posterior viewing portal, and a bursectomy is completed, clearing the anterior and lateral gutters of the subacromial space and exposing the "shoulder" of the greater tuberosity. During bursectomy, care is taken to avoid damaging the biceps tendon.

A space of ~1.0 cm is cleared for placement of the bone socket over the anterolateral aspect of the greater tuberosity, just posterior to the bicipital groove. An 18-gauge spinal needle is used as a guide to determine the appropriate position and angle of approach for the bone socket (Fig. 5-50A). A 2.4-mm guide pin is initially placed (Fig. 5-50B), followed by a cannulated headed reamer (Fig. 5-50C). The bone socket is reamed to the diameter of biceps tendon previously measured (usually 7 or 8-mm in diameter) and to a depth of 25-mm to accommodate a screw length of 23-mm (Fig. 5-50D). In most cases, a previously established portal can be used for guide pin placement and reaming. A separate portal may be necessary, however, to ensure an appropriate approach angle.

A Bio-Tenodesis screw the same size as the reamed hole is then loaded onto the Bio-Tenodesis screwdriver and a loop of #2 FiberWire is fed through the end of the driver tip.

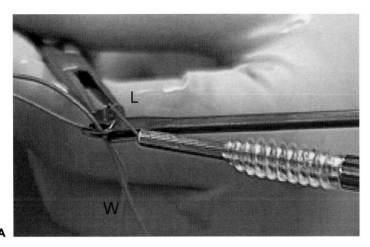
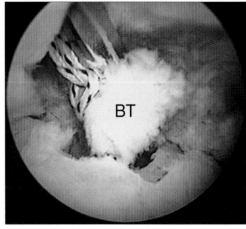

Figure 5-51 **A:** Extracorporeally, the traction sutures and whipstitch are passed through the suture loop at the end of the driver and pulled. **B:** The end of the biceps tendon can now be controlled by the screwdriver tip and manipulated into the bone socket. BT, biceps tendon; W, whipstitch suture ends; L, suture loop threaded through cannulated driver.

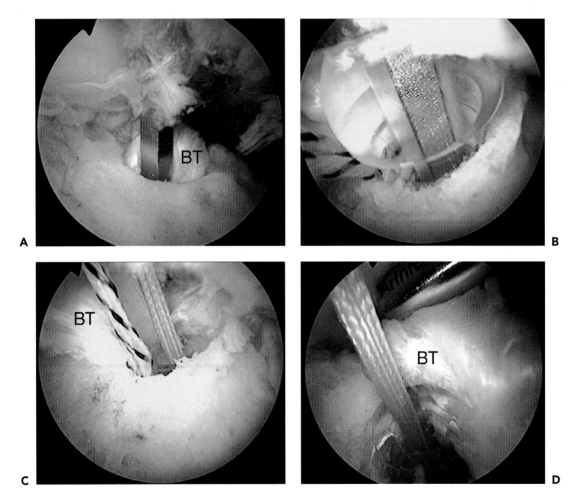

Figure 5-52 Arthroscopic views of a right shoulder demonstrating screw insertion. **A:** After seating the driver tip and biceps tendon into the base of the bone socket, the screw is advanced until flush with the bone **(B)**. The screwdriver is removed, demonstrating excellent placement of the interference screw **(C)**. The biceps tendon-screw–bone interface can be assessed by visualizing the tendon through the transparent cannulated portion of the Bio-Tenodesis (Arthrex, Inc.; Naples, FL) screw **(D)**. BT, biceps tendon.

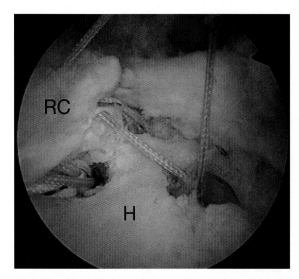

Figure 5-53 Arthroscopic view through a lateral portal of a right shoulder demonstrating the biceps tenodesis and residual rotator cuff defect, with one suture limb from the Bio-Tenodesis (Arthrex, Inc.; Naples, FL) construct having been passed through the rotator cuff. The rotator cuff is repaired, incorporating the sutures from the biceps tenodesis into the repair, in addition to suture anchors, as indicated. H, humerus; RC, rotator cuff.

Extracorporeally, the whipstitch sutures are then advanced through this loop at the end of the screwdriver and the loop is tightened (Fig. 5-51A). (Alternatively, the biceps tendon whipstitch sutures can be fed directly up the cannulated screwdriver by means of a nitinol loop suture passer.) This secures the biceps tendon to the tip of the screwdriver and allows it to be manipulated subacromially (Fig. 5-51B).

The biceps tendon and Bio-Tenodesis screwdriver are then inserted into the base of the bone socket by manipulating the tendon into the socket with the end of the screwdriver (Fig. 5-52A). Care is taken to ensure that the biceps tendon/Bio-Tenodesis screwdriver tip has "bottomed-out." The Bio-Tenodesis screw is then advanced down the shaft of the screwdriver while maintaining the tip of the screwdriver and the end of the biceps tendon at the bottom of the bone socket (Fig. 5-52B,C). Because the cannulated screw is transparent, visualization through the head and shaft of the screw is performed to confirm screw placement and the length of the bone-tendon-screw interface (Fig. 5-52D).

Placement of the Bio-Tenodesis screw along the anterolateral aspect of the footprint allows it to also act as an anchor for rotator cuff repair. The sutures from the whipstitch and half-racking stitch can now be incorporated into the rotator cuff repair (Fig. 5-53).

Operative Technique: Arthroscopic Biceps Tenodesis in the Presence of an Intact Rotator Cuff

If the rotator cuff is intact, a similar technique is used, although it is somewhat more difficult. Instead of a lateral "transrotator cuff tear" portal, an anterosuperolateral portal is created ~1 to 2 cm anterolateral to the anterolateral corner of the acromion, entering the glenohumeral joint through the biceps sheath just above the long head of the biceps as it exits the bicipital groove (Fig. 5-54A). A half-racking stitch is similarly rerouted through this portal and the biceps tendon pulled through the roof of the bicipital sheath, through the subacromial space and skin, so that it is exteriorized (Fig. 5-54B,C,D). The biceps tendon is next prepared using a whipstitch, and the bone socket is drilled at the superior margin of the bicipital groove (Fig. 5-55A,B). After securing the biceps tendon into the humerus, we commonly use one suture to close the residual defect in the rotator interval.

Operative Technique: Arthroscopic-assisted Biceps Tenodesis for Ruptures of the Long Head of the Biceps Tendon: The Cobra Procedure

The Cobra procedure is an uncommon procedure that allows an arthroscopic-assisted approach for biceps tenodesis in acute (<6 weeks) ruptures (16). Following arthroscopic inspection and débridement of the biceps stump, a mini-open incision is used to retrieve the long head of the biceps, followed by an arthroscopic-assisted retrieval of the tendon into the subacromial space where it is arthroscopically tenodesed with a BioTenodesis screw.

First, a 3-cm incision is made over the proximal musculotendinous junction of the retracted biceps, at the proximal end of the biceps lump. This is carried down through subcutaneous tissue to the biceps brachii. The tendon is identified and pulled out through the incision. At this point, the tendon length is assessed by laying the tendon along the upper arm in the direction of its origin (Fig. 5-56). The tendon length must be sufficient to reach the anterolateral corner of the acromion so that it can be retrieved through a high anterolateral portal. If the tendon length is insufficient, then an arthroscopic tenodesis will not be possible and another means of biceps tenodesis at a more distal location must be used. Fixed retraction of the tendon can be a problem in ruptures >6 weeks old. Before passing the tendon proximally, it is whipstitched at its proximal end and the bulbous end of the tendon is débrided, contoured, and sized as described above in the section on operative technique of arthroscopic biceps tenodesis.

The next step is to pass the long head of the biceps tendon proximally beneath the pectoralis major and through the bicipital groove. The pectoralis major insertion and the lower end of the bicipital groove are digitally palpated through the mini-open incision. A switching stick is then carefully passed beneath the pectoralis major tendon, along the bicipital groove and up through the anterior deltoid until the skin is tented. A small (1 cm) skin incision is made over the switching stick to mark the location of the anterolateral portal.

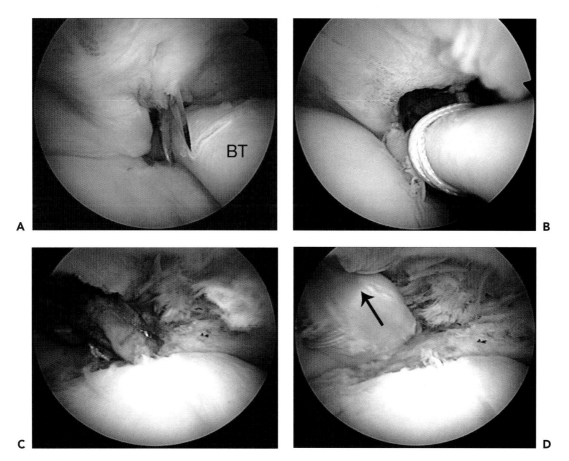

Figure 5-54   Arthroscopic views of a left shoulder through a posterior portal in a patient with biceps degeneration and an intact rotator cuff. **A:** An 18-gauge spinal needle is used to guide placement of the anterosuperolateral portal, which is located above the biceps tendon as it exits the bicipital groove. **B:** The 18-gauge needle is then replaced with a 7-mm clear cannula and a half-racking stitch is placed. **C:** After placement of a half-racking stitch and tenotomy of the biceps tendon, the traction sutures are pulled through the anterosuperolateral portal. Pulling on the traction sutures draws the biceps tendon into the anterosuperolateral cannula. **D:** The traction sutures and cannula are then pulled out of the skin, drawing the tendon through the bicipital roof, into the subacromial space, and out through the skin. Posterior arthroscopic glenohumeral view demonstrating the biceps tendon exiting through the bicipital roof (*arrow*). BT, biceps tendon.

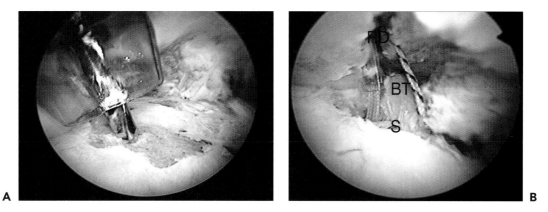

Figure 5-55   Tenodesis of the biceps directly above the bicipital groove. Arthroscopic views through a posterior portal of a left shoulder with a 70° arthroscope. **A:** A 2.4-mm guide pin demonstrates the location of the proposed bone socket just above the superior border of the bicipital groove. **B:** Following placement of the screw, a residual defect (*RD*) is apparent in the bicipital roof and rotator interval. The defect is closed using standard suture passing and knot tying. BT, biceps tendon; RD, residual defect; S, screw.

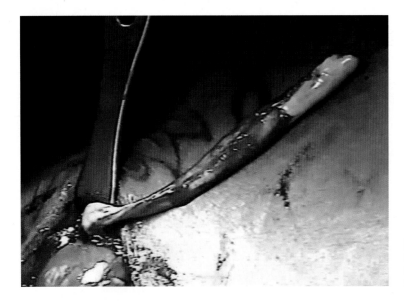

Figure 5-56 Clinical photo. The tendon length is assessed by laying it on the arm in the direction of its origin. The length should be sufficient for the tendon to reach a high anterolateral portal.

To create a safe enclosed tunnel to pass the long head of the biceps tendon proximally, an arthroscopic sheath is inserted over the proximal end of the switching stick (Fig. 5-57) while a 7-mm clear cannula is inserted over the distal end of the switching stick (Fig. 5-58). The cannulas are inserted so that the 7-mm cannula telescopes over the arthroscopic sheath, creating an enclosed tunnel for safe passage of a suture passer. In particular, this enclosed tunnel prevents inadvertent medial penetration of the suture passer, protecting the neurovascular structures.

The switching stick is then removed and a long suture passer or Beath pin is inserted through the two cannulas. The clear cannula is removed and the whipstitch sutures are fed through the suture passer or the hole in the end of the Beath pin. The long head of the biceps tendon is then passed retrograde through its anatomic tract, beneath the pectoralis major, and out through the anterolateral portal (Fig. 5-59). The mini-open incision can now be closed.

The arthroscope is inserted through a posterior portal and into the subacromial space. Bursectomy is performed to

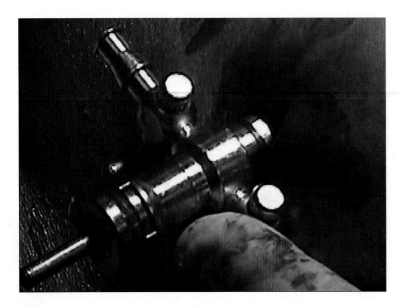

Figure 5-57 Clinical photo. An arthroscopic sheath is inserted over the proximal end of the switching stick as it exits the anterolateral portal.

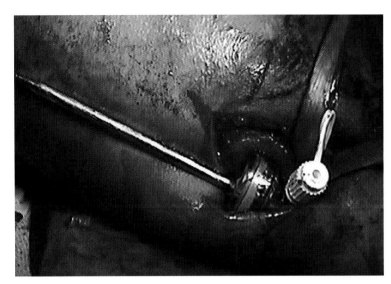

Figure 5-58 Clinical photo. A 7-mm clear cannula is inserted over the distal end of the switching stick as it exits the incision over the biceps deformity.

identify the long head of the biceps tendon in the subacromial space. The bicipital roof is then opened along the lateral aspect of the rotator interval to expose the upper portion of the bicipital groove. The anterolateral portal usually provides the correct angle of approach for tenodesis; however, a separate portal can be used. The biceps tendon is then tenodesed as described above (Fig. 5-60) (see *Arthroscopic Biceps Tenodesis in the Presence of an Intact Rotator Cuff*).

COMBINED SUBSCAPULARIS, SUPRASPINATUS, AND INFRASPINATUS TENDON TEARS

Massive contracted immobile rotator cuff tears are rare lesions that usually require interval slide techniques, as described above, for repair. In complex cases involving tears of the supraspinatus (± the infraspinatus) tendon

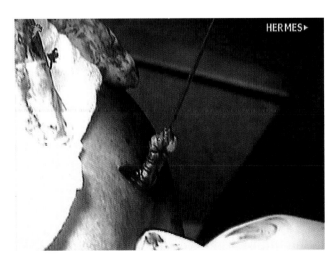

Figure 5-59 Clinical photo. The long head of the biceps brachii is passed retrograde through its anatomic tract beneath the pectoralis major, until the tendon passes out of the high anterolateral portal.

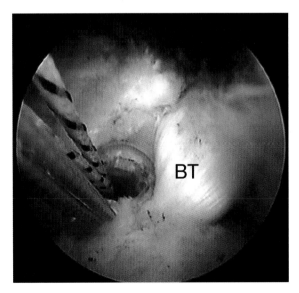

Figure 5-60 Arthroscopic view of a right shoulder from a posterior portal demonstrating visualization of the tenodesed long head of the biceps brachii tendon within the subacromial space. BT, biceps tendon.

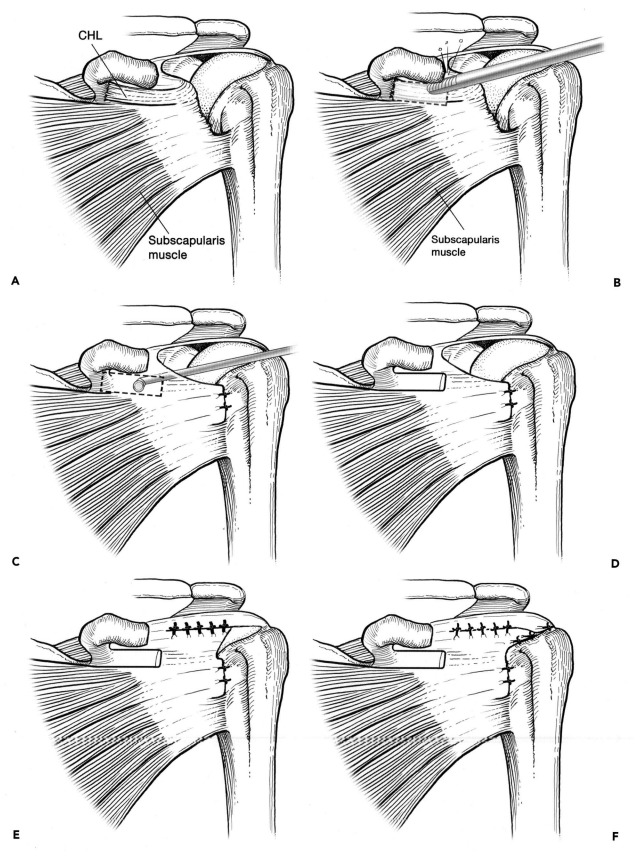

Figure 5-61 Schematic representation of the interval slide in continuity. Anterior view of a left shoulder. **A:** An anterosuperior rotator cuff tear involving 50% of the subscapularis tendon and a massive tear of the supraspinatus and infraspinatus tendons. **B:** A coracoplasty is performed to resect the posterolateral aspect of the coracoid tip. The *dotted box* outlines the proposed area for resection of a portion of the rotator interval for the *interval slide in continuity*. **C:** An *interval slide in continuity* is performed by first exposing the posterolateral aspect of the coracoid all the way to the coracoid neck, releasing any adhesions between the subscapularis tendon and the inferolateral coracoid. Then, the medial rotator interval tissue is excised, creating a

(Continued)

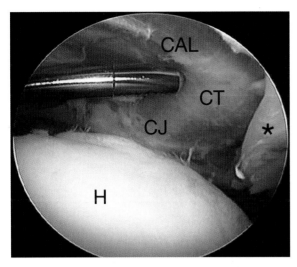

Figure 5-62 Arthroscopic view of a left shoulder from a posterior viewing portal using a 70° arthroscope demonstrating a torn retracted subscapularis tendon with attached "comma sign." In this case, the subscapularis is retracted so far medially that it is not visible, and the comma sign (*) must lead the surgeon to the superolateral border of the subscapularis. In the background are the coracoid tip with attached coracoacromial ligament and conjoint tendon. H, humerus; CT, coracoid tip; CAL, coracoacromial ligament; CJ, conjoint tendon.

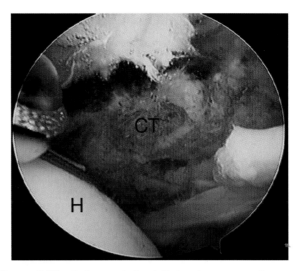

Figure 5-63 Arthroscopic "aerial" view from a posterior portal using a 70° arthroscope demonstrating an increase in the coracohumeral space following coracoplasty. A traction suture has been placed through the subscapularis tendon. CT, coracoid tip; H, humerus.

and the subscapularis tendon, however, an anterior interval slide will create two separate flaps of tissue: (a) an anterior flap consisting of the subscapularis and rotator interval and (b) a posterior flap consisting of the supraspinatus, infraspinatus, and teres minor tendons. Although repair of these two flaps of tissue is technically possible, it is difficult because of the "floppy" nature of the tissue flaps.

As an alternative, we commonly now perform an interval slide in continuity (17). An interval slide in continuity releases and resects a portion of the coracohumeral ligament and rotator interval while maintaining the lateral margin of the rotator interval (Fig. 5-61). This technique improves the mobility of both the subscapularis and supraspinatus tendons without creating two separate flaps of tissue, thereby allowing a simplified repair of the posterosuperior rotator cuff.

Technique

Cases that require an interval slide in continuity are generally large and massive anterosuperior rotator cuff tears involving retracted tears of the subscapularis tendon and posterosuperior rotator cuff. In cases involving chronic retracted adhesed subscapularis tears, identifying the superior and lateral borders of the subscapularis tendon can be difficult. In particular, the lateral margin of the tendon can be obscured by scar tissue or synovial "leaders" attached to the tendon. The comma sign is identified, again to define the superolateral border of the subscapularis tendon (Fig. 5-62).

Subcoracoid impingement is a common associated finding in these tears and, therefore, the coracohumeral space is carefully evaluated. If subcoracoid impingement is present and symptomatic, an arthroscopic coracoplasty is performed (Fig. 5-63).

Massive contracted immobile rotator cuff tears demonstrate minimal mobility from a medial to lateral direction of both the subscapularis tendon and the posterosuperior rotator cuff. To improve the mobility of these tears, an *interval slide in continuity* can be performed. We begin by

◀━━

Figure 5-61 *(continued)* "window" through the rotator interval, partially releasing and excising the coracohumeral ligament. Care is taken to ensure that the lateral margin of the rotator interval remains intact, maintaining the continuity between the subscapularis and the supraspinatus tendons. Then, soft tissues are débrided and released from the posterolateral base of the coracoid while viewing through the "window" with a 70° arthroscope. This completes the release of the coracohumeral ligament without creating separate tissue flaps. **D:** Following an *interval slide in continuity*, mobility of the subscapularis tendon is improved. The subscapularis tear can now be repaired to bone, leaving a U-shaped posterosuperior rotator cuff tear to be repaired. **E:** The residual U-shaped posterosuperior rotator cuff tear is repaired with side-to-side sutures using the principle of margin convergence. **F:** The converged margin is then repaired to bone in a tension-free manner. CHL, coracohumeral ligament.

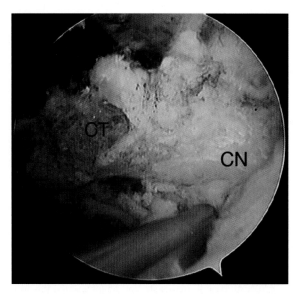

Figure 5-64 Coracohumeral ligament release and coracoid dissection. Arthroscopic view of a left shoulder from a lateral portal. A shaver has been introduced through an accessory lateral portal and, in conjunction with electrocautery and arthroscopic elevators, is used to dissect and expose the coracoid neck, releasing adhesions between the subscapularis and the inferolateral coracoid. CT, coracoid tip; CN, coracoid neck.

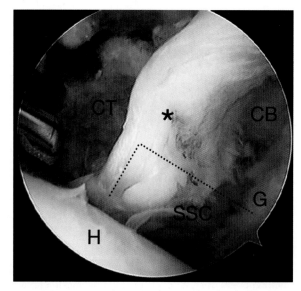

Figure 5-66 Completed interval slide in continuity. Arthroscopic view of a left shoulder from a posterior portal demonstrating a completed interval slide in continuity. Note: A lateral bridge of rotator interval tissue has been maintained, which contains the comma sign (*) and leads to the superolateral aspect of the torn subscapularis tendon. The coracoid tip and coracoid base are visible on either side of the comma sign. CT, coracoid tip; CB, coracoid base; SSc, subscapularis tendon; H, humerus; G, glenoid; ---, superolateral border of subscapularis tendon.

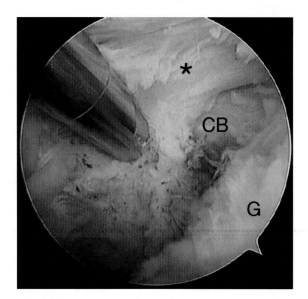

Figure 5-65 Rotator interval resection and release. Arthroscopic view of a left shoulder from a lateral portal. While lateral traction is being applied to the subscapularis tendon, a shaver has been introduced through an accessory lateral portal and a "window" has been created by excising the medial rotator interval while preserving an intact lateral bridge of rotator interval tissue containing the comma sign (*). In this photograph, the coracoid base (CB) can be seen through the window in the rotator interval. Care is taken to completely release and excise the coracohumeral ligament from the lateral aspect of the base of the coracoid. CB, coracoid base; G, glenoid.

first skeletonizing the posterolateral coracoid to safely reach the lateral aspect of the coracoid neck. After the coracoplasty and exposure of the coracoid neck, the posterolateral coracoid base must be exposed. While viewing through a posterior portal with a 70° arthroscope, a shaver or electrocautery probe is introduced through an accessory anterosuperolateral portal, and this instrument completes the dissection of adhesions between the subscapularis and the posteroinferior coracoid neck (Fig. 5-64). Care is taken to avoid dissection inferior and medial to the coracoid, which would place the neurovascular structures at risk.

At this point, by releasing the soft tissues from the lateral aspect of the coracoid neck, a partial coracohumeral ligament release has been performed, which allows greater lateral excursion of the subscapularis. This increased excursion can be demonstrated by applying lateral tension to the traction sutures. A tension-free repair, however, usually requires a more extensive release, which is done next.

Lateral pull on the traction sutures will bring the rotator interval tissue into view. This rotator interval tissue has been medially retracted on a chronic basis because of the contracted coracohumeral ligament. At this point, a shaver or cautery probe is directed to the posterior aspect of the rotator interval and a "window" is created through it by resecting the medial portion of the interval tissue until the lateral aspect of the coracoid base is identified through this

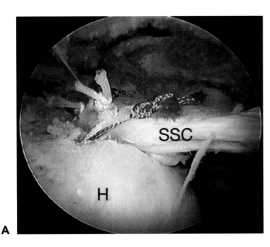 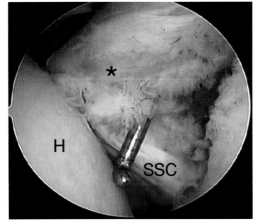

A   B

Figure 5-67 Arthroscopic views demonstrating a completed subscapularis tendon repair. **A:** Posterior portal of a left shoulder using a 70° arthroscope showing "aerial" view of repair. **B:** Posterior portal using a 30° arthroscope showing the intra-articular perspective after subscapularis repair in a left shoulder. Note: The comma sign (*) in this shoulder is still intact. The hooked probe has been placed through the window in the rotator interval, demonstrating the interval slide in continuity. H, humerus; SSc, subscapularis.

defect (Fig. 5-65). The excised tissue includes the coraco-humeral ligament attachment to the coracoid. Care is taken to ensure that the lateral aspect of the rotator interval is preserved, maintaining the continuity of the subscapularis tendon to the supraspinatus tendon (Fig. 5-66). This tissue essentially consists of the lateral rotator interval and the comma sign (i.e., the remnant of the medial sling of the biceps).

Following an interval slide in continuity, the subscapularis tendon mobility will be improved. This will allow a

repair of the torn subscapularis to a bone bed in a tension-free manner (Fig. 5-67). By maintaining the lateral aspect of the rotator interval and comma sign, this tissue can now be incorporated during repair of the posterosuperior rotator cuff (Fig. 5-68). This tissue is essential when repairing U-shaped or L-shaped rotator cuff tears, which require side-to-side sutures for "margin convergence" (Fig. 5-69). Incising or excising this tissue during a standard interval slide would preclude placement of side-to-side sutures, making repair much more difficult.

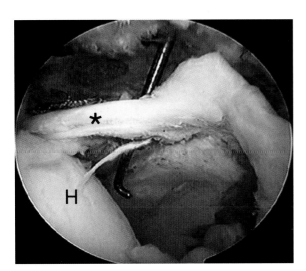 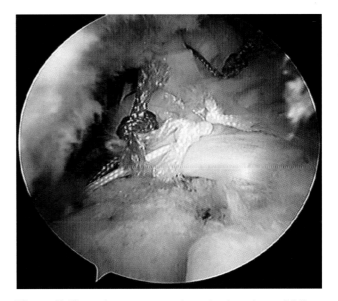

Figure 5-68 Arthroscopic view through a posterolateral portal demonstrating a residual U-shaped posterosuperior rotator cuff defect which can be closed by margin convergence principles. The intact lateral portion of the rotator interval serves as the anterior leaf and can be repaired to the posterior leaf of the rotator cuff. A hooked probe has been placed within the defect created by the interval slide in continuity. H, humeral head; *, comma sign.

Figure 5-69 Arthroscopic view through a lateral portal following rotator cuff repair. The intact lateral portion of the rotator intervals including the tissue of the comma sign, has been incorporated into the side-to-side sutures used during repair of this U-shaped rotator cuff tear. Suture anchors secure the "converged margin" of the tendon to bone.

REFERENCES

1. Lo IK, Burkhart SS. Arthroscopic repair of massive, contracted, immobile rotator cuff tears using single and double interval slides: technique and preliminary results. *Arthroscopy.* 2004;20(1):22–33.
2. Burkhart SS, Tehrany AM. Arthroscopic subscapularis tendon repair: technique and preliminary results. *Arthroscopy.* 2002;18:454–463.
3. Lo IKY, Burkhart SS. Subscapularis tears: arthroscopic repair of the forgotten rotator cuff tendon. *Tech Shoulder Elbow Surg.* 2002;3:282–291.
4. Bennett WF. Subscapularis, medial and lateral coracohumeral ligament insertion anatomy. Arthroscopic appearance and incidence of "hidden" rotator interval lesions. *Arthroscopy.* 2001;17:173–180.
5. Lo IKY, Burkhart SS, Parten PM. Surgery about the coracoid: neurovascular structures at risk. *Arthroscopy.* 2004; 20: 591–594.
6. Warner JJ, Higgins L, Parsons IM 4th, et al. Diagnosis and treatment of anterosuperior rotator cuff tears. *J Shoulder Elbow Surg.* 2001; 10: 37–46.
7. Barth JRH, Burkhart SS, DeBeer JF. The Bear Hug Test: the most sensitive test for diagnosing a subscapularis tear. *Arthroscopy.* In press.
8. Goutallier D, Postel JM, Bernageau J, et al. Fatty muscle degeneration in cuff ruptures. Pre- and postoperative evaluation by CT scan. *Clin Orthop.* 1994;304:78–83.
9. Goutallier D, Postel JM, Bernageau J, et al. Fatty infiltration of disrupted rotator cuff muscles. *Rev Rheum Engl Ed.* 1995;62:415–422.
10. Burkhart SS, Morgan CD, Kibler WB. Current concepts: the disabled throwing shoulder: spectrum of pathology. Part I: Pathoanatomy and biomechanics. *Arthroscopy.* 2003;19:404–420.
11. Resch H, Povacz P, Ritter E, et al. Transfer of the pectoralis major muscle for the treatment of irreparable rupture of the subscapularis tendon. *J Bone Joint Surg.* 2000;82A:372–382.
12. Galatz LM, Ball CM, Teefey SA, et al. The outcome and repair integrity of completely arthroscopically repaired large and massive rotator cuff tears. *J Bone Joint Surg.* 2004;86A:219–224.
13. Lo IK, Burkhart SS. Arthroscopic biceps tenodesis: indications and technique. *Operative Techniques Sports Med.* 2002;10:105–112.
14. Lo IK, Burkhart SS. Arthroscopic biceps tenodesis using a bioabsorbable interference screw. *Arthroscopy.* 2004;20(1):85–95.
15. Richards DP, Burkhart SS, Lo IK. Arthroscopic biceps tenodesis with interference screw fixation: the lateral decubitus position. *Operative Technique Sports Med.* 2003;11:15–23.
16. Richards DP, Burkhart SS. Arthroscopic-assisted biceps tenodesis for ruptures of the long head of biceps brachii: the Cobra procedure. *Arthroscopy.* 2004;20(6):201–207.
17. Lo IK, Burkhart SS. The interval slide in continuity: a method of mobilizing the anterosuperior rotator cuff without disrupting the tear margins. *Arthroscopy.* 2004;20(4):435–441.

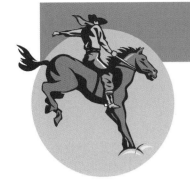

Exposing the Hidden Arthroscopic Landmarks

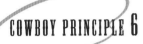

COWBOY PRINCIPLE 6

A man who tells you he's no fool has his suspicions.

The cowboy is at home in his world. On cattle drives, his landmarks are rock formations, hills, and rivers. He knows that clues from the land will help him find his way. He recognizes signs in nature, he learns by observing the natural world around him, and he knows not to drink downstream from the herd.

The advent of arthroscopic repair techniques for small, medium, and large rotator cuff tears has led to the development of new arthroscopic techniques to repair massive rotator cuff tears. Although many massive tears can be repaired with minimal mobilization, some cases of massive immobile contracted rotator cuff tears require considerable dissection and delineation for adequate mobilization and repair. In particular, arthroscopic revision repair of failed open, mini-open, or arthroscopic rotator cuff repair can be demanding because of the tremendous amount of scar tissue that sometimes forms within the subacromial space (1). This scar tissue can completely obliterate all identifiable tissue planes and anatomic landmarks, making rotator cuff repair extremely difficult and tedious. Exposure of consistent landmarks is particularly important when performing single or double interval slides, as well as interval slides in continuity, where identification and delineation of the

coracoid and scapular spine are essential for safe and effective slides (2).

DEMARCATING THE MARGINS OF THE ROTATOR CUFF TEAR

Determining the margins of a rotator cuff tear is an important step during arthroscopic rotator cuff repair. Although this is often a simple, routine task, many cases present in which delineation and dissection of the margins of the rotator cuff can be difficult, time-consuming procedures. This is particularly true in revision rotator cuff repair.

Delineation of the cuff tear margins begins with portal placement. Portals include a standard posterior subacromial viewing portal; a lateral working portal; and an accessory anterior portal for inflow and for use as a secondary working portal. All overlying bursal and fibrofatty tissue is removed by a shaver through a lateral working portal while viewing through a posterior portal (Fig. 6-1). Often, the demarcation between adventitial bursal leader and rotator cuff tissue is difficult to determine. Bursal leaders are poor-quality sheets of adventitial tissue that can look like lateral extensions of cuff tissue. It is important, however, to recognize that bursal leaders insert laterally into the deltoid muscle fascia, whereas rotator cuff tissue inserts into bone. Rotating the arm can help determine whether the tissue is rotator cuff tissue versus fibrofatty bursal leader by bringing into view an intact area of cuff insertion into bone. Recognizing these features, the uppermost intact tendon insertion into the lateral aspect of the humerus is identified (Fig. 6-2) and all adjacent fibrous tissue attaching to

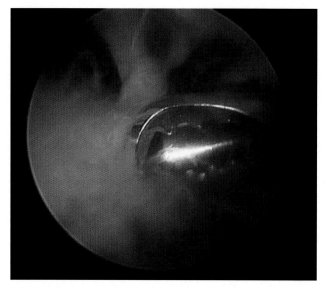

Figure 6-1 Arthroscopic view through a posterior portal of a right shoulder demonstrating débridement of the bursa initially through a lateral working portal.

Figure 6-3 Arthroscopic view through a lateral portal demonstrating débridement of the posterior bursa and posterior gutter.

the deltoid fascia can be safely removed, because this tissue represents bursal leader rather than tendon. The bursal leader is débrided from lateral to medial until the characteristic parallel collagen bundles of rotator cuff tendon are identified.

First, the lateral and anterior margins of the rotator cuff are delineated, and then the posterior margin of the tear is exposed. The posterior margin of the rotator cuff tear is most easily identified while viewing through a lateral portal and introducing a shaver through a posterior portal (Fig. 6-3). A judicious bursectomy or débridement that exposes the anterior, lateral, and posterior subacromial

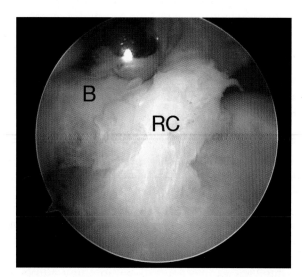

Figure 6-2 Arthroscopic view through a posterior portal of a right shoulder demonstrating débridement of the bursa leader (*B*) overlying the residual intact rotator cuff tendon insertion (*RC*). Internally rotating the arm aids in bringing into view the uppermost of the posterior cuff attachments.

gutters is essential because adventitial swelling during arthroscopic repair can obscure visualization of the tear margins.

EXCAVATING THE ADHESED ROTATOR CUFF

In some cases, particularly in previously operated cases, adhesions can occur between the rotator cuff and deltoid muscle as well as between the rotator cuff and acromion. In such cases, the rotator cuff might be obscured entirely. These adhesions must be lysed or excised not only to define the tear margins but also to obtain sufficient mobility to allow a tension-free repair to bone. We commonly use one of two techniques to identify and mobilize the rotator cuff margins.

First, in most cases of adhesed rotator cuffs, the anterior and posterior borders of the rotator cuff margins are scarred to the inner deltoid muscle fascia, making them difficult to identify. In most of these adhesed cases, the medial margin of the rotator cuff tear is either preserved or easily identifiable by arthroscopic dissection. We begin the dissection medially at the apex of the tear, beneath the medial acromion just posterior to the acromioclavicular (AC) joint. In this area is a consistent fibrofatty layer that separates the rotator cuff below from the acromion, the deltotrapezial fascia, and the deltoid above. In performing this dissection, we commonly view through a lateral portal and introduce our instruments through a posterior portal. The fibrofatty pad posterior to the AC joint is first located medially (Fig. 6-4A) and then followed posteriorly to dissect the posterior leaf of the rotator cuff tear from the acromion and the deltoid (Fig. 6-4B). The anterior rotator

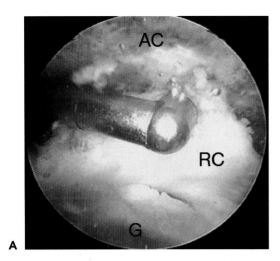

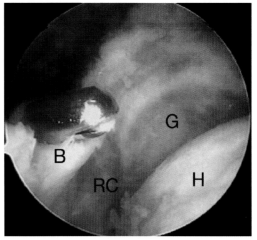

A

B

Figure 6-4 Arthroscopic views through a lateral portal of a right shoulder during rotator cuff mobilization in adhesed rotator cuff tears. **A:** The rotator cuff is initially dissected beneath the medial acromion and the fibrofatty layer is identified above the rotator cuff. This fibrofatty layer identifies the plane between the rotator cuff and acromion. **B:** The same layer is then followed posteriorly to identify the posterior margin of the tear. The synovialized bursal "leader" is débrided until the margins of the rotator cuff are exposed. The key to distinguishing the bursal "leader" from the true rotator cuff tendon is that the bursal "leader" inserts into the deltoid muscle fascia, whereas the cuff tendon inserts into bone (greater tuberosity). G, glenoid; RC, rotator cuff; AC, acromion; H, humeral head; B, bursal "leader."

cuff can be dissected using a similar technique. Even in chronic adhesed tears, this fibrofatty layer usually separates the deltoid and acromion from the rotator cuff and thus can be used as a guide in dissecting the peripheral tear margins from the deltoid and acromion.

In some cases, however, the margins of the rotator cuff tear anteriorly, posteriorly, and medially are completely

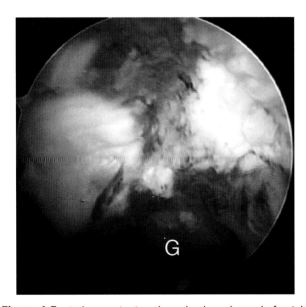

Figure 6-5 Arthroscopic view through a lateral portal of a right shoulder demonstrating a chronically inflamed, adhesed rotator cuff tear where the anterior, posterior, and medial tear margins are completely obscured and indistinguishable from the deltoid. G, glenoid.

obscured and scarred to the deltoid muscle and acromion, and it initially appears as though there is no rotation cuff to repair (Fig. 6-5). In addition, when attempting to insert instruments through the posterior portal, the instruments are restricted by the combined layers of the adhesed deltoid and rotator cuff. This confluent adhesion precludes dissection by the technique described above.

In such cases, we first introduce the arthroscope sheath through the posterior portal, directing the sheath just inferior to the anteromedial acromion, and locate the plane between the acromion and rotator cuff. The arthroscope is then inserted and the arthroscopic view observed.

If the proper plane of dissection (between the acromion and the rotator cuff) has been found, the typical yellow-white, fatty bursa will come into view. If, however, muscular fibers are observed, this indicates that the tip of the scope is within the substance of the deltoid muscle or rotator cuff muscle, and the arthroscope must be redirected. Once the proper plane of dissection has been located, a shaver is introduced through a lateral portal in the same plane as the arthroscope. To assist in triangulating into this restricted space, we commonly use an 18-gauge spinal needle as a guide and then follow this with a shaver (Fig. 6-6).

We then alternately use a shaver and an electrocautery wand to resect the fibrofatty tissue and create a space between the rotator cuff and acromion initially (Fig. 6-7A). This plane is then extended into the interval between the rotator cuff and deltoid muscle. In general, resection directly against the undersurface of the acromion is safe. Care is taken, however, to avoid resection of any muscular tissue. Eventually, the plane between the rotator cuff and

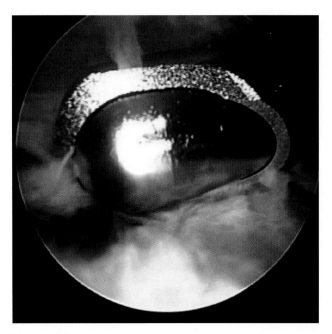

Figure 6-6 Arthroscopic view through a posterior subacromial portal. After triangulating into the very restricted and scar-filled subacromial space, a shaver is introduced through a lateral portal in the same plane as the arthroscope and needle.

deltoid muscle will be revealed and the space can then be enlarged (Fig. 6-7B).

With continued dissection, the humeral head will eventually come into view (Fig. 6-8A), signifying that exposure of the posterior margin of the rotator cuff tear (often with a bursal "leader") has been achieved (Fig. 6-8B), with an increase in the space between the posterior rotator cuff and overlying acromion and deltoid muscle (Fig. 6-8C). Instruments can

now be easily inserted through the posterior portal while viewing through a lateral portal (Fig. 6-8D).

To expose the medial and anterosuperior rotator cuff, a similar dissection proceeds as above by dissecting the soft tissues off the medial acromion until the fat pad behind the AC joint is visible, then progressing anteriorly (Fig. 6-9). The fat pad posterior to the AC joint is always present. It is particularly important during dissection to release all the white fibrous scar tissue until this normal yellowish fat pad appears overlying the medial rotator cuff (Fig. 6-10). This release not only exposes the rotator cuff but also greatly enhances its mobility.

To expose the anterior margin of the rotator cuff tear, dissection is continued anteriorly over the medial margin of the cuff tear and then directed inferiorly toward the rotator interval (Fig. 6-11).

EXPOSING THE CORACOID FOR SAFE ANTERIOR INTERVAL SLIDE

An anterior interval slide consists of releasing the leading edge of the supraspinatus tendon from the rotator interval, coracohumeral ligament, and coracoid. The base of the coracoid lies anteromedial to the root of the biceps tendon and can be identified and palpated through either a subacromial or a glenohumeral approach. Subacromially, the coracoid base can be palpated along with the attached coracohumeral ligament. Coracoid identification is easily done in cases of massive tears where the tendon margin is medial to the glenoid.

The coracoid base can also be identified through a glenohumeral approach. In a glenohumeral approach,

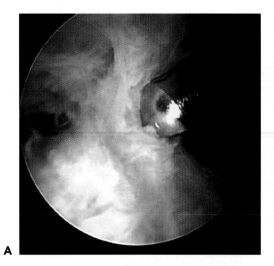

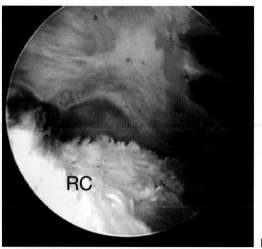

A   B

Figure 6-7 Defining the interval between the rotator cuff and acromion, and the plane between the rotator cuff and deltoid muscle. Arthroscopic views through a posterior subacromial portal. **A:** A shaver is used to initially create a space between the rotator cuff and acromion, and this plane is then followed to the interval between rotator cuff and deltoid muscle, being careful to stay within the confines of the bursal space and avoiding intramuscular tissue. **B:** With continued shaving, the plane of dissection becomes apparent and the space is enlarged. RC, rotator cuff.

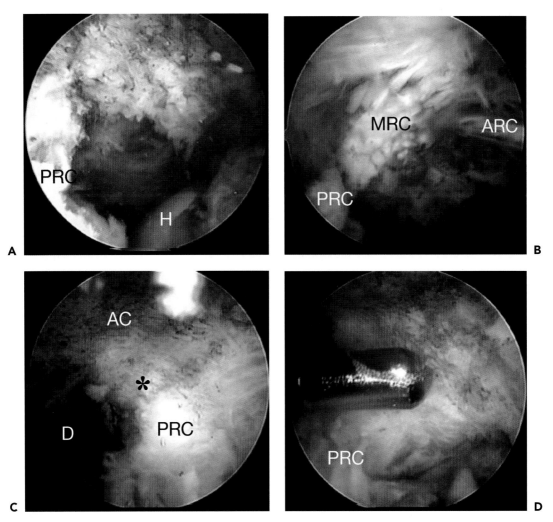

Figure 6-8 Exposure of the posterior margin of the rotator cuff tear of a right shoulder. **A:** Arthroscopic view through a posterior subacromial portal. Dissection is continued with the shaver and electrocautery until the humeral head is visualized. This signifies that the posterior margin of the rotator cuff (frequently with a bursal "leader") has been exposed. **B:** Arthroscopic view through a lateral portal demonstrating that the posterior margin of the rotator cuff has been exposed. **C:** Arthroscopic view through a lateral portal demonstrating an increase in the space *(*)* between the posterior rotator cuff and the overlying deltoid muscle and acromion. Scar tissue still adheres the rotator cuff to the medial acromion. **D:** Arthroscopic view through a lateral portal. Instruments can now be easily inserted through the posterior portal. Note: The posterior rotator cuff is labeled in approximately the same location in each figure. Compare Figure 6-5 with Figure 6-8B. PRC, posterior rotator cuff; ARC, anterior rotator cuff; MRC, medial rotator cuff; H, humeral head; AC, acromion; D, deltoid.

however, the coracoid and coracoid base are "hidden" by the overlying rotator interval and a window must be created through the rotator interval to visualize the coracoid. To locate the coracoid tip, a shaver or switching stick is placed intra-articularly through an anterosuperolateral portal and then directed in an anterior direction while viewing through the posterior portal. The coracoid tip can be clearly felt as a hard, bony protuberance through the rotator interval just anterior to the upper border of the subscapularis tendon (Fig. 6-12). Once the coracoid tip is located, a shaver is introduced through the anterosuperolateral portal and the portion of the rotator interval that is directly over the coracoid tip is resected (Fig. 6-13). The coracoid can be identified within this rotator interval defect along with the attachments of the coracoacromial ligament and conjoint tendon. In the case of a retracted subscapularis tendon tear, a traction stitch along the lateral margin of the subscapularis tendon can be used to pull the rotator interval into view (see anterior interval slide in continuity Chapter 5).

The anterior interval slide begins at the free margin of the rotator cuff that is directly above the root of the biceps and ends at the base of the coracoid. The anterior interval slide typically increases the lateral excursion of the

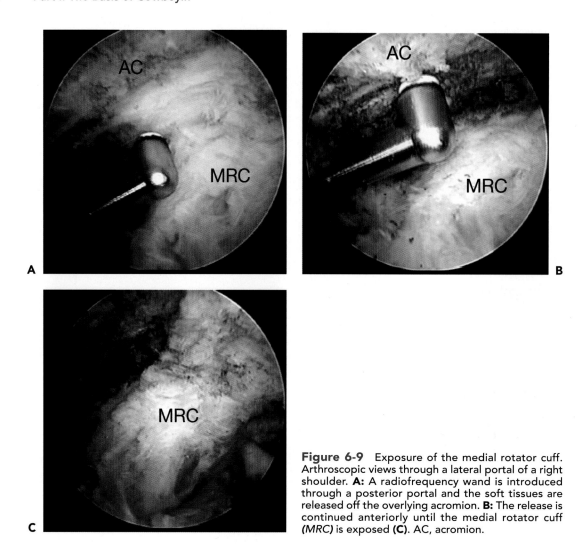

Figure 6-9 Exposure of the medial rotator cuff. Arthroscopic views through a lateral portal of a right shoulder. **A:** A radiofrequency wand is introduced through a posterior portal and the soft tissues are released off the overlying acromion. **B:** The release is continued anteriorly until the medial rotator cuff (*MRC*) is exposed **(C)**. AC, acromion.

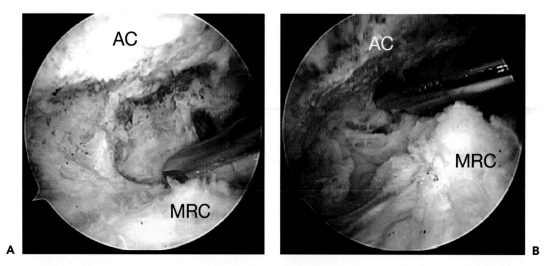

Figure 6.10 Resection of the fibrous scar tissue. Arthroscopic views from a posterior portal of a right shoulder. **A:** The medial rotator cuff is bound by overlying fibrous scar tissue. **B:** The scar tissue is resected using a shaver until the typical yellowish fat is demonstrated overlying the muscular fibers of the rotator cuff. MRC, medial rotator cuff; AC, acromion.

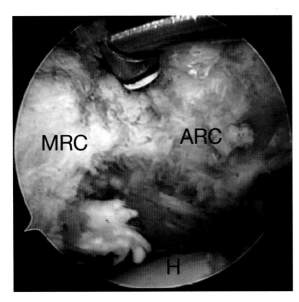

Figure 6-11   Exposure of the anterior rotator cuff. Arthroscopic view through a posterior portal of a right shoulder. The dissection is continued anteriorly over the medial rotator cuff and the anterior rotator cuff margin is then released from the overlying deltoid. ARC, anterior rotator cuff; MRC, medial rotator cuff; H, humeral head.

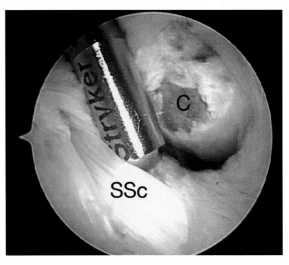

Figure 6-13   Arthroscopic view from a posterior glenohumeral portal of a left shoulder. The overlying rotator interval has been resected revealing the coracoid. SSc, subscapularis; C, coracoid.

supraspinatus tendon by 1 or 2 cm. If further excursion is required to reach the bone bed, a posterior interval slide (see below) may be required.

When performing an anterior interval slide, we prefer to view through a posterolateral subacromial portal and introduce arthroscopic instruments or scissors through a lateral portal. Before initiating the slide, it is important to place a traction suture in the leading edge of the

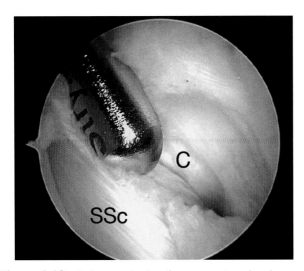

Figure 6-12   Arthroscopic view from posterior glenohumeral portal of a left shoulder. A shaver has been introduced through an anterosuperolateral portal and the coracoid can be palpated as a hard, bony protuberance through the rotator interval just anterior to the superior border of the subscapularis tendon. SSc, subscapularis; C, coracoid.

supraspinatus tendon and to make the release just anterior to the traction stitch. We prefer to use a either a Viper or Scorpion suture passer (Arthrex, Inc.; Naples, FL) to insert a traction suture through the anterior portion of the supraspinatus tendon just posterior to the biceps root. The traction suture is retrieved through an accessory lateral subacromial portal. The traction suture is used to progressively open the apex of the anterior slide incision as it is made, enhancing visualization, and to provide a method of stabilizing the supraspinatus tendon for suture passage during later repair.

The anterior interval slide is begun at the leading edge of the supraspinatus tendon, just above the root of the biceps tendon, and progresses toward the base of the coracoid (Fig. 6-14). The root of the biceps tendon serves as a landmark to identify the border between the leading edge of the supraspinatus tendon and rotator interval. Furthermore, the root of the biceps lays just posterolateral to the base of the coracoid. When performing an anterior interval slide, tension is applied to the traction sutures in a posterior direction. This tension creates an apex at the junction between released and unreleased tissue, facilitating an accurate and precise release. Without tension, the released portion of the supraspinatus tendon becomes floppy, obstructing and obscuring the blades of the arthroscopic scissors and making an accurate release extremely difficult.

EXPOSING THE SCAPULAR SPINE FOR SAFE POSTERIOR INTERVAL SLIDE

When performing a posterior interval slide, it is essential to identify the point along the margin of the tear at which to begin and direct the release. The initial step is to remove all

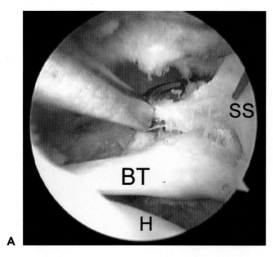

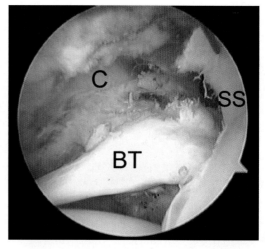

Figure 6-14 Arthroscopic view through a posterolateral portal showing an anterior interval slide of a left shoulder. **A:** Release of the supraspinatus tendon from the rotator interval tissue using an arthroscopic scissor. A traction suture in the supraspinatus tendon progressively opens the apex of the anterior slide as it is made. Care is taken to avoid injury to the biceps tendon. **B:** Completed release of the anterior margin of the supraspinatus tendon. SS, supraspinatus tendon; BT, biceps tendon; C, coracoid; H, humerus.

the soft tissues and periosteum from the undersurface of the acromion, beginning anterolaterally and progressing posteriorly and medially. This portion of the procedure is performed while viewing through a posterior portal and is initially similar to a standard subacromial decompression. The location of the AC joint posteromedially is generally heralded by the presence of a thick fibrofatty tissue pad in the subacromial space lying posteroinferior to the AC joint. Once the fibrofatty tissue is removed, the arching column of the scapular spine will come into view just posterior to the AC joint (Fig. 6-15). This bony arch leads to the keel-shaped base of the scapular spine.

The keel-shaped base of the scapular spine is easiest to view from a lateral portal and is the essential landmark for performance of a posterior interval slide. It is important to clear all fibrofatty tissue and adhesions to completely expose the base of the scapular spine. Once exposed, the base of the scapular spine serves to delineate the border between the muscle bellies of the supraspinatus and the infraspinatus tendons. The posterior interval slide then begins at the junction between the supraspinatus and infraspinatus tendons just lateral to the keel of the scapular spine.

When performing a posterior interval slide, we prefer to view from a lateral portal. Two traction sutures are placed.

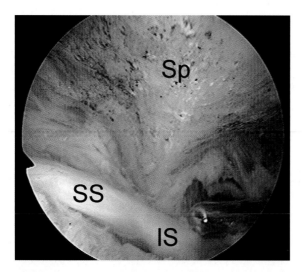

Figure 6-15 Arthroscopic view from a lateral portal of a left shoulder showing the "keel" of the scapular spine, which delineates the junction between the supraspinatus tendon and the infraspinatus tendon. Sp, scapular spine; SS, supraspinatus tendon; IS, infraspinatus tendon.

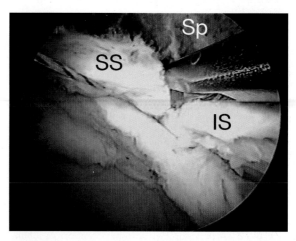

Figure 6-16 Arthroscopic view from a lateral viewing portal of a left shoulder showing the location for a posterior interval slide. The incision for the posterior interval slide is directed toward the keel of the scapular spine. SS, supraspinatus tendon; Sp, scapular spine; IS, infraspinatus tendon.

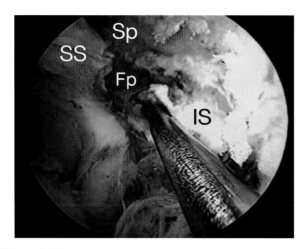

Figure 6-17 Arthroscopic view from a posterolateral portal of a left shoulder demonstrating a completed posterior interval slide. Note: The traction sutures have been placed into each tendon. Care is taken to avoid injury to the underlying suprascapular nerve. Sp, scapular spine; SS, supraspinatus tendon; IS, infraspinatus tendon; Fp, fat pad.

One traction suture is placed at the posterior aspect of the supraspinatus tendon and another traction suture is placed at the anterior aspect of the infraspinatus tendon. The supraspinatus traction suture is retrieved through an anterior subacromial portal, whereas the infraspinatus traction suture is retrieved through a posterior or posterolateral portal. While viewing through a lateral portal, we introduce arthroscopic scissors through a posterolateral portal

and begin the release between the traction sutures in the interval between the supraspinatus and infraspinatus tendons (Fig. 6-16). By applying anterior tension on the supraspinatus tendon and posterior tension on the infraspinatus tendon by means of the traction sutures, an apex is created between released and unreleased tissue. Tension allows clear visualization of the tips of the arthroscopic scissors, which then allows for a precise and safe posterior interval slide (Fig. 6-17).

When performing a posterior interval slide, care is taken to lift the tips of the scissors away from the bony glenoid to avoid injury to the suprascapular nerve. The suprascapular nerve is located along the bony edge of the glenoid neck at the base of the keel of the scapular spine, ~2 cm medial to the corner of the glenoid, protected by a surrounding fat pad. This fat pad will pop into view as soon as the posterior interval slide is complete, and the scissors are withdrawn to avoid injury to the nerve. Traction on the two sutures as the release is performed will further protect the nerve by pulling the tendon margin away from the nerve. Once the double interval slide has been completed, usually both the supraspinatus and infraspinatus tendons have gained up to 4- to 5-cm of addition lateral excursion.

REFERENCES

1. Lo IK, Burkhart SS. Arthroscopic revision of failed rotator cuff repairs: technique and results. *Arthroscopy.* 2004;20(3):250–267.
2. Klein JR, Burkhart SS. Identification of essential anatomic landmarks in performing arthroscopic single- and double-interval slides. *Arthroscopy.* 2004;20(7):765–770.

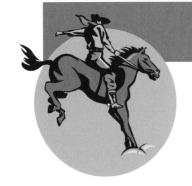

Insurmountable Problems—Bone Deficiency

THE ORIGIN OF THE SIGNIFICANCE OF BONE DEFICIENCY

In 2000, Burkhart and DeBeer (1) reported on 194 consecutive arthroscopic Bankart repairs using a suture anchor technique. In this study, despite surgery performed by very experienced arthroscopic surgeons, 21 patients had recurrent instability (10.8% recurrence rate) at 14 to 79 months follow-up. A superficial glance at this study might lead to the conclusion that these results would condemn arthroscopic Bankart repairs. The authors demonstrated, however, that arthroscopic Bankart repair, in fact, had no inherent technical weakness; instead, the recurrent instability rate stemmed from a failure to recognize significant concomitant pathology that was not amenable to arthroscopic treatment—a failure to recognize significant bone loss.

The authors demonstrated a 4% recurrence rate (7 recurrences in 173 patients) in patients having no significant bone defects. In patients with significant bone defects, however, a 67% recurrence rate (14 recurrences in 21 patients) was noted. Clearly, bone defects or the failure to identify and address them had a significant impact on the outcome following arthroscopic Bankart repair. In fact, in this situation we believe that patients with significant instability and bone defects should be treated with a bone-restoring procedure (e.g., Latarjet procedure) and not a standard arthroscopic Bankart repair.

This study also demonstrated that careful arthroscopic Bankart repair using suture anchors in patients without significant bone defects could lead to excellent results with recurrence rates comparable to open Bankart repairs.

Because of our disappointment with our results using arthroscopic Bankart repair in the face of significant bone defects (as defined below), we began doing open Latarjet reconstructions in 1996 in patients with severe bone loss. By December 2002, Burkhart and DeBeer (2) had accumulated 102 patients with instability and severe bone deficiency who had had open Latarjet reconstruction of the shoulder, with an average follow-up of 39 months. In this group were seen four recurrent dislocations and one recurrent subluxation, for a 4.9% recurrence rate. This was far better than the unacceptable high recurrence rate (67%) after arthroscopic repair in this same category of patients. This study (2) gave objective justification for the open coracoid bone-grafting approach in cases of severe bone deficiency.

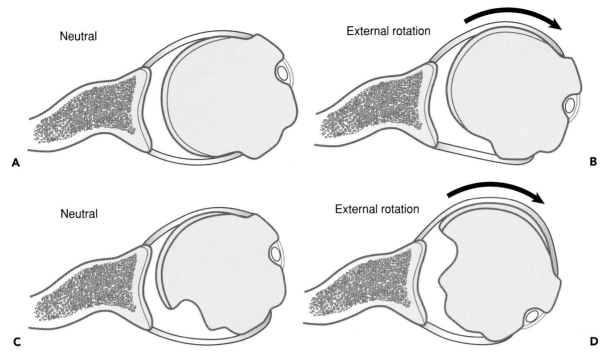

Figure 7-1 **A:** Normal relationship of the glenoid and humeral articular surfaces. **B:** Full external rotation still maintains contact between the humeral and glenoid articular surfaces. **C:** Large Hill-Sachs lesions cause an articular arc length mismatch. **D:** A small amount of external rotation will cause the Hill-Sachs lesion to engage the anterior corner of the glenoid. (From Burkhart, SS, et al. Articular arc length mismatch. *Arthroscopy.* 2000;16(7):740–744, Fig. 3; with permission.)

BONE DEFECTS

Significant bone defects can occur on the humeral or the glenoid side. These include the engaging Hill-Sachs lesions and the inverted pear glenoid.

Humeral Side Defects: The Engaging Hill-Sachs Lesion

Hill-Sachs lesions occur when the humeral head is impacted against the anterior inferior aspect of the glenoid during dislocation or during traumatic relocation. Although Hill-Sachs lesions can vary in size, what is important is whether the Hill-Sachs lesion engages the anterior rim of the glenoid when the arm is brought into a position of athletic function (i.e., combined abduction and external rotation) (1,3).

An engaging Hill-Sachs lesion is usually a large Hill-Sachs lesion involving a significant portion of the humeral articular surface (Fig. 7-1). When the arm is brought up into a position of athletic function (90° of abduction and 90° of external rotation), the Hill-Sachs lesion engages the anterior inferior aspect of the glenoid rim and can cause symptoms of subluxation, including catching or popping. This situation, which can occur even if the Bankart lesion is repaired, is caused by an articular arc deficit of the humeral head. Symptoms occur when the long axis of the Hill-

Sachs defect presents parallel to the anterior glenoid rim when the arm is brought up into a functional position of abduction and external rotation (Fig. 7-2). In most cases, a large engaging Hill-Sachs lesion occurs in combination with a significant glenoid bone defect.

In contrast, a nonengaging Hill-Sachs lesion presents itself nonparallel or diagonal to the anterior rim of the glenoid when the shoulder is in a position of 90° abduction and 90° external rotation and, therefore, does not engage (Fig. 7-3). Engagement of these defects only occurs with the arm in a nonfunctional position (for athletics), such as shoulder extension or abduction <70°. Because the defect is presented diagonal to the anterior rim of the glenoid with the arm in a functional position, continual contact of the humeral head with the glenoid (i.e., no articular arc deficit) occurs and the defect does not engage. Nonengaging Hill-Sachs lesions, therefore, are amenable to arthroscopic Bankart repair.

It is important to remember that the creation of engaging and nonengaging Hill-Sachs lesions is purely dependent on the position of the arm when the defect was created. Once the shoulder has dislocated, the humeral head can impact against the glenoid rim in any degree of abduction, with the arm at the side or with the arm in extension. For example, although the shoulder can dislocate with the arm in abduction and external rotation, it may immediately

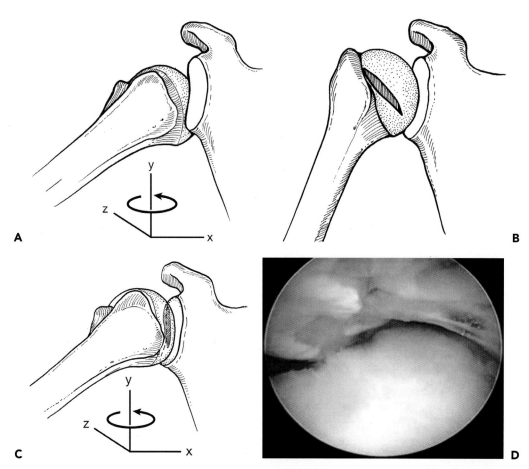

Figure 7-2 Engaging Hill-Sachs lesion. In a function position of abduction and external rotation, the long axis of the Hill-Sachs lesion is parallel to the glenoid and engages its anterior corner. **A:** Creation of lesion in a left shoulder with arm in abduction and external rotation. **B:** Orientation of Hill-Sachs lesion. **C:** Engagement of Hill-Sachs lesion in functional position of abduction and external rotation. **D:** Arthroscopic photograph of an engaging Hill-Sachs lesion in a right shoulder as it approaches its engagement position with the anterior glenoid rim. (From Burkhart SS, DeBeer JF. Traumatic glenohumeral bone defects and their relationship to failure of arthroscopic Bankart repairs: significance of the inverted-pear glenoid and the humeral engaging Hill-Sachs lesion. *Arthroscopy.* 2000;16(7):677–694, Fig. 2; with permission.)

revert to a position of 0° of abduction (i.e., the arm at the side) after dislocation and during impaction against the glenoid. This would create a Hill-Sachs lesion that is vertically oriented and would be a nonengaging Hill-Sachs lesion when the arm is brought up into abduction and external rotation.

Once a large engaging Hill-Sachs lesion has been identified, it should be recognized that an isolated arthroscopic Bankart repair will likely be insufficient to provide stability to the glenohumeral joint. Several options exist, including (a) restricting the external rotation of the arm sufficiently to prevent the Hill-Sachs lesion from engaging (Fig. 7-4); (b) restoring the articular arc defect of the humerus by bone grafting with allograft (Fig. 7-5); or (c) performing a rotational proximal humeral osteotomy. We do not recommend these procedures, however, because of the significant problems that can occur with them. For example, we have

seen open capsular shift procedures stretch out, allowing recurrent engagement of the Hill-Sachs lesion. We have seen resorption of allograft bone grafts to the humeral head, resulting in humeral articular arc incongruity. Potential problems with proximal humeral osteotomy include nonunion, neurovascular injury, and over- or undercorrection. It is our preference, therefore, to lengthen the articular arc of the glenoid to prevent engagement of the Hill-Sachs defect. We achieve this by performing a modified Latarjet procedure (Fig. 7-6) (see below).

Inverted Pear Glenoid

When the glenoid is viewed *en face*, it normally has the shape of a pear (i.e., the inferior half of the glenoid is significantly wider than the upper half of the glenoid) (Fig. 7-7A). With recurrent instability, however, the shape of the glenoid

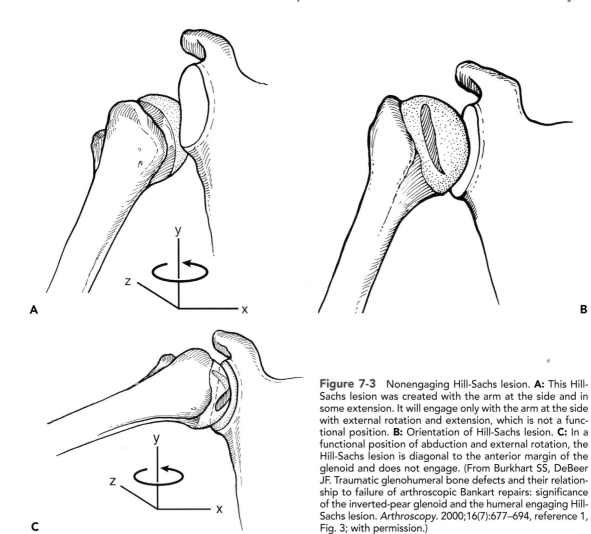

Figure 7-3 Nonengaging Hill-Sachs lesion. **A:** This Hill-Sachs lesion was created with the arm at the side and in some extension. It will engage only with the arm at the side with external rotation and extension, which is not a functional position. **B:** Orientation of Hill-Sachs lesion. **C:** In a functional position of abduction and external rotation, the Hill-Sachs lesion is diagonal to the anterior margin of the glenoid and does not engage. (From Burkhart SS, DeBeer JF. Traumatic glenohumeral bone defects and their relationship to failure of arthroscopic Bankart repairs: significance of the inverted-pear glenoid and the humeral engaging Hill-Sachs lesion. *Arthroscopy.* 2000;16(7):677–694, reference 1, Fig. 3; with permission.)

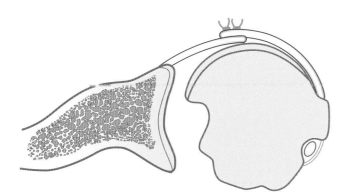

Figure 7-4 Capsular plication or imbrication will restrict external rotation, thereby preventing engagement of the Hill-Sachs lesion with the anterior corner of the glenoid. (From Burkhart SS, DeBeer JF, Barth JR, et al. Results of modified Latarjet reconstruction in patients with anteroinferior instability and significant bone loss. Accepted for publication in *Arthroscopy*, Fig. 4; with permission.)

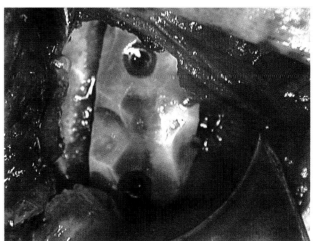

Figure 7-5 Clinical photo demonstrating restoration of the articular arc defect with matched humeral head allograft.

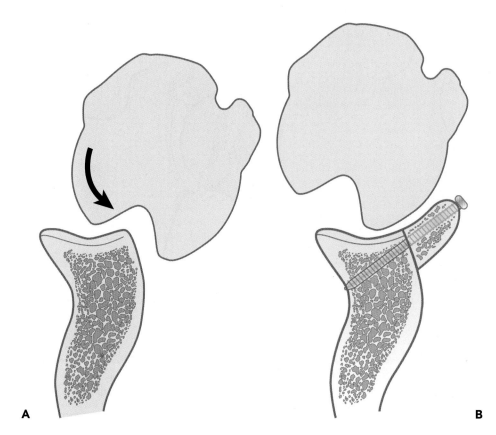

Figure 7-6 Schematic drawing demonstrating the use of a modified Latarjet procedure to lengthen the glenoid articular arc to prevent engagement of an engaging Hill-Sachs lesion. **A:** Engagement of Hill-Sachs lesion. **B:** Prevention of engagement by lengthening the glenoid articular arc.

A

B

can be converted to an inverted pear, whereby the inferior half of the glenoid appears narrower than the superior half of the glenoid. This can occur with a large bony Bankart lesion; with a Bankart lesion without a bone fragment, but with a compression defect of the anterior inferior glenoid; or a combination of both (Fig. 7-7B,C). The inverted pear glenoid is easily recognizable through an anterosuperolateral viewing portal, which allows the glenoid to be viewed *en face* (Fig. 7-8). The presence of an inverted pear glenoid usually indicates glenoid bone loss of ≥25% (4). In general, a difference of >6 mm between the anteroinferior gle-

noid radius and the posteroinferior glenoid radius indicates >25% bone loss. (See Chapter 4 for a complete discussion of accurately measuring glenoid bone loss.)

In the situation of a bony Bankart lesion, one option is to excise the bone fragment and repair the capsulolabral complex to the residual anterior glenoid rim. In small bony Bankart lesions (e.g., <12% loss of the inferior diameter of the glenoid), this excision combined with capsular repair may be sufficient to restore stability, but we generally prefer to repair the small bony Bankart fragment to the glenoid (Fig. 7-9).

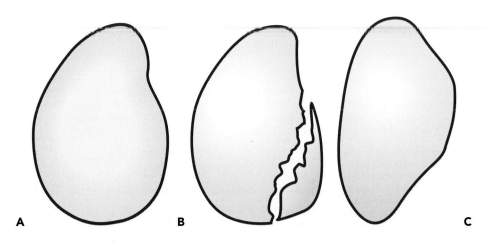

A

B

C

Figure 7-7 **A:** The normal shape of the glenoid is that of a pear, larger below than above. **B:** A bony Bankart lesion can create an inverted-pear configuration. **C:** A compression (impression) Bankart lesion can also create an inverted pear.

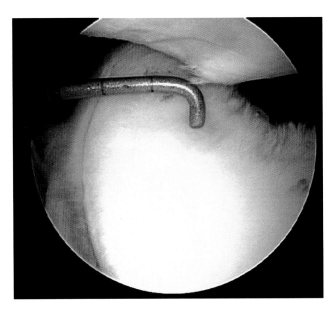

Figure 7-8 Arthroscopic view of a left shoulder through an anterosuperolateral portal demonstrating an inverted pear glenoid. Note: The inferior aspect of the glenoid appears narrower than the superior aspect of the glenoid and it narrows to an apex.

The bony glenoid provides two major mechanisms to contain the humeral head. First, the anterior glenoid rim "deepens" the glenoid because of the longer arc of its concave surface (Fig. 7-10A). Thus, an inverted pear glenoid will have lost a significant portion of the glenoid surface and the glenoid, therefore, will be shallower and less resistant to shear or translational forces that might cause dislocation (Fig. 7-10B).

Second, the glenoid provides bony resistance to axial and off-axis humeral forces. That is, axial forces generated intrinsically by the musculature or extrinsically by applied external loads are normally resisted by the bony glenoid until the direction of the force vector exceeds the anatomic limit of the glenoid (Fig. 7-11). At that point, the force is resisted primarily by the bone-labrum-ligament interface and can result in a Bankart lesion if sufficient force is applied. With an inverted pear glenoid, however, the normal arc through which the bony glenoid can resist axial forces (i.e., the safe zone) is reduced (Figs. 7-12 and 7-13). Thus, in an inverted pear configuration, axial forces which would normally be resisted by the bony glenoid are now being resisted by soft tissues (i.e., capsulolabral complex), a clearly unfavorable scenario.

In the case of an inverted pear configuration, we prefer to perform a modified Latarjet procedure, which restores the anterior glenoid bone stock and enlarges the arc through which the bony glenoid can resist axial forces (the safe zone).

MODIFIED LATARJET PROCEDURE

Our preference for restoring the anterior inferior bone deficiency (i.e., correcting an inverted pear glenoid) or for lengthening the articular arc of the glenoid (i.e., restoring stability in an engaging Hill-Sachs defect) is to perform a modified Latarjet procedure. This procedure differs from the classic Bristow procedure in that a significantly larger fragment of bone (~2–3 cm in length) is harvested from the coracoid. This large bone graft can be used to create an impressive lengthening of the articular arc of the anterior inferior aspect of the glenoid. Furthermore, because the conjoined tendon attachments remain on the coracoid graft, they further help to stabilize the shoulder by virtue of their sling effect as the arm goes into abduction and external rotation.

Text continues on page 164.

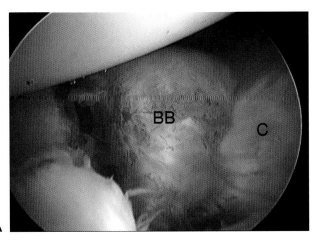
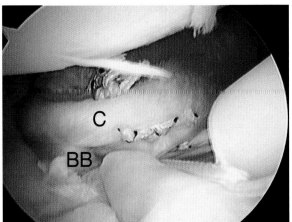

Figure 7-9   A: Arthroscopic view of a left shoulder through an anterosuperolateral portal demonstrating a small bony Bankart lesion representing <12.5% of the glenoid width. **B:** The bony Bankart lesion is repaired by passing sutures from the anchors through the capsule and the bone fragment (by means of a Sidewinder suture passer), and are then tied as a means of repairing the bone fragment to the glenoid. BB, bony Bankart fragment; C, capsule.

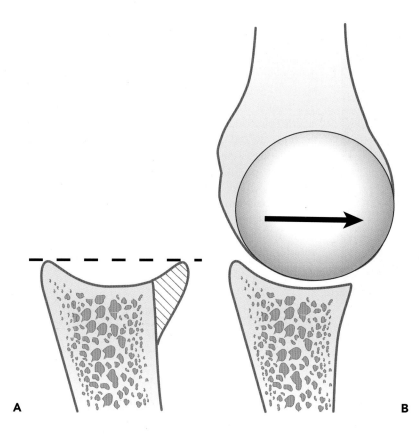

Figure 7-10 A: The anterior glenoid rim serves to "deepen the dish" of the glenoid and acts as a buttress to resist dislocation. **B:** A shoulder with a bony Bankart lesion has a shallower "dish" anteriorly with less resistance to shear forces. (From Burkhart SS, DeBeer JF. Traumatic glenohumeral bone defects and their relationship to failure of arthroscopic Bankart repairs: significance of the inverted-pear glenoid and the humeral engaging Hill-Sachs lesion. *Arthroscopy.* 2000;16(7):677–694, Fig. 6; with permission.)

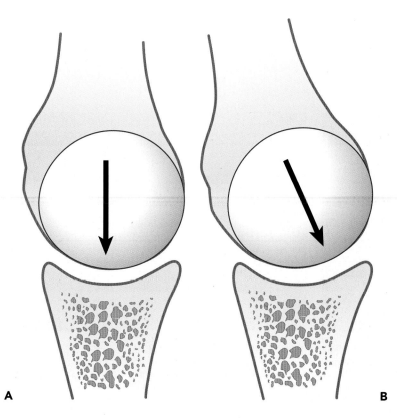

Figure 7-11 Effect of glenoid arc length. The glenoid resists angles from the humerus throughout the glenoid arc length **(A** and **B)**. Force vectors that pass beyond the edge of the glenoid can create Bankart lesions. Loss of a part of the glenoid articular surface (e.g., a bony Bankart lesion) shortens the arc through which the glenoid can resist humeral forces). (From Burkhart SS, DeBeer JF. Traumatic glenohumeral bone defects and their relationship to failure of arthroscopic Bankart repairs: significance of the inverted-pear glenoid and the humeral engaging Hill-Sachs lesion. *Arthroscopy.* 2000;16(7):677–694, Fig. 7; with permission.)

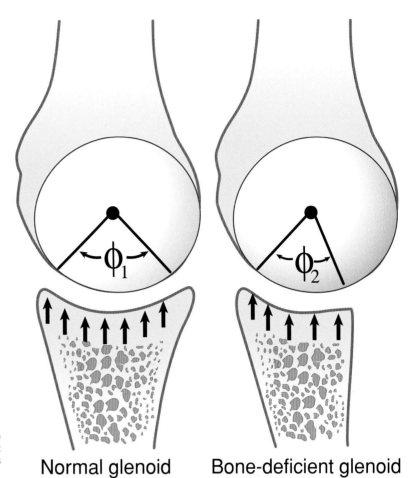

Figure 7-12 Glenoid bone loss shortens the "safe arc" through which the glenoid can resist axial forces. Φ_2 (bone-deficient condition) is less than Φ_1 (normal glenoid).

Normal glenoid   Bone-deficient glenoid

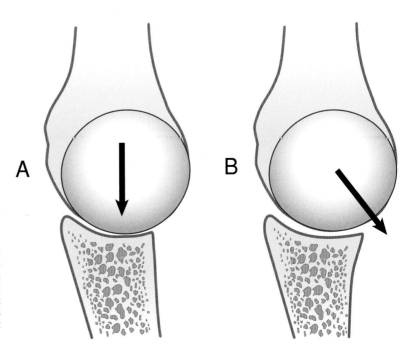

Figure 7-13 **A:** Axial force from the humerus applied centrally on the glenoid will not create a Bankart lesion or cause a failure of a soft tissue Bankart repair. **B:** If an axial force is applied through a point beyond the edge of the deficient glenoid, failure of a soft tissue Bankart repair is likely because the load must be borne by the soft tissues.

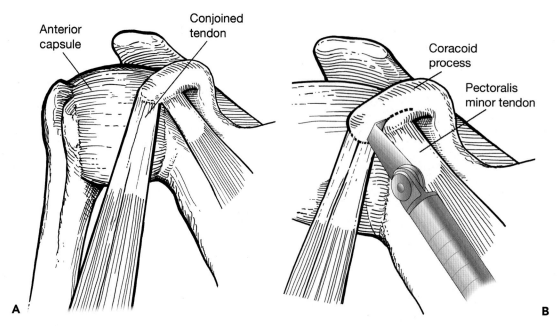

Figure 7-14 **A:** Tendon attachments onto the coracoid process before coracoid osteotomy **B:** Pectoralis minor (*insertion at dotted line*) is removed with a small piece of bone so that the final coracoid osteotomy can be made proximal to the "elbow" of the coracoid.

Although we have performed bone grafting procedures of the glenoid arthroscopically, they are extremely difficult to do and specific instrumentation for these procedures does not exist at this time. Therefore, we currently prefer an open approach for easy, reproducible reconstruction.

Preoperative Imaging

All patients having instability surgery have standard anteroposterior glenohumeral joint, transscapular lateral, and axillary radiographic studies performed preoperatively. Although these views can sometimes suggest significant glenoid deficiency, the degree of bone loss cannot be quantified on plain x-ray films. We do not currently employ specific imaging or sequencing protocols for quantifying bone loss, although our initial experience with three-dimensional computed tomography (3D CT) scanning (in which we utilize a "glenoid index" to compare the involved glenoid dimensions with the uninvolved glenoid dimensions) has been encouraging.

Surgical Technique

We always perform arthroscopy first, even when we are certain that we are going to do an open Latarjet procedure, because we have noted about a 20% incidence of superior labrum anterior and posterior (SLAP) lesions in these cases of significant bone loss. Obviously, the SLAP component of the injury is best repaired arthroscopically. The arthroscopy also provides us the opportunity to measure directly the size of the glenoid and to calculate the size of

the defect, as well as to assess dynamically whether an engaging Hill-Sachs lesion exists.

We have not found that an expeditious arthroscopy has made the subsequent open procedure more difficult.

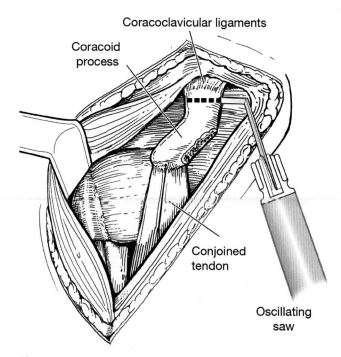

Figure 7-15 Osteotomy of coracoid. Note: The osteotomy is made proximal to the neck of the coracoid. An angled saw blade simplifies the osteotomy by more easily achieving the proper angle of approach.

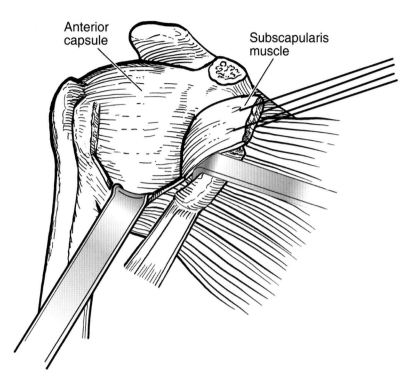

Figure 7-16 Management of the subscapularis tendon. Detach the superior half of the tendon, then develop a plane between the inferior half of the subscapularis and the capsule.

After doing the arthroscopy with the patient in the lateral decubitus position, we reposition the patient in a semibeach chair position with the arm draped free for manipulation during surgery.

In performing the modified Latarjet procedure, a standard deltopectoral approach is used. The cephalic vein is protected and retracted laterally with the deltoid muscle. The coracoid is exposed from its tip to the insertion of the coracoclavicular ligaments at the base of the coracoid. The coracoacromial ligament is sharply dissected from the lateral aspect of the coracoid, and the pectoralis minor tendon insertion on the medial side of the coracoid is

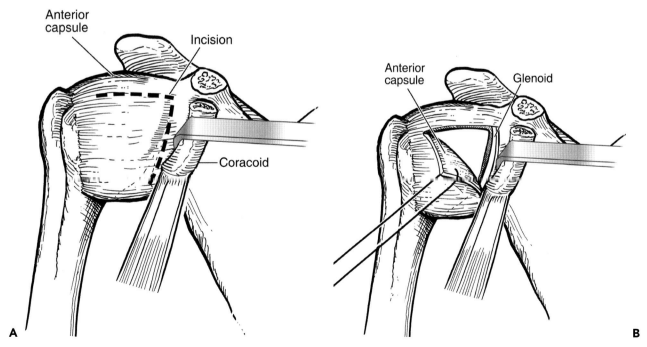

Figure 7-17 A: Outline of capsulotomy. **B:** Dissect the capsule 1-cm medial to the glenoid rim before detaching it from the glenoid neck to preserve as much capsular length as possible for later reattachment.

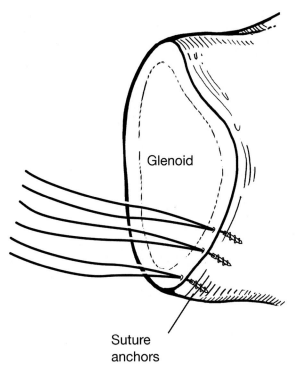

Figure 7-18   Suture anchors are placed for later reattachment of the capsulolabral complex.

removed along with a small piece of attached bone using an angled saw blade or an osteotome (Fig. 7-14). This medial cut surface of the coracoid is usually the surface that conforms best to the contour of the anterior glenoid where the bone graft will be placed.

Next the angled saw blade is used to osteotomize the coracoid just anterior to the coracoclavicular ligaments at the coracoid base (Fig. 7-15). If osteotome is used to perform the coracoid osteotomy, all medial retractors are removed to allow the osteotome's angle of approach to be anterior to the glenoid, thereby avoiding intra-articular glenoid fracture. An angled saw blade greatly simplifies this osteotomy by allowing an angle of approach that makes intra-articular glenoid fracture much less likely. Neurovascular structures are protected by retractors medial and inferior to the coracoid. The conjoined tendon is left attached to the coracoid graft because this provides some blood supply to the coracoid and makes it a vascularized graft (1–3); the transferred coracoid graft continues to serve as a stable attachment point for the conjoined tendon. After mobilization of the coracoid and the attached conjoined tendon, the musculocutaneous nerve is protected by retracting the coracoid medially, thereby preventing any stretch injury to the nerve.

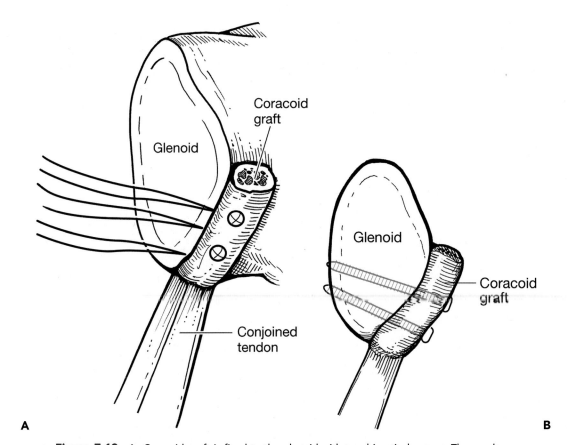

Figure 7-19   **A:** Coracoid graft is fixed to the glenoid with two bicortical screws. The raw bone surface where the pectoralis minor was removed usually provides the best fit against the glenoid, and the graft can be further contoured with a power burr to fit the curve of the anterior-inferior glenoid. **B:** Note: The coracoid graft restores the pear shape of the glenoid by widening its inferior diameter.

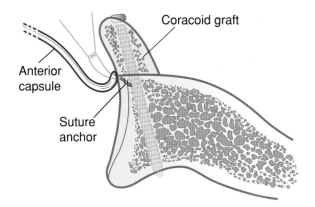

Figure 7-20 A graft is placed so that it becomes an extra-articular platform that acts as an extension of the articular arc of the glenoid.

Once the coracoid has been osteotomized, there is a clear view of the anterior shoulder. The upper half of the subscapularis tendon is detached distally and reflected medially in these patients (Fig. 7-16). The insertion of the lower half of the subscapularis tendon is preserved. After detachment of the upper subscapularis tendon, the plane between lower subscapularis tendon and anterior joint capsule is developed.

The capsular incision is begun 1 cm medial to the rim of the glenoid by subperiosteal sharp dissection to preserve enough capsular length for later reattachment (Fig. 7-17). The anterior glenoid neck is prepared as the recipient bed for the coracoid bone graft by means of a curette or a burr, being careful to preserve as much native glenoid bone as possible. "Dusting" of the anterior glenoid neck to a bleeding surface is performed with a high-speed burr without actually removing bone. Next, three suture anchors (BioFASTak or BioSutureTak; Arthrex, Inc.; Naples, FL) are placed in the native glenoid at 3, 4, and 5 o'clock (in a right shoulder) for later capsular repair (Fig. 7-18).

Proper position of the coracoid bone graft relative to the glenoid is critical. The long axis of the coracoid graft is aligned in a superior to inferior orientation and positioned against the anterior glenoid neck. The graft is rotated as necessary and trimmed as necessary for a good fit, and the best fit usually involves placing the medial surface of the coracoid (where the pectoralis minor insertion had been) against the glenoid neck (Fig. 7-19). Care is taken not to place the graft too far laterally or medially. It is not intended to be a bone block and, therefore, it is placed so that it functions as an extension of the glenoid articular arc (Fig. 7-20). In fact, Allain et al. (5) have shown that placement of the bone graft too far laterally, where it acts as a bone block, leads to an increased rate of postoperative degenerative arthritis. On the other hand, fixation of the graft too far medially places the shoulder at increased risk for recurrent subluxation or dislocation (Fig. 7-21).

The coracoid graft is fixed in place with two cannulated AO 4.0-mm cancellous screws (Synthes; Paoli, PA). These usually measure 34 to 36 mm in length. The capsule is then repaired to the native glenoid by means of the previously placed suture anchors, thereby making the coracoid graft an extra-articular structure and preventing its articulation directly with the humeral head. This precludes any abrasive effect of the graft against the articular cartilage of the humerus (Fig. 7-22).

Next, the upper subscapularis is repaired. The conjoined tendon, still attached to the coracoid graft, passes through the split between the upper and lower halves of subscapularis tendon (Fig. 7-23). The detached pectoralis minor is not reattached to the residual coracoid base or adjacent soft tissues because it does not retract. We have not observed any residual symptoms or cosmetic deformity relative to the unrepaired pectoralis minor. After subscapularis repair, a standard skin closure is performed.

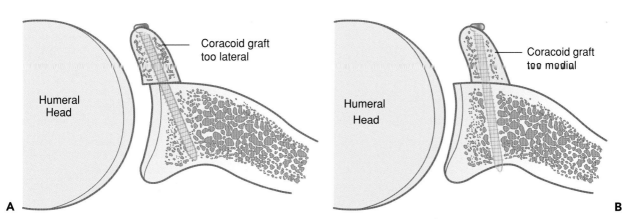

Figure 7-21 Incorrect placement of coracoid bone graft. **A:** The graft must not be placed so that it protrudes lateral to the joint surface and acts as a bone block. Such placement produces a high incidence of late osteoarthritis. **B:** Conversely, it is important also to avoid medial placement of the graft because this can predispose to recurrent dislocation.

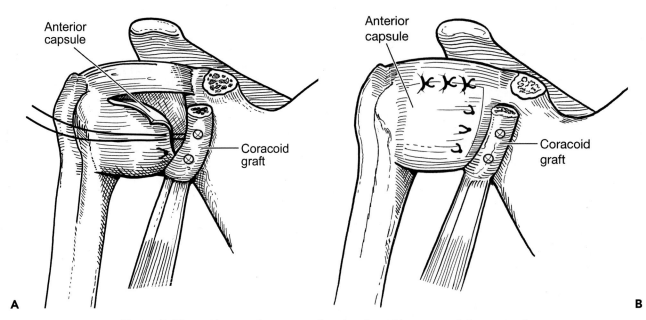

Figure 7-22   A: The capsule is repaired to the glenoid by means of the previously placed suture anchors. **B:** Completed capsular repair with graft in place. Note: The coracoid graft is extra-articular.

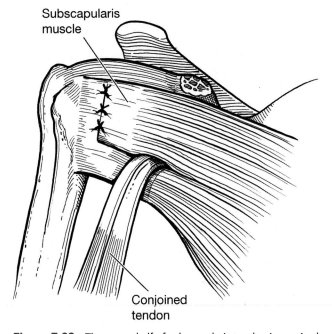

Figure 7-23 The upper half of subscapularis tendon is repaired to its stump. The conjoined tendon, attached to the coracoid bone graft, exits anteriorly between the upper and lower subscapularis.

Postoperative Rehabilitation

The patient uses a sling for 3 to 4 weeks, with external rotation restricted to 0°. At this point, the sling is discontinued and overhead motion is encouraged. Gentle external rotation stretching is begun at 6 weeks postoperative. Our goal at 3 months postoperative is for the external rotation on the operated shoulder to be half that of the opposite side. Strengthening exercises are delayed until 3 months postoperative, at which time the bone graft usually shows radiographic evidence of consolidation with the glenoid. Contact sports or heavy labor are generally allowed at 6 months postoperative.

REFERENCES

1. Burkhart SS, DeBeer JF. Traumatic glenohumeral bone defects and their relationship to failure of arthroscopic Bankart repairs: significance of the inverted-pear glenoid and the humeral engaging Hill-Sachs lesion. *Arthroscopy.* 2000;16(7):677–694.
2. Burkhart SS, DeBeer JF, Barth JR, et al. Results of modified Latarjet reconstruction in patients with anteroinferior instability and significant bone loss. Accepted for publication in *Arthroscopy.*
3. Burkhart SS, Danaceau SM. Articular arc length mismatch as a cause of failed Bankart repair. *Arthroscopy.* 2000;16(7):740–744.
4. Lo IK, Parten PM, Burkhart SS. The inverted pear glenoid: an indicator of significant glenoid bone loss. *Arthroscopy.* 2004;20(2):169–174.
5. Allain J, Goutallier D, Glorion C. Long-term results of the Latarjet procedure for the treatment of anterior instability of the shoulder. *J Bone Joint Surg Am.* 1998; 80(6):841–852.

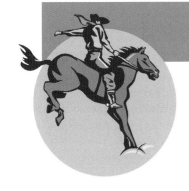

Gaining Speed and Tricks of the Trade

COWBOY PRINCIPLE 8

Set your pace by the distance you've got to ride.

Cowboys on cattle drives are keenly aware that they have to maintain a certain pace on the trail if they are ever going to get their cattle to market. They can't stop and dwell on how far they've come; they always have to be thinking ahead to how far they have to go. Forward progress occurs only when the cowboy is in the saddle and pushing the herd.

COROLLARY TO COWBOY PRINCIPLE 8

Tossin' a rope before buildin' a loop don't catch the calf.

Cowboy skills are built on progression. A cowboy ropes, then throws, then brands a steer—always in that order. Maybe that's why a cowboy's favorite recreation is playing pool. A good pool player is simultaneously doing two things with each shot: pocketing the shot he's playing, and setting up his next shot. This strategy is good not only for pool—it's good for just about everything in life that's worthwhile.

SECOND COROLLARY TO COWBOY PRINCIPLE #8

Lightning does the work; thunder takes the credit.

Things aren't always as they seem. Tricks can make the effort seem effortless. It's fun to listen to the thunder, but we can only learn by watching the lightning.

Any arthroscopic procedure performed properly and precisely can be time-consuming. In the shoulder, however, prolonged operating time can be particularly disconcerting because it can result in massive shoulder swelling, decreased visualization, and inability to complete the procedure. When learned correctly, however, every arthroscopic shoulder procedure should be within the reach of most arthroscopists as long as a thoughtful, expeditious surgical strategy is used. Furthermore, along the way are various principles and "tricks" that can be used to improve the speed of surgery and maintain a steady working pace.

VISUALIZE, VISUALIZE, VISUALIZE

As described in Chapter 1, you must visualize the pathology. This cannot be overemphasized. When we have visiting

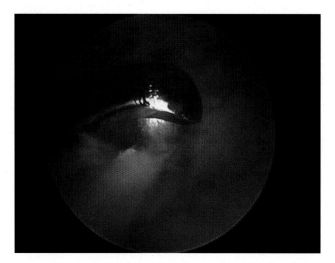

Figure 8-1 Arthroscopic view from a lateral subacromial portal of a right shoulder demonstrating débridement of the posterior rotator cuff and overlying bursa by means of a shaver introduced through a posterior portal. The posterior gutter must be cleared.

surgeons attend our operating theaters to observe arthroscopic shoulder surgery, most are surprised by the consistently clear visualization we routinely achieve. When one cannot see clearly or if one begins to cut corners (e.g., tying knots blind without visualization), the case begins to fall apart. When first attempting any shoulder reconstructive procedure, it is certainly easier and less frustrating if clear, unobstructed visualization is obtained before beginning the reconstructive portion of the procedure.

REMOVE ALL OVERLYING SOFT TISSUES ON THE FIRST PASS

Nowhere is soft tissue débridement more important than when trying to master arthroscopic rotator cuff repair. Nothing is more frustrating than repetitively débriding the subacromial bursa to permit visualization during an already difficult procedure. It is paramount when first evaluating the subacromial space and bursa to perform a thorough bursectomy of the anterior, posterior, medial, and lateral aspects of the subacromial space. Repeating the bursectomy at a later date is both time consuming and potentially disastrous when anchors are already placed and sutures have been passed, because the sutures will be at risk for damage by the shaver.

It is particularly important to remove the bursa overlying the posterior rotator cuff (Fig. 8-1) and the lateral subacromial gutter around the shoulder of the greater tuberosity (Fig. 8-2). When passing, retrieving, and tying sutures through the posterior cuff or the far lateral cuff (toward the end of the case), it often seems that visualization can be difficult. For this reason, we spend more time performing a complete bursectomy in these regions. In addition, when sequentially tying sutures (all other things being equal),

we will tie the side-to-side and posterior sutures first (where visualization can be more difficult) and then advance anteriorly and laterally (where visualization is usually easier) (Fig. 8-3).

When performing the bursectomy, particularly when débriding tissue overlying the rotator cuff muscle, it is important to avoid violating the muscle fascia or muscle belly. If a repeat bursal débridement is needed for visualization (which the surgeon must do if unable to see) after sutures have been passed, then placing traction on the sutures can protect them from being entangled and damaged by the shaver.

MULTIPLE PORTALS FOR MULTIPLE DIRECTIONS

One of the distinct advantages to arthroscopic surgery over open surgery is an ability to evaluate and approach multiple pathologies simultaneously from an almost limitless selection of angles of approach with minimal disruption to the overlying soft tissues. This is true for both visualization and instrumentation and has allowed the arthroscopic surgeon to better understand shoulder pathology. In addition, the arthroscopist can now repair pathology that otherwise would be "irreparable" from a standard single incision open approach (e.g., triple labral lesions, massive rotator cuff tears involving subscapularis, supraspinatus, and infraspinatus tendons).

Some arthroscopists have interpreted the arthroscopic minimally invasive approach to mean that a minimal number of incisions or portals must be used. Although in general, the fewer portals required to repair a shoulder condition, the better, never compromise angle of approach to spare a small

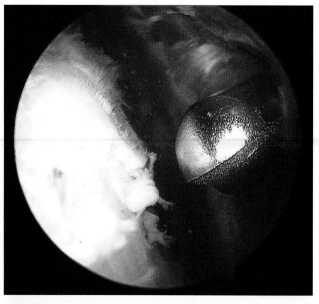

Figure 8-2 Arthroscopic view from a posterior subacromial portal of a right shoulder demonstrating débridement of the lateral gutter.

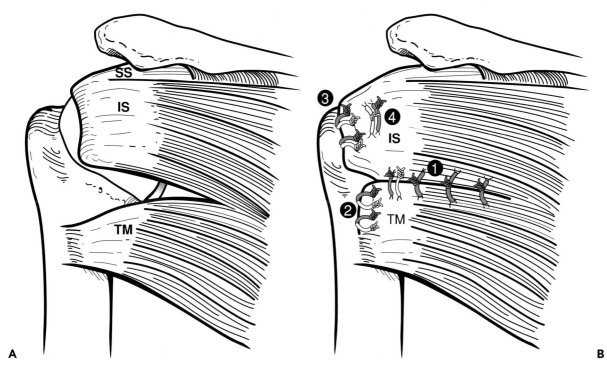

Figure 8-3 Schematic diagram demonstrating the general sequence of tying knots for arthroscopic rotator cuff repair. This is a reverse-L tear **(A)** in a left shoulder, repaired with a double-row technique **(B)**. The side-to-side sutures *(1)* are tied first, followed by the posterolateral sutures *(2)*, then next progressing anterolaterally *(3)*. If a double row repair is performed, then the medial row is tied last *(4)*. SS, supraspinatus; IS, infraspinatus; TM, teres minor.

puncture through skin. We never hesitate to make an additional portal to ensure the correct angle of approach. This may even include making separate 2-mm incisions for each anchor during rotator cuff repair. The addition of an extra portal to guarantee the correct angle of approach both minimizes technical errors and results in a faster procedure. Some traditional open surgeons argue that arthroscopic surgery and open surgery are both minimally invasive; that is, they suggest that when the lengths of all the portal punctures are added, the total equals the length of their open incision. They fail to realize that the puncture through skin is irrelevant as long as the soft tissue below is preserved. The advantages of smaller incisions are only the "tip of the iceberg."

MAINTAINING DIRECTION: THE SECRET OF THE SPINAL NEEDLE

Whenever we are creating portals for either instrumentation or anchor placement, we always preliminarily place a spinal needle to ensure the correct angle of approach. This is a simple and routine "trick" with which most arthroscopic surgeons are familiar. We, however, have also noted that many arthroscopic surgeons will place the spinal needle, incise the skin, and then remove the needle before placing the actual instrument through the soft tissues. Then, the arthroscopist has to visualize and recreate the

correct angle of approach mentally. We prefer to leave the needle in place after incising the skin, to act as a guide to the correct angle of approach. Only after the instrument or implant has been placed in the proper location do we remove the spinal needle. In this fashion, the spinal needle continually reminds us of the correct angle of approach and makes reproduction of this angle easy. In the case of anchor insertion, we do not remove the spinal needle until the anchor has been seated into bone, after all punching and tapping have been performed (Fig. 8-4).

PASSING SUTURES BEFORE TYING: MAXIMIZING FIXATION

Suture passage is a vitally important technical step to master when performing arthroscopic shoulder reconstructions. With repetition, this can become one of the easiest parts of the procedure, particularly with new instrumentation. A tendency exists, however, particularly for the novice arthroscopist, to "tie as you go." That is, before a second anchor is placed, sutures from the first anchor are tied after suture passage. This is especially tempting during complex reconstructions requiring multiple suture anchors.

The major advantage of tying as you go is that it limits the number of free suture limbs in the glenohumeral or subacromial space at one time, simplifying suture management.

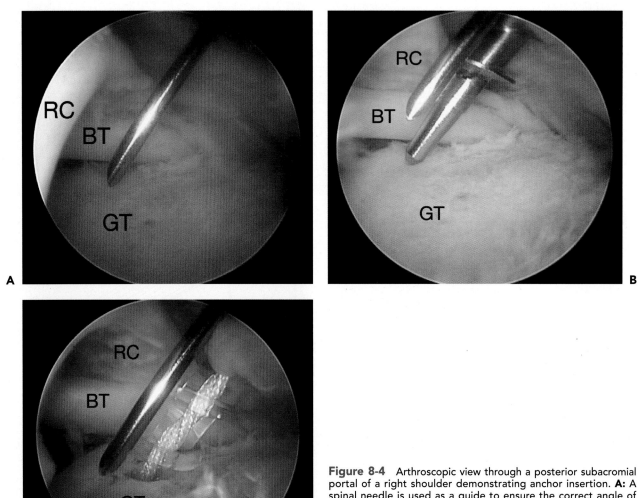

Figure 8-4 Arthroscopic view through a posterior subacromial portal of a right shoulder demonstrating anchor insertion. **A:** A spinal needle is used as a guide to ensure the correct angle of approach for a proper dead-man angle. **B:** Using the spinal needle as a guide, the bone is punched and tapped. **C:** The spinal needle is kept in place while the anchor is inserted. It is removed only after the anchor is seated, so that it can serve as a guide for the entire procedure of anchor insertion. RC, rotator cuff; GT, greater tuberosity; BT, biceps tendon.

Tying as you go, however, tends to bind the soft tissue to the bone bed, making subsequent suture passage more difficult (Fig. 8-5). This is because most instruments require a certain amount of space between the bone bed and soft tissue for easy suture passage. The consequence of tying as you go may be twofold. First, initial soft tissue fixation can loosen if subsequent suture passage is difficult and manipulative. This is particularly relevant if soft tissue quality is poor and can result in tearing of the tied sutures through soft tissue. Second, if the soft tissue is tightly bound, a tendency exists to redirect the next fixation point further away from the first anchor site. Although this simplifies suture passage, by moving the next anchor and suture loop further away, this eventually results in fewer anchors and fewer sutures for fixation of the entire construct. The result is few fixation points, a weaker construct, and more force per unit fixation point. This can result in an unstable construct.

As a general rule, we prefer to insert all anchors and pass all sutures before tying. This maximizes fixation and ensures placement of anchors and sutures at their ideal positions. Although this approach complicates suture management, we generally use one of the techniques described below for easy, reproducible suture management. The major exception to placing all sutures before tying any sutures is that, when performing a U- or L-shaped rotator cuff repair, we tie the side-to-side sutures first (once they have all been placed), before placing our lateral fixation. This sequence of repair serves to converge the rotator cuff margin toward the bone bed (margin convergence) and simultaneously to decrease the strain at the "converged" cuff margin, thereby protecting the tendon-to-bone repair.

SUTURE MANAGEMENT

Suture management is a fundamental process that encompasses many steps, including suture organization, retriev-

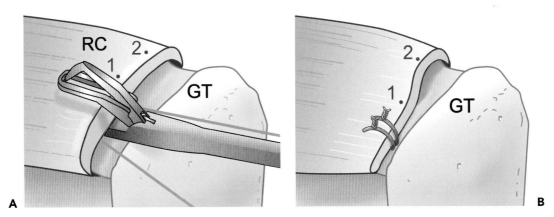

Figure 8-5 Schematic drawing. The effect of "tying as you go" during rotator cuff repair. Tying sutures as they are passed and tied tend to bind the adjacent soft tissues tightly to bone. This makes subsequent suture passage more difficult and can loosen fixation if traumatic manipulation of the soft tissue is required to pass the suture. In **(A)**, the surgeon ideally would like the sutures from the second anchor to be passed through point 1. Tying the initial sutures **(B)** has bound down point 1, however, so that the suture passage there is not possible, and point 2 has to be accepted for suture passage. The effect of this soft tissue tightening is to move the next point of fixation further away from the first, simplifying suture passage but resulting in a less than optimal mechanical construct.

ing sutures, and minimizing tangles. Many novice arthroscopists find this one of the most difficult tasks in shoulder arthroscopy. A step-by-step method of organization and retrieval can greatly minimize frustration, however.

Suture Organization

Many different techniques can be used collectively to assist in suture organization. First, when using double-loaded suture anchors, it is preferable to have each of the sutures colored

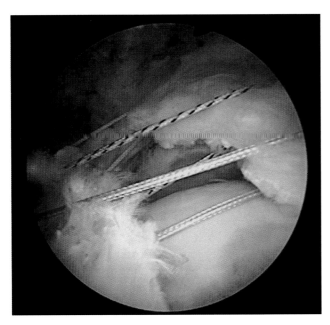

Figure 8-6 Arthroscopic view through a lateral portal of a left shoulder demonstrating alternating colors of side-to-side sutures.

differently. This automatically halves the number of sutures the surgeon has to remember. Second, when passing sutures from each anchor, it is important to use the same protocol every time. For example, if initially the blue suture is passed from the first anchor, on subsequent anchors always pass the blue suture first and the TigerWire (Arthrex, Inc.; Naples, FL) suture second. This separates sutures of the same color and can help with subsequent suture retrieval when tying knots at the end of the case. It is important to alternate suture colors also when passing side-to-side sutures (Fig. 8-6). Fourth, to help organize sutures, it is common practice to use hemostats to match pairs of sutures together or all the sutures from one anchor together. This technique can be helpful, particularly when performing arthroscopic Bankart repair, when many sutures from different anchors are being retrieved and temporarily held through the same cannula. When performing arthroscopic rotator cuff repair, however, we prefer to use a different method.

When performing an arthroscopic rotator cuff repair, it is not uncommon to place five anchors for a large rotator cuff tear. This, of course, means 5 anchors, 10 sutures, or 20 suture limbs. This can be a nightmare if using one portal for all anchor insertions. Alternatively, we generally use a separate 2- to 3-mm skin puncture for each anchor. This ensures an adequate angle of approach during anchor insertion and also assists in suture management. When placing skin punctures, we generally create portal sites that match the footprint we have created on the bone bed. For example, if we have placed a two-medial, two-lateral anchor configuration on the bone bed (Fig. 8-7A), the puncture wounds in the skin will mirror this with two skin punctures immediately adjacent to the acromion and then two puncture wounds slightly more lateral (Fig. 8-7B).

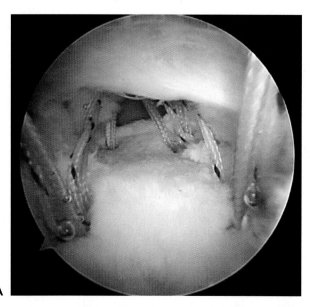 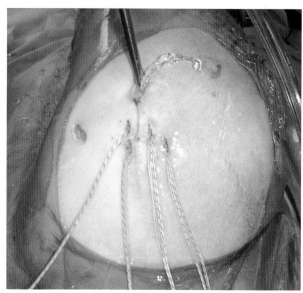

Figure 8-7 The "mirror method" of suture management. **A:** Arthroscopic view through a lateral portal of a right shoulder demonstrating a construct of two medial anchors and two lateral anchors for footprint reconstruction of the rotator cuff. **B:** External view of the same shoulder demonstrating two puncture wounds adjacent to the acromion and two puncture wounds more laterally. Note: The skin puncture wounds "mirror" the suture anchor arrangement on the footprint, simplifying suture management.

It is important to remember that we do place anchors individually, and then pass the suture from the anchor before inserting the next anchor. The key to this technique is that after suture passage and before placing the next anchor, the sutures are retrieved back out from the skin puncture wound used for inserting the anchor. This organizes the sutures together with the corresponding anchor and identifies them with the appropriate skin puncture wound (Fig. 8-8). With subsequent knot tying, it becomes easy to retrieve sutures. For example, if we wish to tie the sutures from the anterolat-

eral anchor, as long as we retrieve the matching pair of suture limbs moving through our anterolateral skin puncture (which mirrors our bone bed footprint), then these are the correct sutures. Using separate skin punctures for each anchor also separates the sutures, making retrieval easier.

Retrieving Sutures

Retrieving suture limbs for suture passage or for tying can occasionally be difficult when multiple sutures are already in the glenohumeral or subacromial space. When retrieving sutures, two scenarios are commonly problematic: (a) when retrieving and pulling one suture limb, it is important to ensure that the sutures are not unloaded from the anchor; and (b) when determining which two suture limbs in the joint match each other, be sure that the two strands retrieved are part of the same suture pair.

Preventing Anchor Unloading

Unloading an anchor, particularly if single loaded or if suture passage has already been completed, can be a disheartening experience. This usually occurs when retrieving and pulling suture limbs out of portals for suture passage or knot tying. The easiest way to prevent unloading of an anchor is consistent viewing of the suture anchor eyelet as the suture is being pulled. As long as the suture is not pulling through the eyelet, the anchor will not unload. For example, suppose an anchor has been placed on the lateral aspect of the greater tuberosity and preparations are being made to pass a suture through the rotator cuff using an

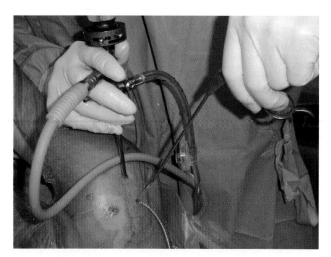

Figure 8-8 To use the skin punctures for suture management after suture passage, the sutures are retrieved back out the skin puncture wound through which the anchor was inserted, organizing the sutures with the suture anchor and the corresponding puncture wound.

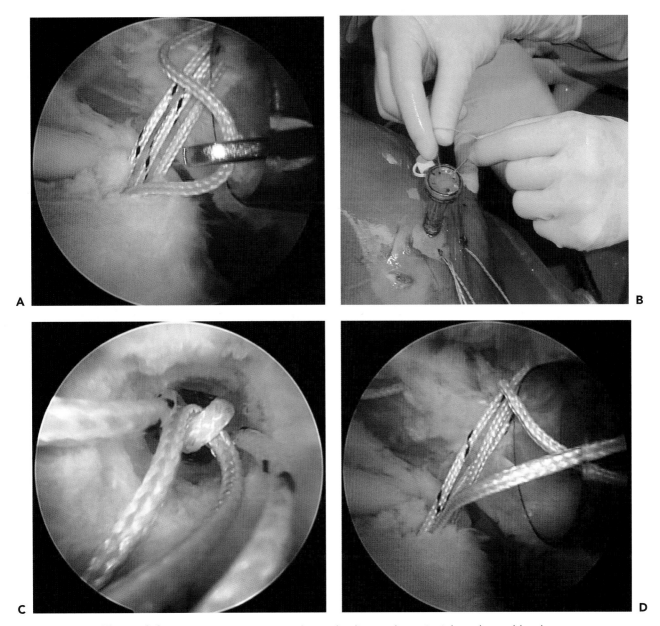

Figure 8-9 Retrieving sutures—avoiding unloading anchors. **A:** A lateral portal has been established and one limb of the suture is retrieved and pulled out the lateral cannula. Arthroscopic view of a right shoulder through a posterior subacromial portal. **B:** After the suture has been retrieved, an assistant grasps each side of the loop with separate hands. **C:** Arthroscopic view through a posterior subacromial portal using a 70° arthroscope. As the assistant alternately pulls each side of the loop, the arthroscopist views the suture eyelet. Pulling on the incorrect side of the loop will cause the suture to run through the eyelet, potentially unloading the anchor **D:** Pulling on the correct side of the loop will not move the suture through the eyelet but will pull the correct limb into the cannula.

antegrade suture passing device (e.g., Viper or Scorpion [Arthrex, Inc.; Naples, FL] suture passer). To perform this maneuver, however, one suture limb must be retrieved from the suture anchor and pulled out the lateral portal (Fig. 8-9A). As the retrieved suture limb exits the cannula extracorporeally, it will appear as a loop of suture. The question, of course, is which side of the suture loop should be pulled? The easiest way to determine the correct side is to ask an assistant to grasp each side of the loop individually with separate hands (Fig. 8-9B). While viewing the suture anchor eyelet, the assistant pulls on either end of the loop (Fig. 8-9C). If the suture is seen to slide through the anchor eyelet, then this is the wrong end of the loop to pull. If the suture remains stationary in the anchor eyelet, however, then the correct end of the loop is being pulled (Fig. 8-9D). As long as the suture remains stationary in the anchor eyelet, the anchor cannot be unloaded. This, of course, assumes the correct anchor eyelet is being observed.

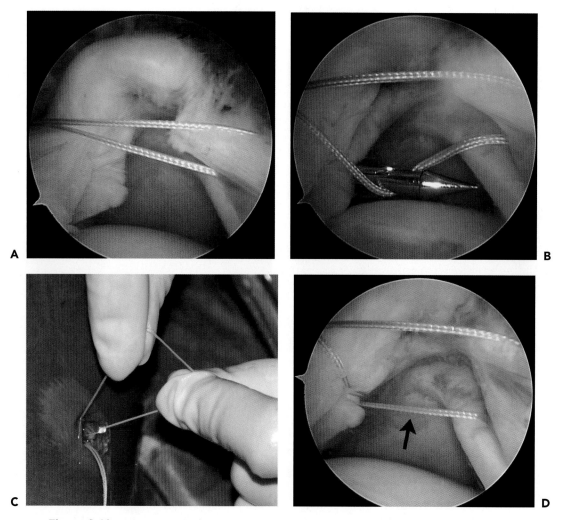

Figure 8-10 Retrieving sutures—preventing unloading of a side-to-side suture. **A:** Arthroscopic view through a lateral subacromial portal of a U-shaped rotator cuff tear in a right shoulder. A suture has already been placed in the anterior leaf. **B:** Arthroscopic view through a lateral subacromial portal. A Penetrator (Arthrex, Inc.; Naples, FL) is then introduced through the posterior portal and passes through the posterior leaf of the rotator cuff to retrieve the undersurface limb of the anterior suture. **C:** Clinical photo of the assistant grasping each side of the loop extracorporeally from the posterior portal. **D:** As the assistant alternately pulls each side of the loop, the arthroscopic surgeon views the portion of the suture that is between the anterior and posterior leaves (arrow), ensuring that this portion of the suture remains stationary.

A similar technique can be used when pulling suture limbs following retrograde suture passage. For example, suppose an arthroscopic rotator cuff repair is being performed and an anchor has been placed in the posterolateral aspect of the footprint. While viewing through a lateral portal, a Penetrator suture passer (Arthrex) is used to pass a suture through the posterior aspect of the rotator cuff in a retrograde fashion. The Penetrator passes through the cuff tissue, captures a suture limb, and then pulls the suture limb back through the cuff. As the Penetrator is pulled out through the posterior portal, a suture loop is seen extracorporeally, which is the suture loop that has been passed through the posterior rotator cuff. While viewing the anchor eyelet, an assistant similarly grabs each side of the loop and alternately pulls each side of the loop. The one that does not

cause the suture to move through the anchor eyelet is the proper side of the loop to pull.

Finally, when placing side-to-side sutures for rotator cuff repair, a similar technique can be used. Suppose a side-to-side suture is being placed for a U-shaped rotator cuff repair and a suture has already been placed through the anterior leaf (Fig. 8-10A). A Penetrator is then used through a posterior portal to puncture the posterior leaf, and the undersurface limb is retrieved (Fig. 8-10B) and passed retrograde through the posterior leaf and out the posterior portal. An assistant then grabs the suture loop, which appears extracorporeally out the posterior portal (Fig. 8-10C). In this situation, instead of looking at an anchor eyelet, it is important to visualize the portion of the suture between the anterior and posterior leaves (Fig. 8-10D). As long as this portion of

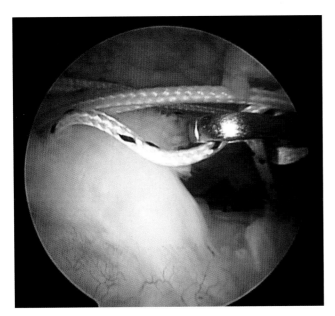

Figure 8-11 Arthroscopic view through a posterior subacromial portal of a right shoulder. Clearing a path for knot tying. When retrieving sutures for knot tying, each suture limb should be retrieved simultaneously as close to the tendon (soft tissue limb) and anchors (free limb) as possible without crossing over any sutures. This creates an unobstructed path for knot tying.

the suture remains stationary as the assistant pulls on the suture limb, the correct limb of the suture loop is being pulled.

Finding Matching Sutures

Occasionally, when a suture "jungle" develops as sutures are placed in the glenohumeral or subacromial space, it can be difficult to determine which suture limbs match each other. Usually, this occurs when tying knots toward the end of the case. The easiest way to match sutures is to first retrieve one limb. Usually, one limb is always easily seen (usually the suture limb on the anchor side) and can be retrieved safely (see section on preventing unloading sutures). To identify the matching suture limb, the retrieved suture is then pulled, allowing a small amount of the suture to run through the anchor eyelet. This maneuver will also exert a pull on the matching limb and then the suture limb that has moved can be identified and retrieved.

Minimizing Tangles and Untangling Sutures

When retrieving sutures, commonly many of the suture limbs will be overlapped and twisted upon one another. It is possible, however, to untangle the limb and retrieve the suture all in one simple step. The key is to retrieve the suture as close to its exit from the cuff or from the anchor eyelet as possible. For example, consider the stage of arthroscopic rotator cuff repair at which all the sutures have been passed, and it is time to begin tying sutures for the lateral fixation. At

this point, the surgeon may see a multitude of sutures, which appear to overlap one another. To minimize entanglement and to avoid tying down other sutures, it is important to perform the retrieval by retrieving both suture limbs simultaneously and grabbing the suture limbs as close to their exit point as possible. In this scenario, the one limb should be grabbed as close to the anchor as possible and then the other suture limb should be grabbed as it exits the rotator cuff without crossing over any other sutures (Fig. 8-11). When the suture is then retrieved through a portal, an unobstructed pathway for subsequent knot tying is created.

If a suture knot is ever inadvertently made, then a suture retriever can be used to untangle the knot. We find the Arthrex suture retriever a valuable instrument when performing this procedure.

Finding the Lost Suture

When swelling becomes significant in the subacromial space, the bursa and fibrofatty tissue can completely obstruct the visualization of some suture limbs. This most commonly occurs with suture limbs exiting through a posterior portal or a modified Neviaser portal. Despite attempts to retrieve the suture, including débridement of soft tissues, the suture cannot be identified. In this case, one can use a single-diameter knot pusher to push the suture into the subacromial space in an area where it is visible. For example, if attempting to retrieve a suture that is exiting the posterior portal, it is easiest to view through a lateral portal. The suture limb is then threaded through a single-diameter knot pusher and then the knot pusher is advanced back into the subacromial space (Fig. 8-12). When performing this, it is important to attempt to reproduce the same angle of approach and to use the same established soft tissue tunnel through which the suture exited. Once the suture is identified, it can be retrieved. When using this technique, if the same angle of approach and the same soft tissue tunnel are not reproduced, then a bridge of tissue will become trapped within the suture loop (Fig. 8-13). This will bind (in this example) the deltoid muscle or deltoid fascia against the rotator cuff. It is important to recognize this and either attempt to reproduce the correct soft tissue tunnel again or to débride the intervening soft tissue bridge.

RELOADING ANCHORS

Occasionally, if one is not careful, an anchor can be unloaded. It is possible to reload anchors *in situ*, however, particularly if using anchors with a suture loop eyelet design (e.g., 5.0-mm BioCorkscrew [Arthrex] suture anchor).

If one suture still remains in the anchor eyelet, then reload the anchor (to make it double loaded again) by using the remaining suture as a shuttle. First, retrieve one end of the suture out of the shoulder so that most of the

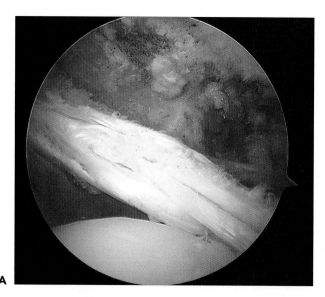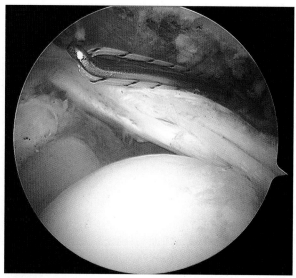

Figure 8-12 Arthroscopic view through a lateral subacromial portal of a right shoulder, looking toward the posterior leaf of the rotator cuff. **A:** The suture limb cannot be identified in the fat overlying the posterior leaf of the rotator cuff because, during retrograde suture passage, the suture passer did not exit the fat before entering into the tendon. **B:** A single-diameter knot pusher is used to push the suture limb into the field of view and the matching suture can now be retrieved.

suture is outside the cannula (Fig. 8-14A). Be careful not to also unload this suture from the anchor eyelet. Using a straight needle (Graft Preparation Needle [Arthrex]), pass a second differently colored suture through this suture (Fig. 8-14B,C). Then, pull the other end of the intact threaded suture, which is through the anchor, out a separate portal. This will retrieve the original suture and shuttle the second suture through the anchor eyelet (Fig. 8-14D). Pull the

intersection of the two sutures extracorporeally, then disengage the second suture from the first suture and equalize the suture limb lengths (Fig. 8-14E). It is important when performing this technique not to inadvertently unload the last remaining suture. In addition, because a hole has been made in the original suture, remember that a weakness in the suture exists at this level and this weak spot should not be included in the final construct during subsequent suture passage or knot tying.

If no sutures remain in the anchor, the suture anchor can only be reloaded if the suture loop is visible and accessible above the bone. If this situation exists, passing a 0 polydioxanone (PDS) suture through the anchor eyelet by means of a Suture Lasso (Arthrex) (Fig. 8-15A) and shuttling a nonabsorbable suture into place can reload the anchor (Fig. 8-15B). Naturally, we prefer to avoid this scenario, if possible, because it requires that the eyelet be sitting "proud" above the surface of the bone, which is not the optimal situation. It may be possible, however, to drive the anchor deeper below the bone surface by rethreading the sutures through the BioCorkscrew inserter and reseating the inserter tip over the hex head of the anchor to advance it.

INSERTING ANCHORS IN POOR BONE

We have been concerned from the beginning about optimizing the mechanical strength of our rotator cuff repair construct. In our ongoing efforts to improve fixation, the senior author (SSB) has been involved in the development of a modified biodegradable suture anchor, the Bio-

Figure 8-13 Arthroscopic view through a lateral subacromial portal of a right shoulder, looking toward the posterior cuff. It is important to recreate the same angle of approach and the same soft tissue tunnel; otherwise a soft tissue bridge of deltoid muscle will be created as seen in this arthroscopic photo. The soft tissue bridge will bind the deltoid muscle to the rotator cuff.

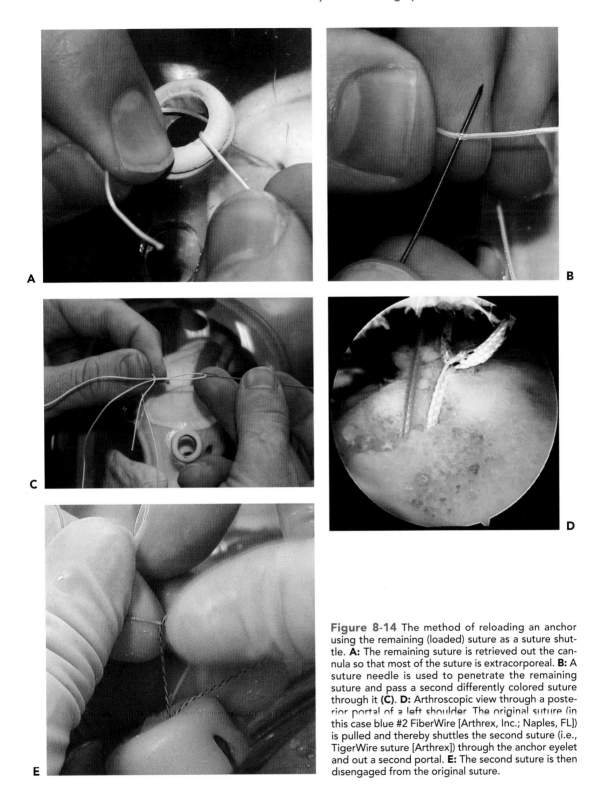

Figure 8-14 The method of reloading an anchor using the remaining (loaded) suture as a suture shuttle. **A:** The remaining suture is retrieved out the cannula so that most of the suture is extracorporeal. **B:** A suture needle is used to penetrate the remaining suture and pass a second differently colored suture through it **(C)**. **D:** Arthroscopic view through a posterior portal of a left shoulder. The original suture (in this case blue #2 FiberWire [Arthrex, Inc.; Naples, FL]) is pulled and thereby shuttles the second suture (i.e., TigerWire suture [Arthrex]) through the anchor eyelet and out a second portal. **E:** The second suture is then disengaged from the original suture.

Corkscrew-FT (fully threaded BioCorkscrew anchor) (Fig. 8-16). This anchor has threads all the way to the top of the suture anchor to maximize fixation. To have the eyelet below the level of the bone, the eyelet had to be recessed within the body of the anchor. As in the BioCorkscrew suture anchor, the eyelet is composed of a flexible suture, except in this case it is made of #4 FiberWire, giving it even greater resistance to failure than the eyelet of the standard BioCorkscrew, which consists of an insert-molded polyester suture. Furthermore, the internal hex drive allows insertional torques of five times those that can be achieved with the standard BioCorkscrew anchor, making it highly unlikely that the anchor will break on insertion, even in very hard bone.

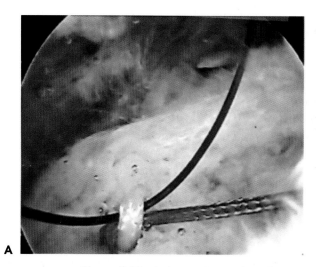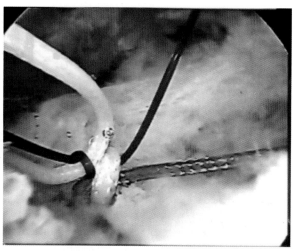

Figure 8-15   Arthroscopic view through a posterior subacromial portal. **A:** The suture anchor eyelet loop has been threaded with a #1 polydioxanone (PDS) suture using a suture lasso. **B:** A nonabsorbable suture is then shuttled through the anchor eyelet.

In poor bone, anchor fixation can be problematic. This usually happens when fixing chronic rotator cuff tears with osteopenic bone in the greater tuberosity. Although anchor pull-out rarely occurs in-line with the direction of insertion (especially when placed at a dead-man's angle), we still test its fixation by an in-line pull. If fixation appears tenuous, one option is to place a larger anchor (e.g., 6.5-mm BioCorkscrew suture anchor). This is easiest when recognizing poor bone quality during punching and tapping and immediately inserting a larger anchor. Usually, if a 5.0-mm BioCorkscrew anchor has already been placed and the anchor partially backs out because of poor bone, a 6.5-mm BioCorkscrew will not provide sufficient fixation either.

In this situation, it is better to push the 5.0-mm BioCorkscrew back slightly below the bone surface, then place a second 5.0-mm BioCorkscrew anchor next to it as a press-fit compressive wedge to achieve an interference fit of an anchor against an anchor. This is done by punching a small pilot hole (through cortex only) directly adjacent to the first anchor, then inserting a second BioCorkscrew without tapping or punching (Fig. 8-17). To prevent simply pushing the first anchor ahead of the second, keep light traction on the sutures of the first anchor as the second anchor is inserted. This second 5.0-mm BioCorkscrew usually provides sufficient interference fit for secure anchor placement. Furthermore, the double-anchor configuration provides four suture pairs for more security of fixation.

Occasionally, the bone will be so osteoporotic that all efforts to obtain good fixation are futile. After trying insertion of various diameter anchors, followed by interference fixation of two side-by-side anchors in which the bone is still inadequate to prevent pullout, a large hole may be seen in the bone, the equivalent of a bone cyst. In such a case, we treat these cavities in the same way that we would treat a large bone cyst, with compaction grafting followed by anchor insertion, as described in the next subsection.

COMPACTION BONE GRAFTING TECHNIQUE FOR BONE CYST AND BONE DEFECTS

Bone defects can occur in the proximal humerus for many different reasons. Degenerative bone cysts of the proximal humerus can be associated with impingement syndrome and rotator cuff pathology. Although these defects are usually small, occasionally they can be sufficiently large to create an area of significant bony deficiency within the proximal humerus. In addition, removal of an implant (e.g., a suture anchor or screw) can leave a significant cavity in the bone as well.

Figure 8-16   The fully threaded BioCorkscrew suture anchor (BioCorkscrew-FT; Arthrex, Inc.; Naples, FL).

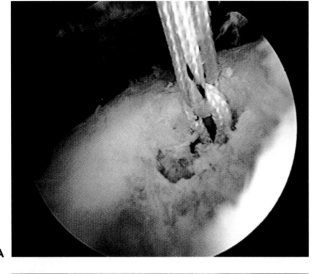

A

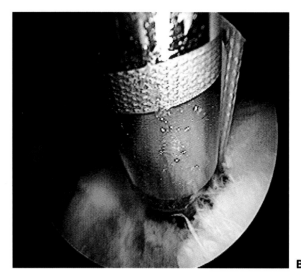

B

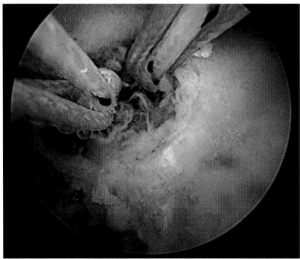

C

Figure 8-17 Arthroscopic view through a posterior subacromial portal of a left shoulder demonstrating the method of interference fixation of an anchor against an anchor in poor bone. **A:** A 5.0-mm BioCorkscrew (Arthrex, Inc.; Naples, FL) suture anchor has been inserted into poor bone and, when tested, pulls out beyond the bone bed. **B:** A second 5.0-mm BioCorkscrew suture anchor is inserted adjacent to the original 5.0-mm BioCorkscrew suture anchor securing both anchors together and to the bone bed via an interference fit. Light traction is applied to the sutures of the first anchor during insertion of the second anchor. **C:** The double-anchor configuration provides four pairs of sutures for fixation.

When a symptomatic rotator cuff tear is associated with a large defect in the bone, arthroscopic treatment of the rotator cuff tear is problematic. These cysts can involve such a large area of the rotator cuff footprint that secure anchor fixation of the rotator cuff cannot be achieved.

The surgical technique begins with a thorough evaluation of the rotator cuff and the cyst. A posterior viewing portal is used and a lateral subacromial working portal is also established. An anterior portal is established for inflow and as an accessory working portal. The rotator cuff is prepared in the usual manner, as previously discussed, and the tear pattern is assessed.

Preparation of the bone bed is carried out in a systematic manner. Even in patients with large bone cysts, a thin rim of intact overlying cortical bone often exists. After clearing the lateral footprint of all soft tissue, the lateral cortex is carefully probed. If an underlying cyst is found, usually an area is seen of soft bone with a springy feel that can be palpated with a probe. A small elevator can then be used to break the overlying cortex of this soft spot, allowing entry to the cyst cavity.

The cyst and its contents are then thoroughly débrided and excavated using an arthroscopic shaver and arthroscopic curettes (Fig. 8-18A). Care is taken to curette the cyst wall of any fibrous tissue. Bone grafting of the cyst is then performed using the disposable osteochondral autograft transfer system (OATS [Arthrex]). We typically use allograft cancellous bone chips or bone croutons and pack them into a 6-mm OATS harvesting tube (or larger-diameter tube if the mouth of the cyst is >6 mm) (Fig. 8-18B). The OATS harvesting tube is then inserted into the subacromial space via an accessory lateral portal that is chosen to give a straight line approach to the mouth of the cyst cavity. Under arthroscopic visualization, the OATS tube is placed at the mouth of the cyst cavity and the cancellous bone graft is inserted into the cyst by means of a screw-in handle on the harvester tube (Fig. 8-18C). This screw-in mechanism compresses the bone graft into the cyst. The bone graft is further compacted using a tamp (Fig. 8-18D). The harvester tube is filled with bone as many times as necessary to fully fill the cystic cavity with compacted bone graft. This process

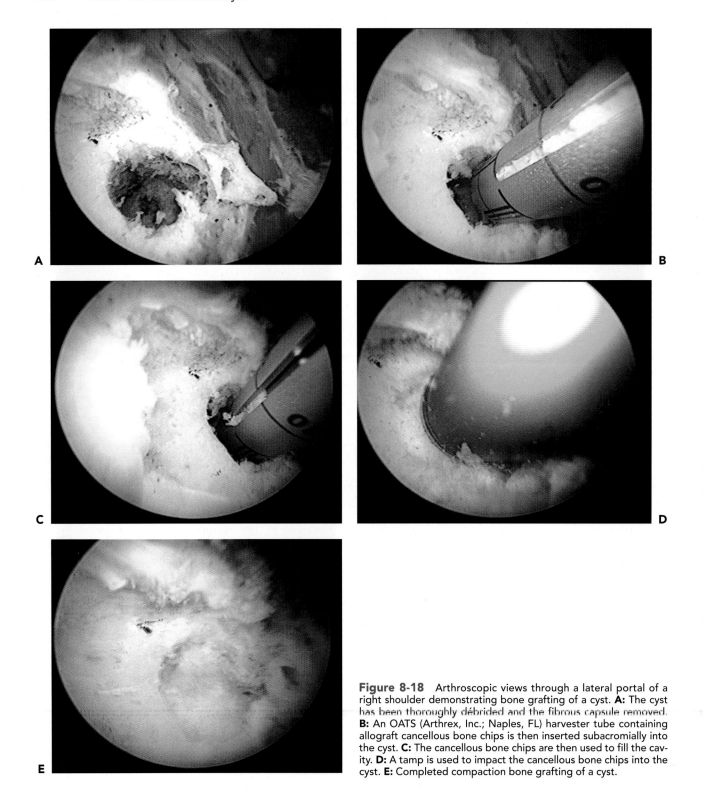

Figure 8-18 Arthroscopic views through a lateral portal of a right shoulder demonstrating bone grafting of a cyst. **A:** The cyst has been thoroughly débrided and the fibrous capsule removed. **B:** An OATS (Arthrex, Inc.; Naples, FL) harvester tube containing allograft cancellous bone chips is then inserted subacromially into the cyst. **C:** The cancellous bone chips are then used to fill the cavity. **D:** A tamp is used to impact the cancellous bone chips into the cyst. **E:** Completed compaction bone grafting of a cyst.

can be repeated as many as seven or eight times until the cyst is completely filled with compacted graft (Fig. 8-18E).

After bone grafting the cyst, a small punch is used to create a starter hole in the packed bone graft and then a standard biodegradable anchor (BioCorkscrew or BioCorkscrew-FT) is placed in the starter hole and screwed into the bone graft. After thoroughly recessing

the suture anchor, the security of fixation is assessed by tugging on the suture limbs that are attached to the suture anchor. Usually, excellent fixation is achieved. If the anchor is felt to be loose, then a second suture anchor can be placed adjacent to the first anchor to achieve interference fixation of an anchor against an anchor within the compacted bone graft. After placement of the anchors,

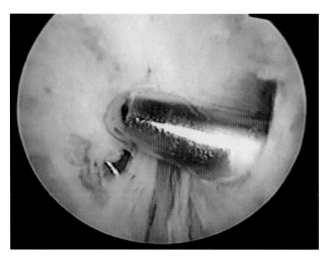

Figure 8-19   The proximal end of a metal anchor is seen above the bone surface of the greater tuberosity.

standard repair of the rotator cuff is completed as previously described.

With very large bone defects, an alternative fixation technique might be chosen in which a larger implant is used to compact the graft maximally for better fixation of

the implant. We have found the Bio-Tenodesis screw (Arthrex) ideal for such an application. After preparing and bone grafting the cyst cavity, #2 FiberWire sutures are placed into the torn rotator cuff margin using the Viper or Scorpion suture passer (Arthrex). Several sutures may be required to adequately reduce the free rotator cuff margin to the edge of the grafted cyst cavity. The Bio-Tenodesis screwdriver is then loaded with the appropriately sized Bio-Tenodesis screw (5.5–9 mm diameter). The traction sutures are then passed through a suture loop that has been threaded through the cannulation of the Bio-Tenodesis screwdriver, so that the loop holds these sutures at the leading edge of the Bio-Tenodesis inserter. A small punch creates a "starter hole" in the grafted bone cyst. The screwdriver tip is then inserted into this channel and the screw is advanced. While inserting the Bio-Tenodesis screw, the rotator cuff sutures are tensioned in such a way that the cuff margin advances snugly against the bone bed adjacent to the Bio-Tenodesis screw. The Bio-Tenodesis screw is advanced until its upper surface is flush with the surface of the bone graft within the bone cyst. Then, the suture ends are passed back through the cuff margin and tied together as a static arthroscopic knot, using a Surgeon's Sixth Finger (Arthrex) knot pusher. In essence, this creates a double row

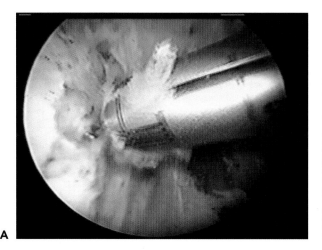

A

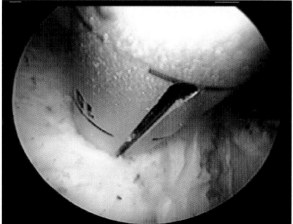

B

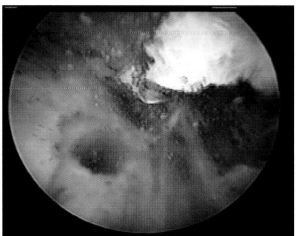

C

Figure 8-20   A: The OATS (Arthrex, Inc.; Naples, FL) harvester is advanced over the anchor, in line with the axis of the anchor. **B:** The OATS harvester is impacted into the bone to a depth of 12 mm. **C:** The screw-in anchor is visible at the base of the OATS harvester as it is removed. Counterclockwise removal of the harvester assures that the screw will withdraw with the bone.

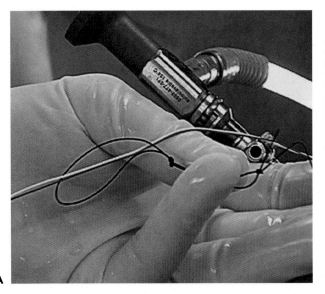

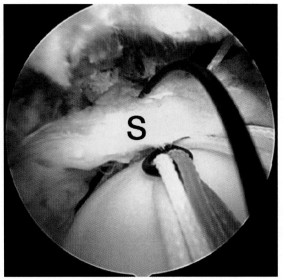

Figure 8-21   Traction shuttle technique. **A:** A loop is tied in the posterior limb of the traction suture and one limb of each # 2 FiberWire suture from the suture anchor is threaded through this loop. Note: The dilator knots are proximal to the loop. **B:** The anterior limb of the traction suture is pulled, advancing the traction loop and anchor sutures through the subscapularis tendon (S).

repair around the large diameter Bio-Tenodesis screw. This technique will give excellent footprint reconstruction.

REMOVING A BROKEN OR "PROUD" METAL SUTURE ANCHOR

On occasion, a situation presents in which a "proud" metal anchor exists in either the glenoid or the proximal

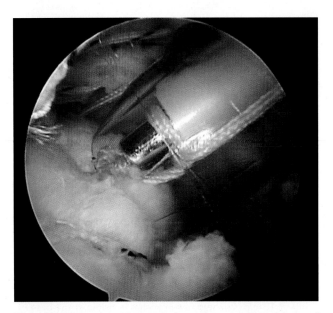

Figure 8-22   Arthroscopic view through a posterior subacromial portal demonstrating knot tying completely within a clear 7.0-mm cannula that has been placed through a lateral portal.

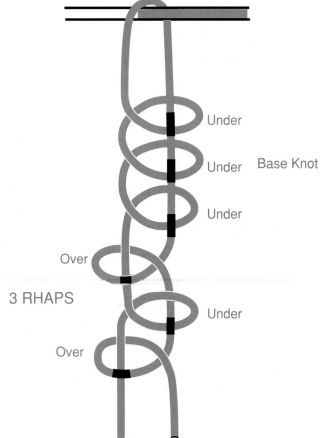

Figure 8-23   Schematic drawing of the Surgeon's knot consisting of a base knot of three half-hitches in the same direction followed by three reversing half-hitches on alternating posts (RHAP).

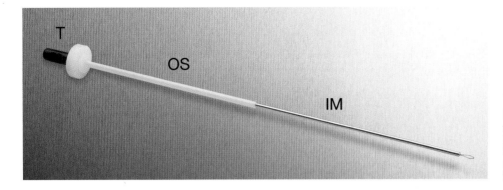

Figure 8-24 Clinical photo of the Surgeon's Sixth Finger (Arthrex, Inc.; Naples, FL) knot pusher. IM, inner cannulated metal tube; OS, outer plastic sleeve; T, suture threader.

humerus. This can occur if the anchor has backed partly out, if it had never been fully seated into the bone, or if it broke during insertion and a portion of it was left above the surface of the bone or the articular cartilage. Such anchors need to be removed before continuing with rotator cuff, Bankart, or superior labrum anterior and posterior (SLAP) lesion repair. This situation is particularly problematic in the case of a Bankart repair because this hard metallic point can rapidly destroy the articular surface on the humeral head if it is not properly addressed. The problems that can occur in extraction of such an anchor vary. In the case of a broken anchor, no way exists to engage an inserter or an extraction tool over the anchor because it no longer has the geometric end that will fit into the inserter. In the case of an anchor that has partly backed out, it may be possible to use an inserter to remove it if it is a screw-in anchor and if the proper inserter is available. The exact type of anchor that has been placed is

not always known, however, and that type of inserter may not be available (Fig. 8-19).

In the case of a push-in anchor, particularly one with barbs, the barbs can prevent extraction with any type of instrument.

The technique that we have found most useful in removing these devices has been to use an OATS harvesting tube to remove a core cylinder of bone that includes the anchor. In the case of a small screw-in anchor, after the cylinder of bone has been removed, the anchor can be unscrewed from the bone and the cylinder of bone can be reinserted as its own graft. In using the OATS harvesting tube as an extractor, be careful to create a portal in which the angle of approach is exactly in line with the axis of the anchor. A spinal needle is used to determine that angle of approach

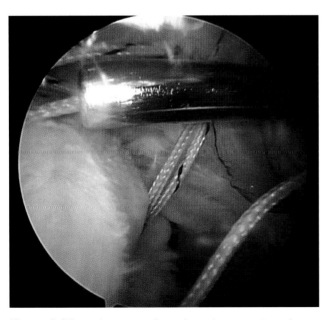

Figure 8-25 Arthroscopic photo through a posterior subacromial viewing portal of a right shoulder as the inner metallic tube is pushed through the cannula and down to the rotator cuff tissue.

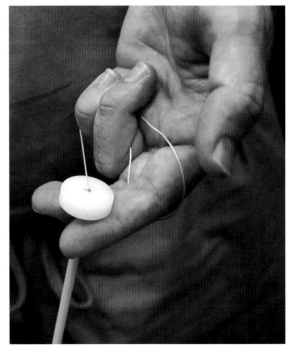

Figure 8-26 Clinical photo demonstrating use of the Surgeon's Sixth Finger (Arthrex, Inc.; Naples, FL) knot pusher. Any excess suture from the post limb is wrapped around the fingers of the hand.

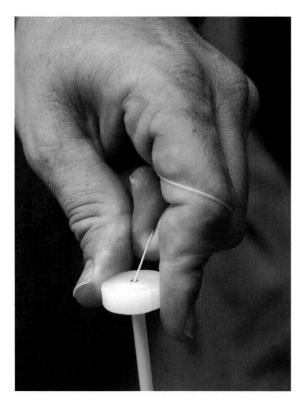

Figure 8-27 Clinical photo demonstrating use of the Surgeon's Sixth Finger (Arthrex, Inc.; Naples, FL) knot pusher. Tension is provided along the post limb by pulling on the post limb while pushing the knot pusher.

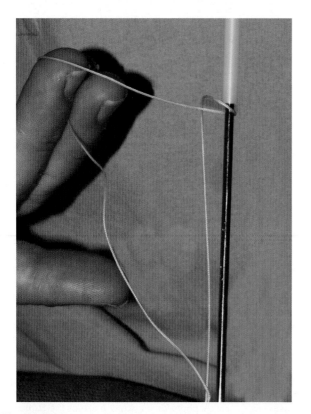

Figure 8-28 Clinical photo demonstrating a half-hitch throw around the inner metallic post.

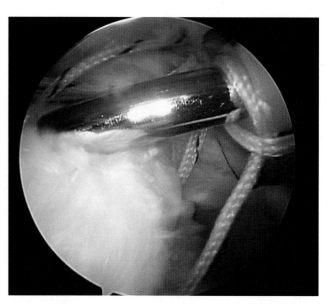

Figure 8-29 Arthroscopic photo through a lateral viewing portal of a right shoulder demonstrating a half-hitch, which is pushed into the joint and against the tissue using the outer plastic sleeve.

and then a portal is established. For all of the standard glenoid anchors, a 5.5-mm OATS harvester tube provides sufficient clearance to go around the anchor. In the proximal humerus, a larger harvester tube may be necessary, depending on the type of anchor that has been used. The OATS harvester tube is impacted around the anchor for a depth of 12 to 15 mm, which is the length of most suture anchors (Fig. 8-20). In the case of a screw-in anchor, the OATS harvester should be removed by rotating it in a counterclockwise direction, which is the same direction as would be used to unscrew the anchor. In this way, in the event that the screw threads extend beyond the core of bone that the OATS harvester has encompassed, the remaining threads will simply be unscrewed from the bone. If the anchor can be extracted in such a way that an intact cylinder of bone remains to place in the cylindrical cavity that has been created, this extracted bone can be reinserted as its own graft. If the anchor cannot be removed in such a way as to preserve the bone as a graft, we prefer to use bone chips or bone croutons, inserting them by means of a disposable OATS harvester tube into which these bone chips have been compacted. This method is explained in further detail under the preceding section entitled *Compaction Bone Grafting Technique for Bone Cyst and Bone Defects.*

In the case of extraction of a glenoid anchor, we prefer to place additional anchors above and below the defect created by extraction of the anchor. If necessary, an anchor can be placed back into that defect after compaction grafting has been accomplished.

In the case of extraction of an anchor from the proximal humerus, the subsequent anchors can be placed within the grafted area, if necessary. The geometry and pattern of the tear will determine where the anchors must be placed.

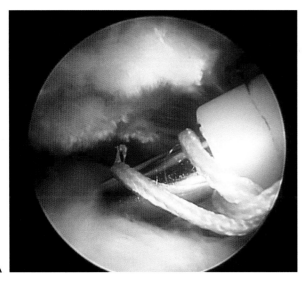 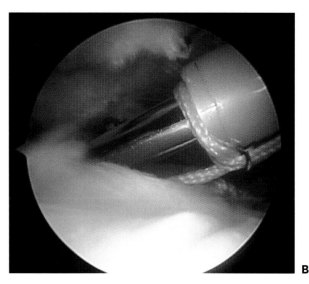

A   B

Figure 8-30 Arthroscopic photo through a lateral viewing portal. **A:** A half-hitch has been pushed down into the joint, but is twisted. **B:** The half-hitch is untwisted by turning the outer plastic sleeve (clockwise in this case), allowing the half-hitch to be advanced without twists, eliminating slack between throws.

SHUTTLE SUTURES USING A NONABSORBABLE SUTURE: THE DILATOR KNOT

Occasionally, it is necessary to shuttle sutures through soft tissue when various direct-passage instruments are not able to pass directly through tissue. One option is to use a Suture Lasso (Arthrex) and a suture passing wire. Another option is to use a "traction shuttle technique." In this technique, a braided suture from the anchor is passed through the tendon by threading the suture through a loop on a previously placed traction suture and then pulling the traction suture through the tendon (Fig. 8-21). In this way, the traction suture becomes a shuttle for the anchor suture. To aid in passage of this large bulk of suture through the tendon, two progressively larger "dilator knots" are tied in the traction suture proximal to the loop. This progressively enlarges the hole in the tendon so that the traction suture will not break when its bulky knot is pulled through the tendon. This essentially "shuttles" the braided suture through the tendon.

TYING KNOTS IN A CANNULA

When tying knots, it is not just the arthroscopist who must be facile with the procedure but also an assistant. After retrieval of sutures through the cannula, an assistant must be able to stabilize the camera so that visualization of knot tying is complete. In addition, it is exceptionally helpful if the same assistant (or another assistant) can stabilize the cannula through which knot tying is being performed. Furthermore, the cannula should be directed toward the sutures being tied and should be stabilized so that the cannula does not move or fall out as the knot is being tied. Be careful that the suture does not abrade against the edge of the cannula. This can groove the cannula and damage the suture, weakening the final construct.

Tying through a clear cannula is also advantageous. A clear cannula expands the working space during knot tying such that in cases of significant swelling, a knot can be tied completely within the cannula itself (Fig. 8-22).

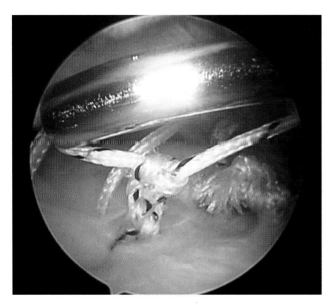

Figure 8-31 Arthroscopic photo through a lateral viewing portal of a right shoulder demonstrating past-pointing to maximize knot security.

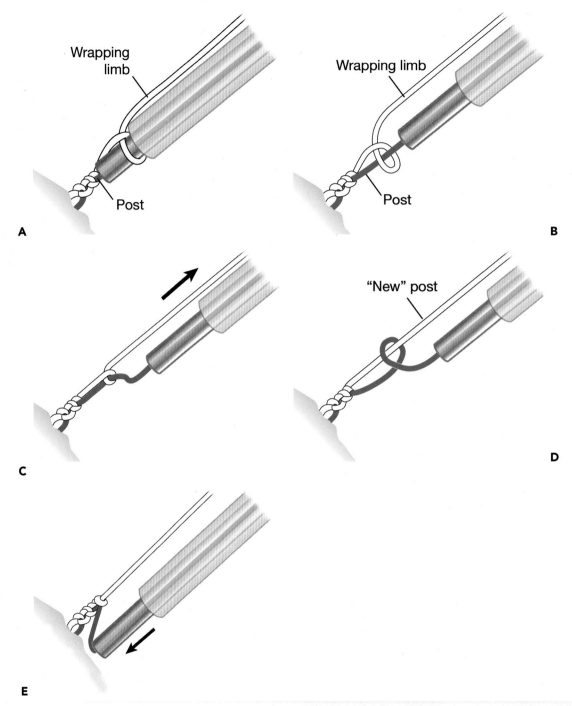

Figure 8-32 Switching posts without rethreading. **A:** Advance the half-hitch with a double-diameter knot pusher. **B:** Back off the knot pusher by ~10 to 15 mm and **(C)** then advance the knot pusher. While advancing the knot pusher, pull on the wrapping limb. **D:** This flips the post and converts the wrapping limb to the new post limb. **E:** Past-point to tighten the knot.

Tying Knots with the Sixth Finger Knot Pusher

To ensure both loop security and knot security, we prefer to tie an arthroscopic knot composed of six stacked half-hitches with a double-diameter knot pusher (Surgeon's Sixth Finger) (Fig. 8-23)(see Chapter 3: *Achieving a Stable Construct*). By using the Surgeon's Sixth Finger knot pusher (Fig. 8-24), continuous tension can be maintained on the post limb as sequential half-hitches are thrown. This prevents loosening of the soft tissue loop between throws (maximizing loop security). Furthermore, the tissue to be secured can be manipulated into place using the end of the Surgeon's Sixth Finger.

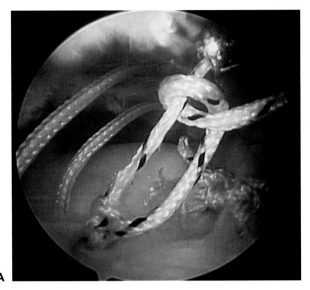
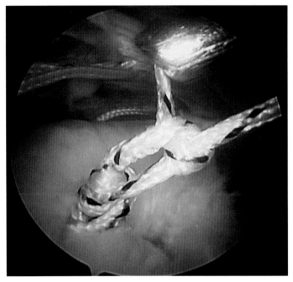

A   B

Figure 8-33 Arthroscopic view through a posterior subacromial portal demonstrating reversing the half-hitch and alternating the posts by tensioning the wrapping limb. **A:** Over-under half-hitch has been advanced down the post limb with the knot pusher. The knot pusher is backed off the knot. **B:** Then, the wrapping limb is tensioned, reversing the half-hitch and alternating the post. The new configuration is an under-over half-hitch, with the knot pusher now on the wrapping limb, and the post limb being the one without the knot pusher.

The Surgeon's Sixth Finger knot pusher consists of an inner cannulated metallic post and an outer plastic sleeve, which freely slides along the inner metallic post to push sequential half-hitches down the metallic post (see Fig. 8-24). To tie an arthroscopic knot, we first retrieve both suture limbs out a separate cannula with equal length on both limbs. All other sutures are held out of the way in temporary holding portals. One limb of the suture (i.e., the post limb) is threaded through the inner metallic tube using the suture threader and the inner metallic tube of the knot pusher is pushed through the cannula down to the tissue (Fig. 8-25). We usually choose the limb that penetrates the soft tissue, so that when the knot is tied it is tied on the tissue portion of the repair construct. Any excess suture from the post limb is wrapped around the fingers of the hand to provide tension along the post limb (Fig. 8-26). While tying, tension can be applied to the post limb by pulling on the post limb while pushing on the knot pusher (Fig. 8-27).

While maintaining tension on the post limb, we tie a base knot consisting of three stacked half-hitches in the same direction. The opposite hand is used to throw sequential half-hitches around the inner metallic post (Fig. 8-28), which are then pushed down the inner metallic post using the outer plastic sleeve (Fig. 8-29). When pushing half-hitches down the inner metallic sleeve, any twists in the half-hitch are unraveled by turning the outer plastic sleeve (Fig. 8-30). Past-pointing is used to tighten each throw (Fig. 8-31), minimizing slack between throws and maximizing knot security. This initial base knot is followed by three additional half-hitches in which the post is reversed for each throw using the technique described below. Thus, when tying a surgeon's knot, using a

Surgeon's Sixth Finger knot pusher, we throw the same half-hitch around the inner metallic sleeve six times. We "flip" the fourth and sixth throws, however.

REVERSING THE HALF-HITCH AND ALTERNATING THE POST WITHOUT RETHREADING: FLIPPING THE KNOT

All knots, whether stacked half-hitches or sliding knots, should be secured with a series of three reversing half-hitches on alternating posts. This configuration increases both knot and loop security of static or sliding knots. One method to do this is to rethread the knot pusher to the opposite suture limb after each throw, reversing the next half-hitch. Rethreading three consecutive half-hitches, however, can be a time-consuming process.

Instead, the half-hitch can be reversed and the post simultaneously alternated by tensioning the wrapping limb (1). This can be performed whether using a standard knot pusher or a double-diameter knot pusher (Surgeon's Sixth Finger). To "flip the post" using a double-diameter knot pusher, first tie a base knot (either a sliding knot or a series of three half-hitches) (Figs. 8-32 and 8-33). Then, advance the next half-hitch down the double-diameter knot pusher, using the outer plastic sleeve. As the half-hitch approaches the tip of the double-diameter knot pusher, the knot pusher is backed off by ~10 to 15 mm. Then, release the tension in the post limb and pull the tension in the wrapping limb. This differential tensioning "flips" the knot so that the knot pusher, which had been threaded on the post suture limb, is now threaded on the

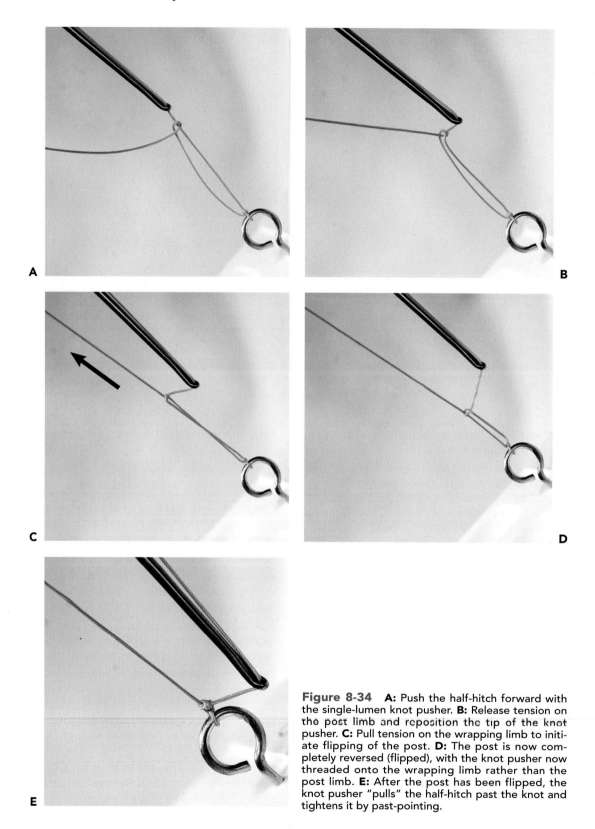

Figure 8-34 A: Push the half-hitch forward with the single-lumen knot pusher. **B:** Release tension on the post limb and reposition the tip of the knot pusher. **C:** Pull tension on the wrapping limb to initiate flipping of the post. **D:** The post is now completely reversed (flipped), with the knot pusher now threaded onto the wrapping limb rather than the post limb. **E:** After the post has been flipped, the knot pusher "pulls" the half-hitch past the knot and tightens it by past-pointing.

wrapping limb. Then advance the knot pusher to "pull" the half-hitch onto the top of the knot stack by past-pointing beyond the knot. This maneuver simultaneously alternates the post and reverses the half-hitch. "Flipping" the post can also be performed using a single-diameter knot pusher along with the same maneuvers of differential tensioning (Fig. 8-34).

REFERENCE

1. Chan KC, Burkhart SS. How to switch posts without rethreading when tying half-hitches. *Arthroscopy.* 1999;15:444–450.

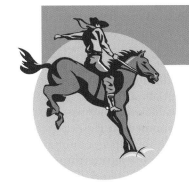

9

Order of Steps

COWBOY PRINCIPLE 9

Before you go into a canyon, know how you'll get out.

On the trail, the cowboy starts every day with a plan. The plan is always flexible enough to adapt to unanticipated challenges, but the basic structure of daily goals is always there. The cowboy is adaptable, thinking his way to a better solution. Unlike most of his pompous city-dwelling detractors, he knows there is a clear-cut difference between horse sense and mule-headedness. After all, every jackass thinks he has horse sense.

Shoulder arthroscopy allows the simultaneous treatment of multiple disorders. This can include multiple pathologies related to the same diagnosis (e.g., type II superior labrum anterior and posterior [SLAP] lesion and Bankart lesion) and differing pathologies related to different diagnoses (e.g., Bankart lesion and rotator cuff tear). When faced with multiple pathologies, the order in which to proceed with each diagnosis can become critical. Treatment order becomes a factor because certain procedures are "timed" procedures where shoulder swelling will compromise an effective repair or where fixation of certain pathologies will make other repairs more difficult.

ROTATOR CUFF TEARS

In general, soft tissue swelling will compromise the tight anterior portion of the joint before it affects other areas. We, therefore, usually approach any subscapularis tendon or anterior joint pathology first. This can include subscapularis tendon tears, biceps tendinopathy or instability, and subcoracoid process impingement. Any biceps pathology identified is treated initially. The biceps is tagged with one or two racking sutures. Then, it is released and brought out extracorporeally. A whipstitch is placed to securely tag the biceps tendon, which is then tucked out of the way into the anterolateral subacromial space for later tenodesis. If only a tenotomy is to be performed, the biceps tendon is released without tagging.

The subscapularis tendon can now be evaluated thoroughly again without the long head of the biceps (particularly if dislocated) obstructing visualization. We observe the subscapularis tendon through a posterior viewing portal using both 30° and 70° arthroscopes to obtain an "aerial view." If evidence is seen of subcoracoid impingement in addition to a subscapularis tear, arthroscopic coracoplasty is performed next. Performing an arthroscopic coracoplasty will increase the working space available anteriorly for subscapularis tendon repair. In addition, in the process of dissecting the coracoid and performing a coracoplasty, the coracohumeral ligament is partially released. This begins the process of mobilizing the subscapularis tendon for later repair. Following arthroscopic coracoplasty and subscapularis tendon release, arthroscopic subscapularis repair is performed next.

After arthroscopic subscapularis tendon repair, we perform a subacromial decompression and the superior and posterior rotator cuff is repaired, if necessary. We usually perform a subacromial decompression (modified to preserve the coracoacromial arch in cases of massive rotator cuff tear), plus or minus distal clavicle excision before biceps tenodesis and repair of the superior and posterior rotator cuff. Next, we tenodese the biceps tendon along the anterolateral corner of the supraspinatus footprint adjacent to the bicipital groove. The tenodesis is performed where we would normally place an anterolateral suture anchor and, therefore, we use the tenodesis screw to replace this anchor. We use the extra sutures from the tenodesis (whipstitch suture ends and racking-hitch suture ends) for suture passage through the rotator cuff. This saves both an anchor and space on the limited anterolateral aspect of the supraspinatus footprint.

If performing a double row rotator cuff repair to reconstruct the footprint, we insert anchors and pass sutures for the medial row first. Then, we proceed with lateral row anchor insertion and suture passage. The lateral row of anchors is then tied first with the arm in 30° to 45° of abduction. This lateralizes the rotator cuff to the lateral aspect of the footprint. The arm is then brought down into adduction and the medial row is tied, compressing the rotator cuff against the footprint.

LABRAL TEARS

Triple labral lesions involving tears of the anterior, posterior, and superior labra are the most complex labral tears. In the case of triple labral lesions, we first place anchors and pass sutures for the superior labral tear. We do not tie the sutures down initially, however. Tying the superior labral sutures early will tighten the glenohumeral joint, making subsequent repair of the anterior and posterior labra more difficult. In addition, waiting to pass sutures through the superior labrum until after anterior and posterior labral repair is usually difficult because the superior sulcus (overlying the superior labrum) will have become swollen and obliterated. This makes suture passage and visualization of the superior labrum difficult.

After suture passage through the superior labrum, the anterior labrum is repaired while viewing through an anterosuperolateral portal. Again, we do not tie the anterior sutures until after the posterior pathology has been addressed by anchor insertion and suture passage. We tie sutures sequentially, starting anteroinferiorly and progressing anterosuperiorly, then going posteroinferiorly and progressing posterosuperiorly. Finally, we tie the sutures for the superior labrum.

ROTATOR CUFF AND LABRAL TEARS

In the event of a combined rotator cuff and labral repair, the pathologies are addressed in this sequence.

1. Biceps tendon release and whipstitch placed
2. Subcoracoid decompression
3. Subscapularis repair
4. Superior labrum anchor insertion and suture passage
5. Anterior labral anchor insertion and suture passage
6. Posterior labral anchor insertion and suture passage
7. Tying of anterior labral sutures, posterior labral sutures, and superior labral sutures
8. Biceps tenodesis
9. Superior and posterior rotator cuff repair

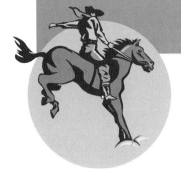

Rotator Cuff Tear Patterns: Repairing a Tear the Way It Ought to Be

10

COWBOY PRINCIPLE 10

There are usually two ways to do things: the easy way and the cowboy way.

Cowboys know that simple-minded solutions are usually not the best ones, and that logic must be at the core of every decision. Although simple solutions can be profound, simple-minded ones are shallow and often ill-advised. The easy way is not necessarily the right way.

Traditional open surgical management of rotator cuff tears has historically been limited by an anterolateral exposure. This restricted "window of visualization," however, has created a bias toward medial to lateral repair of the torn rotator cuff to bring the tendon into the window of visualization. In contrast, arthroscopy is not restricted by spatial constraints and, because of this, rotator cuff tears can now be assessed and treated arthroscopically from several different angles with minimal disruption to the overlying deltoid muscle. This new perspective on evaluating and treating rotator cuff tears refutes routine medial to lateral repair of the rotator cuff and emphasizes the importance of understanding and recognizing rotator cuff tear patterns. Repairing the tear according to its natural mobility decreases repair tension, limits tension overload (a common cause of failure of rotator cuff repairs), and improves the results of treatment.

ASSESSING MOBILITY

The key element in identifying rotator cuff tear patterns is a complete and accurate assessment of the intrinsic (i.e., before release) mobility of the rotator cuff tear. This assessment is performed precisely in a step-wise progression to ensure proper identification and, therefore, repair of the rotator cuff tear (Fig. 10-1). While assessing the mobility of the rotator cuff tendon tear, we begin the process of mentally visualizing the proposed rotator cuff repair construct (including tendon, anchor, and suture placement). This simultaneous integration of tear pattern recognition and repair construct formulation will ensure rapid and reproducible rotator cuff repair.

Medial to Lateral Mobility

Medial to lateral mobility of the rotator cuff tear is assessed first. Some tears, even though massive, can have significant mobility in the medial to lateral direction. To assess the medial to lateral mobility of a rotator cuff tear, a tendon grasper is introduced through a lateral portal while viewing through a posterior portal (Fig. 10-2A). The medial aspect of the rotator cuff tendon tear is then grasped and pulled to the bone bed laterally (Fig. 10-2B). If the rotator cuff tendon tear is reducible under minimal tension to (or close to) the lateral aspect of the footprint, the tear is a crescent-shaped rotator cuff tear. Because of their significant medial to lateral mobility, crescent-shaped rotator cuff tears can be repaired anatomically by direct tendon-to-bone repair. In particular, these tears are highly amenable

Text continues on page 197.

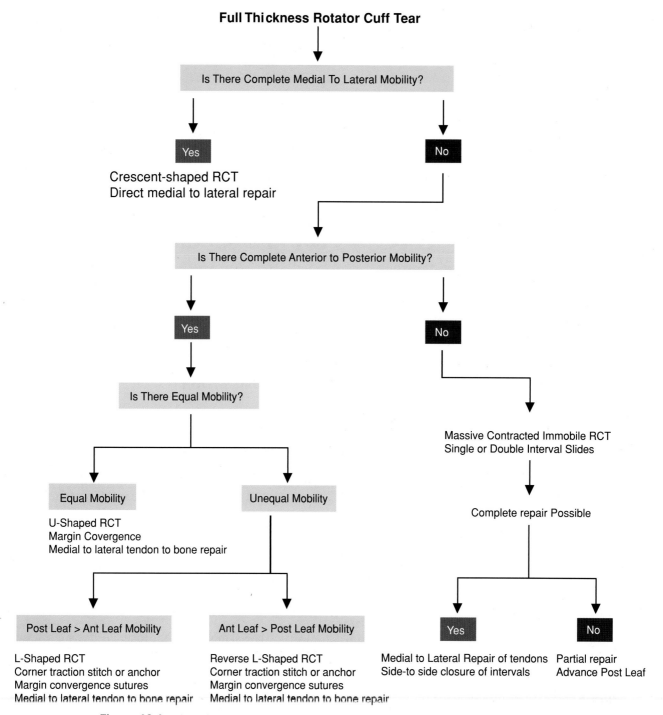

Figure 10-1   Chart demonstrating the step-wise progression of mobility assessment of rotator cuff tears.

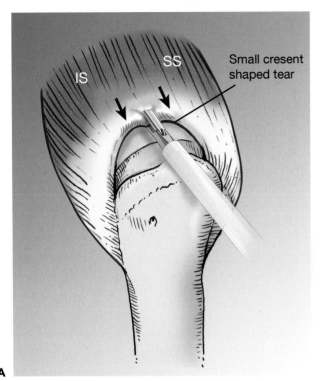

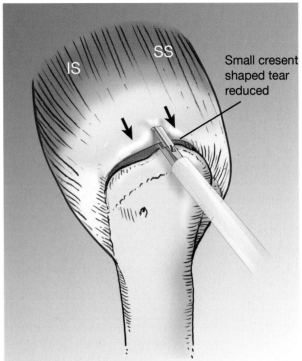

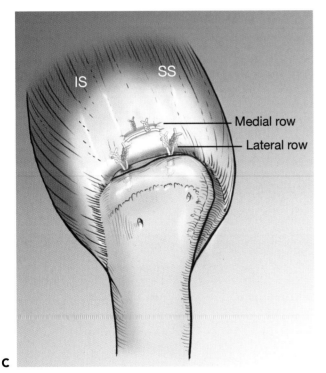

Figure 10-2 Assessment of medial to lateral mobility. **A:** A tendon grasper introduced through a lateral portal is used to grasp the medial aspect of the rotator cuff tendon tear while viewing through a posterior portal. **B:** The rotator cuff tendon tear is then pulled laterally toward the bone bed, and the medial to lateral mobility of the tendon is assessed. **C:** Double row rotator cuff repair construct of a crescent-shaped rotator cuff tear viewed through a lateral portal. IS, infraspinatus tendon; SS, supraspinatus tendon.

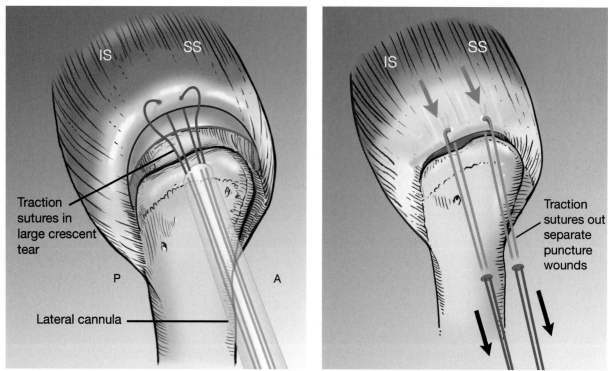

Figure 10-3 Large crescent-shaped rotator cuff tear. **A:** Traction sutures are placed along the medial margin of the rotator cuff tear. **B:** Lateral traction allows reduction of the tendon margin toward the bone bed as an assessment of cuff tear mobility. IS, infraspinatus tendon; SS, supraspinatus tendon; P, posterior; A, anterior.

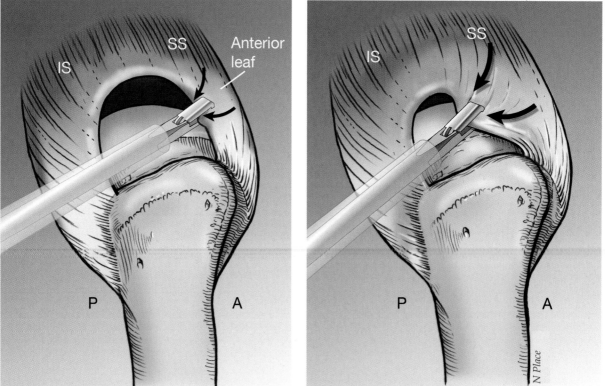

Figure 10-4 Posterior mobility of the anterior leaf. **A:** While viewing through a lateral subacromial portal, a tendon grasper is introduced through the posterior portal to grasp the anterior leaf of the rotator cuff tear. **B:** Traction is applied in a posterior direction to determine the posterior mobility of the anterior leaf. IS, infraspinatus tendon; SS, supraspinatus tendon; P, posterior; A, anterior.

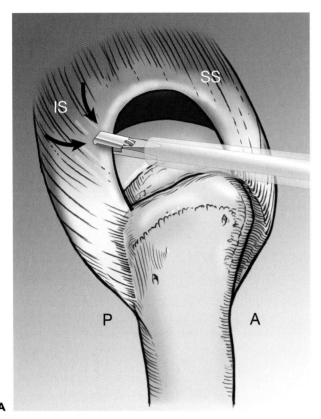

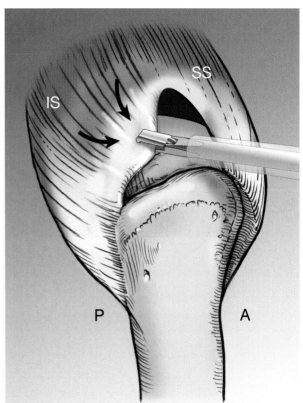

A   **B**

Figure 10-5   Anterior mobility of the posterior leaf. **A:** A tendon grasper is introduced through an anterior portal to grasp the posterior leaf of the rotator cuff tear. **B:** Traction is applied in an anterior direction to determine the anterior mobility of the posterior leaf. IS, infraspinatus tendon; SS, supraspinatus tendon; P, posterior; A, anterior.

to double-row repair to reconstruct the footprint of the rotator cuff (Fig. 10-2C).

In larger crescent-shaped rotator cuff tears, it can be difficult to reduce the entire rotator cuff tear completely with a single tendon grasper. In this situation, traction sutures placed along the margin of the rotator cuff can assist in tendon reduction and assessment of mobility along the tendon margin (Fig. 10-3A,B). It is important when placing traction sutures to place them in the correct position in the tendon *and* to retrieve them out the appropriate portal to apply the proper direction of tension.

Anterior to Posterior Mobility

If the tear is not completely reducible under minimal tension in a medial to lateral direction, then the anterior to posterior mobility of the tear is assessed. Assessment of anterior to posterior mobility is performed while viewing through the lateral "50 yard line" portal. While viewing through this portal, the tendon grasper is introduced through the posterior portal to grasp the anterior leaf of the rotator cuff tear (Fig. 10-4A). Traction is applied in a posterior direction to determine the mobility of the anterior leaf

of the rotator cuff tear (Fig. 10-4B). Similarly, to determine the anterior mobility of the posterior leaf, a tendon grasper is introduced through an anterior portal and the posterior leaf of the rotator cuff tear is grasped (Fig. 10-5A). Traction is then applied in an anterior direction to determine the anterior mobility of the posterior leaf (Fig. 10-5B).

Significant and equal mobility of the tendon margins in an anterior to posterior direction (i.e., anterior mobility of the posterior leaf equals posterior mobility of the anterior leaf) represents a U-shaped rotator cuff tear. U-shaped tears are amenable to initial side-to-side suturing of the anterior and posterior leaves to accomplish margin convergence of the rotator cuff laterally toward the bone bed (Fig. 10-6A,B). Following margin convergence of the rotator cuff tear, tendon-to-bone fixation can be performed. These tears may be amenable to a double row repair. Advanced mental visualization of the repair construct is necessary, however, because placement of the medial row can be difficult if margin convergence sutures have already been placed and tied. Tying these side-to-side sutures early in the repair construct phase can inadvertently tension the rotator cuff tendon against the bone bed, obstructing placement of the

Text continues on page 200.

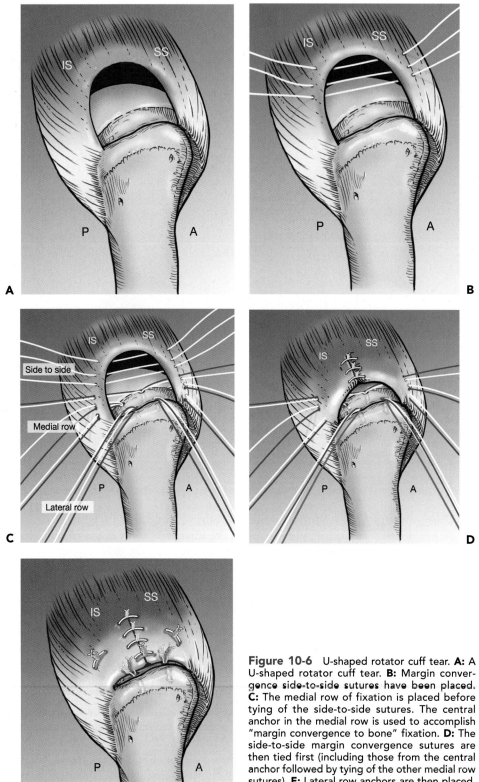

Figure 10-6 U-shaped rotator cuff tear. **A:** A U-shaped rotator cuff tear. **B:** Margin convergence side-to-side sutures have been placed. **C:** The medial row of fixation is placed before tying of the side-to-side sutures. The central anchor in the medial row is used to accomplish "margin convergence to bone" fixation. **D:** The side-to-side margin convergence sutures are then tied first (including those from the central anchor followed by tying of the other medial row sutures). **E:** Lateral row anchors are then placed, and their sutures provide a complete double row rotator cuff repair construct for this U-shaped rotator cuff tendon tear. IS, infraspinatus tendon; SS, supraspinatus tendon; P, posterior; A, anterior.

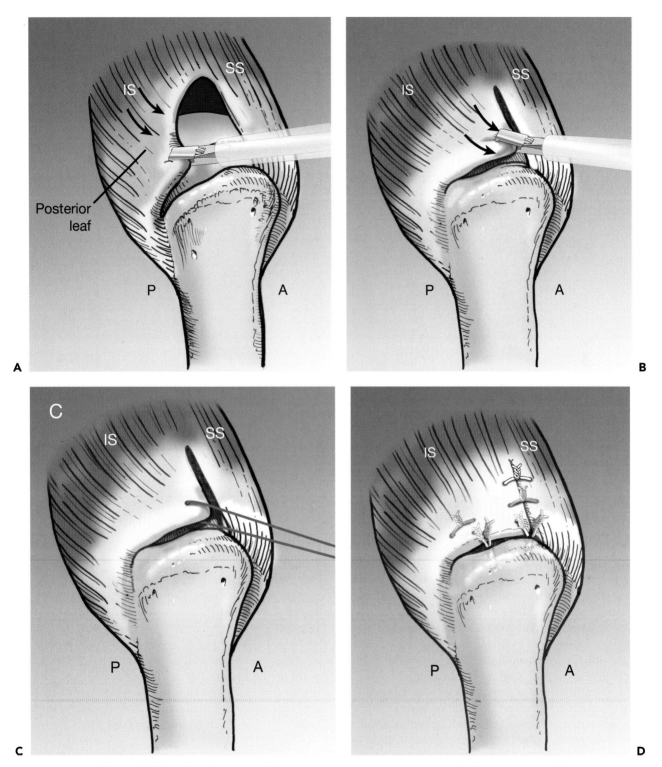

Figure 10-7   L-shaped rotator cuff tendon tear. Arthroscopic views through a lateral subacromial portal. **A:** A tendon grasper is introduced through an anterior portal to grasp a point on the posterior leaf of the rotator cuff tendon tear. **B:** The tendon margin is then pulled anteriorly and laterally toward the bone bed, reducing the tear. **C:** A traction stitch is placed at the corner of the tear to temporarily reduce the tendon during creation of the rotator cuff repair construct. **D:** Double row rotator cuff repair construct of an L-shaped rotator cuff tear. IS, infraspinatus tendon; SS, supraspinatus tendon; P, posterior; A, anterior.

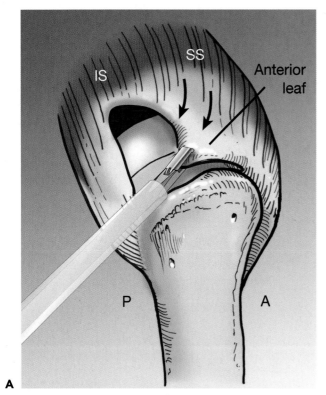
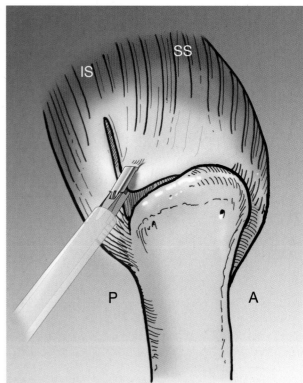

Figure 10-8 Reverse L-shaped rotator cuff tendon tear. **A:** A tendon grasper is introduced through a posterior portal to grasp a point on the anterior leaf of the rotator cuff tendon tear. **B:** The tendon margin is then pulled posteriorly and laterally toward the bone bed, reducing the tear. IS, infraspinatus tendon; SS, supraspinatus tendon; P, posterior; A, anterior.

medial row of anchors and sutures. In this situation, medial row suture anchor placement and suture passage are usually performed after side-to-side margin convergence suture placement, but before tying the side-to-side sutures. The middle anchor of the medial row is used to accomplish "margin convergence to bone" by using its sutures for side-to-side repair. After the medial row has been tied, lateral anchors are placed and their sutures are passed and tied as simple sutures (Fig. 10-6C,D,E). This sequence of tying the medial row before tying the lateral row for U-shaped tears is just the opposite of what we do for large crescent-shaped tears (where we tie the lateral row sutures first).

With significant but unequal medial to lateral mobility, the tear pattern is that of an L-shaped or reverse-L rotator cuff tear. These tears have significant longitudinal splitting between the leading edge of the supraspinatus tendon and the rotator interval (i.e., L-shaped rotator cuff tear) or between the supraspinatus and infraspinatus tendons (i.e., reverse L-shaped rotator cuff tear). In this situation, it is very important to determine the corner of the L-shaped tear, which is usually best determined while viewing through the lateral portal.

If the tear is an L-shaped tear, a tendon grasper is introduced through an anterior or accessory anterolateral portal and a point on the posterior leaf of the rotator cuff is grasped (Fig. 10-7A) and pulled anteriorly and laterally

toward the bone bed (Fig. 10-7B). Different points along the posterior leaf are evaluated for their anterolateral mobility to determine the point with the most mobility (i.e., the corner of the tear) to allow anatomic reconstruction. It is helpful to place a traction stitch at the corner of the tear to reduce the tear so that placement of anchors and passage of sutures can be performed accurately (Fig. 10-7C). These tears can also be amenable to double row repair (Fig. 10-7D).

Similarly, if the tear is a reverse L-shaped tear, the tendon grasper is introduced through a posterior portal and a point on the anterior leaf of the rotator cuff is grasped and pulled posteriorly and laterally toward the bone bed. Once the corner of the tear is identified, it is repaired in the same sequence as an L-shaped tear (Fig. 10-8A,B).

Minimal or No Medial to Lateral and Anterior to Posterior Mobility

With minimal medial to lateral and anterior to posterior mobility of the tendon, the tear usually represents a massive contracted immobile rotator cuff tear (Fig. 10-9A,B,C). These tears are not amenable to direct medial to lateral repair or margin convergence. They are usually only amenable to repair by interval slide techniques (see Chapter 5 for a complete discussion of the techniques

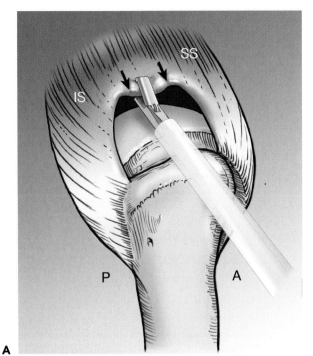

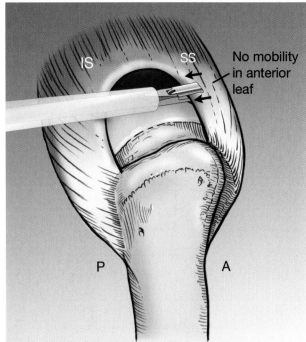

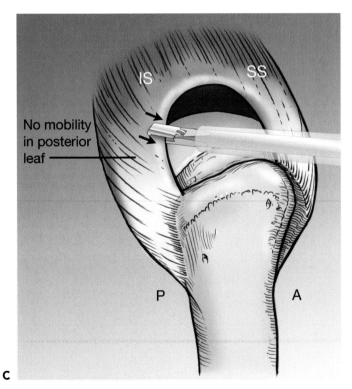

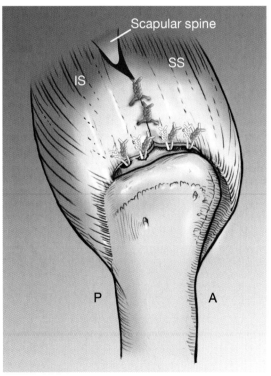

Figure 10-9   Massive adhesed contracted immobile rotator cuff tear. **A:** Traction in a medial to lateral direction demonstrates minimal mobility in that direction. **B:** Posterior traction applied to the anterior leaf demonstrates minimal posterior mobility. **C:** Anterior traction applied to the posterior leaf demonstrates minimal mobility of that leaf. **D:** Rotator cuff repair construct following double interval slide of a massive contracted immobile rotator cuff tear. IS, infraspinatus tendon; SS, supraspinatus tendon; P, posterior; A, anterior.

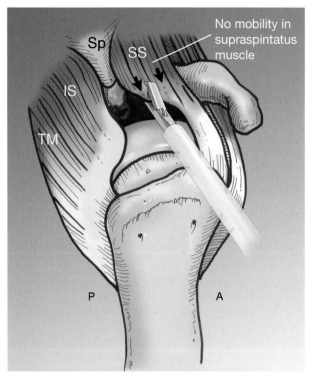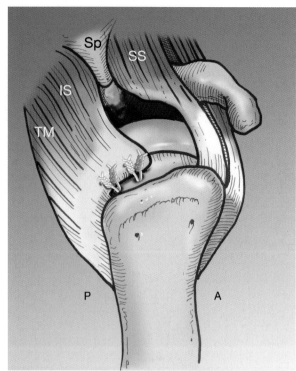

Figure 10-10 Partial repair of a massive contracted immobile rotator cuff tear. **A:** Following double interval slide, the supraspinatus tendon still cannot be brought laterally to the bone bed. **B:** A partial repair is performed, advancing the posterior leaf (infraspinatus, teres minor *(TM)* tendons) superiorly and laterally. IS, infraspinatus tendon; Sp, scapular spine; SS, supraspinatus tendon; P, posterior; A, anterior.

of single and double interval slide as well as interval slide in continuity). With development of the interval slide techniques, particularly the double interval slide, we now find that most rotator cuff tears are fully repairable (Fig. 10-9D).

Although rotator cuff repair is possible using these interval slide techniques, a double row repair may not be possible. By using the double interval slide, however, irreparable tears are distinctly unusual and the indications

for partial repair are diminishing. Partial repair is performed in the situation that, despite an anterior and posterior interval slide, the supraspinatus tendon is still not amenable to repair (Fig. 10-10A). In this scenario, the posterior cuff (i.e., the infraspinatus and teres minor tendons) is advanced superiorly and laterally to a more biomechanically favorable position by tendon-to-bone repair to better balance the anterior forces from the subscapularis tendon (Fig. 10-10B).

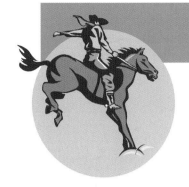

Postoperative Rehabilitation

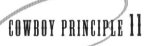

11

COWBOY PRINCIPLE 11

Never spur a horse when he's swimming.

A cowboy with horse-sense never confuses pain with persuasion. Equanimity and ego travel different trails.

REHABILITATION AFTER ARTHROSCOPIC ROTATOR CUFF REPAIR

The senior author (SSB) has long believed that early range of motion after rotator cuff repair is contraindicated in most cases. This belief was based on personal observations of intraoperative knot failure during open rotator cuff repair when patients had their shoulder taken through a range of motion. In fact, at the time of open repair, if the surgeon takes the patient's arm up to 180° of elevation six or seven times in a row, the last throw of the knot will typically come untied because of the generation of large torsional forces within the knot. If the arm is then taken through another six or seven overhead elevations, the second throw of the knot will come untied and the knot will sequentially fail in this manner. Furthermore, if one looks arthroscopically at a single row repair in which the rotator cuff is nicely apposed to the rotator cuff footprint with the

arm at the side, and then brings the arm into overhead elevation, the medial portion of the footprint lifts off the prepared greater tuberosity bone bed. If this is occurring repetitively, no chance for healing exists at this interface because of the continual motion between tendon and bone. We, therefore, have generally attempted to immobilize our rotator cuff repairs for the first 6 weeks after surgery to achieve secure biologic healing before starting range of motion maneuvers.

More recently, additional basic science information suggests that immobilization is beneficial to rotator cuff healing. Soslowsky and associates have presented information that significant increases in strain occur at the repaired rotator cuff margin if the arm is brought passively into the overhead position (personal communication 2003).

A recent study by Gerber (1) showed that, with early passive motion after rotator cuff repair, the collagen fibers tended to align in a random fashion, whereas with immobilization for several weeks, the collagen fibers aligned in a parallel array, giving stronger resistance to applied forces. Based on the above information, it seems evident that a period of immobilization to allow healing of the rotator cuff to bone would be beneficial.

One of the most appealing features of shoulder arthroscopy in comparison with open surgery is that little scarring occurs between the deltoid muscle and underlying tissues with the arthroscopic approach. For that reason, immobilization for 6 weeks does not result in the extreme stiffness that would occur with a similar period of immobilization after open repair.

In general, following arthroscopic rotator cuff repair, our rehabilitation protocol is as follows:

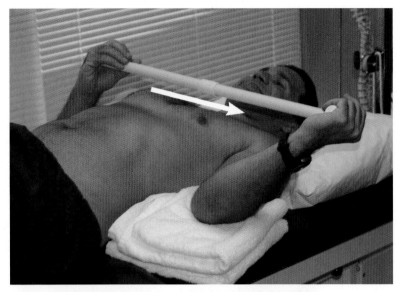

Figure 11-1 The patient uses a plastic T-bar while supine to perform passive external rotation while keeping the elbow of the involved shoulder at the side. Folded towels should be placed beneath the involved elbow to raise it to the midcoronal plane of the body.

1. First 6 weeks: The patient wears a sling and does passive external rotation stretches, as tolerated, and the patient is encouraged to achieve at least 45° of external rotation (Fig. 11-1). The exception to this protocol is in the patient with a subscapularis tendon repair. If the subscapularis tendon is repaired as a part of the overall cuff repair, external rotation is restricted to 0° for the first 6 weeks, and then increased as tolerated.
2. Weeks 7 through 12: The patient begins passive elevation, as tolerated, using a rope and pulley (Fig. 11-2) as well as supine overhead stretches using the opposite arm (Fig. 11-3). The patient also continues with passive external rotation stretches.
3. Week 13 and thereafter: The patient begins a strengthening program using Thera-Band with our standard "four-pack" exercises (Fig. 11-4). The four-pack includes

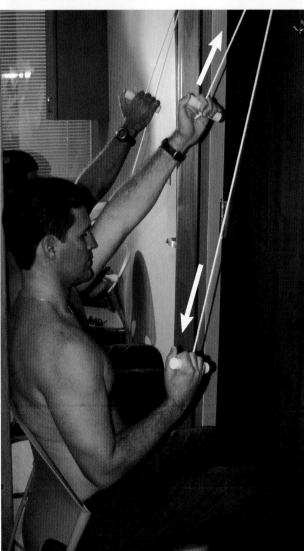

Figure 11-2 A rope and pulley draped over a door is used for passive overhead elevation.

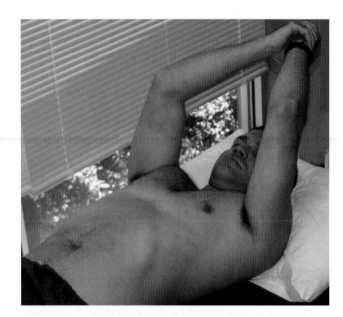

Figure 11-3 Supine passive elevation is accomplished by using the opposite arm to stretch the involved shoulder.

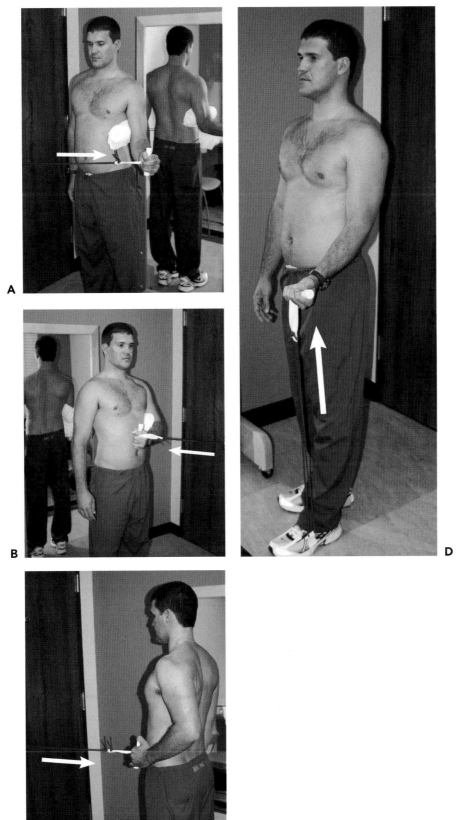

Figure 11-4 The "four-pack" exercises. **A:** Resisted external rotation. **B:** Resisted internal rotation. **C:** One-armed row. **D:** Biceps curl.

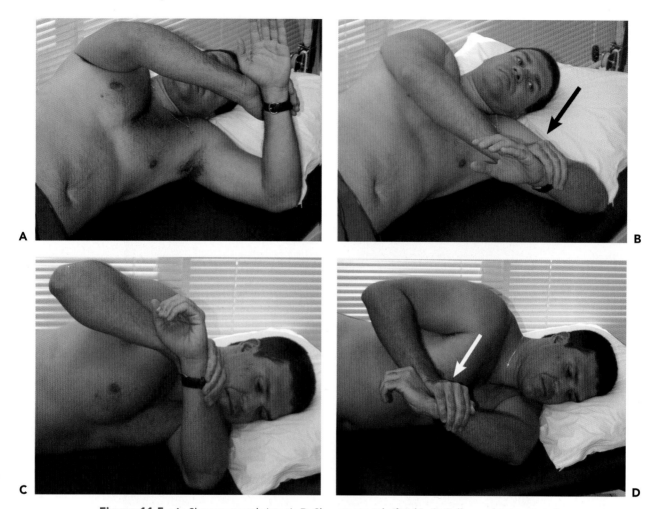

Figure 11-5 **A:** Sleeper stretch (start). **B:** Sleeper stretch (finish). **C:** Rollover sleeper stretch (start). **D:** Rollover sleeper stretch (finish).

resisted external rotation, resisted internal rotation, one-armed row, and biceps curl. The patient starts with the smallest diameter Thera-Band, which is a red Thera-Band, and is encouraged to do four sets of ten repetitions twice a day. The patient progresses up to the green Thera-Band and then the blue Thera-Band, as tolerated.

4. In the case of a revision rotator cuff repair or repair of a rotator cuff tear >5 cm in diameter, we do not begin strengthening until 17 weeks (4 months) postoperative. The reason for this more extended period of immobilization is that we believe that more time is needed for vascular ingrowth in these massive and revision repairs than in smaller repairs to achieve strong mechanical healing before stressing these repairs.

5. Month 6 and thereafter: The patient may resume full unrestricted activities if this is a primary repair <5 cm in diameter. If it is a revision repair or has a diameter >5 cm, we have the patient wait until 12 months postoperative to resume full unrestricted activities, which could include golf or overhead sports.

Currently, two exceptions exist to the initial 6-week period of immobilization that we employ in our practice. The first exception is the patient with calcific tendonitis. We have observed that such patients are likely to develop profound chemical synovitis and chemical bursitis from the calcific deposits after the surgery; if early stretching is not instituted, these patients tend to become stiff postoperatively. We, therefore, start immediate postoperative stretching, including passive elevation with a rope and pulley as well as passive external and internal rotation. The other exception is the patient who has a small rotator cuff tear (<3 cm diameter) in association with a superior labrum anterior and posterior (SLAP) lesion that is repaired at the same time. In our practice, we have found that this combination also makes the patient susceptible to stiffness if early passive stretching is not begun, so we now start immediate passive forward elevation as well as passive external and internal rotation. In general, these small rotator cuff tears are amenable to double row fixation and we are confident about starting early passive range of motion because of the high fixation strength of this double row repair.

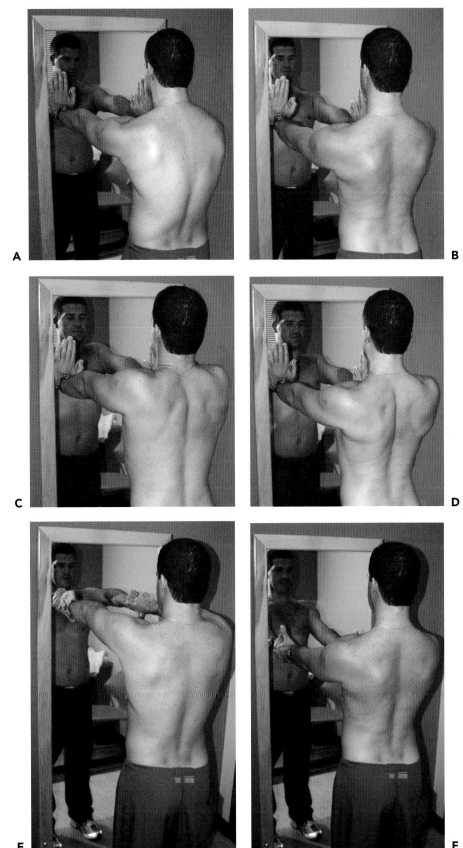

Figure 11-6 Closed-chain scapular control exercises. **A:** Protraction. **B:** Retraction. **C:** Elevation and retraction. **D:** Depression and retraction. **E:** Internal rotation and elevation. **F:** External rotation and depression.

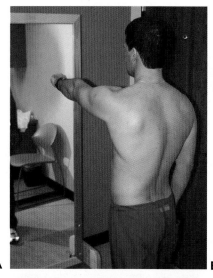
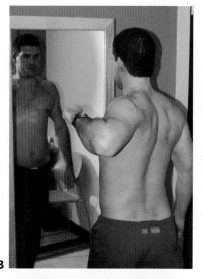
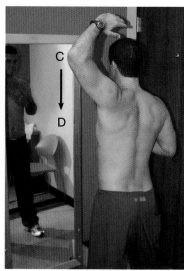

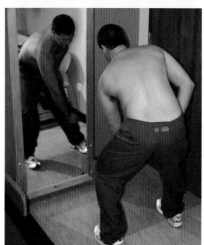
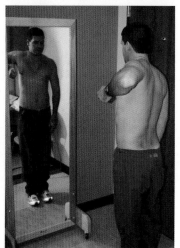

Figure 11-7 Open-chain scapular strengthening exercises. **A,B:** Forward lunges to strengthen scapular protractors **(A)** and retractors **(B)**. **C,D:** Lateral lunge for scapular retractors and upward rotators (upstroke) **(C)** as well as scapular depressors and downward rotators (downstroke) **(D)**. **E,F:** Diagonal pulls (lawnmower pulls) to strengthen scapular protractors and depressors **(E)** as well as retractors and elevators **(F)**.

In general, for all categories of rotator cuff tear, internal rotation stretching is begun 6 weeks postoperatively, but is not particularly emphasized. We simply have the patient begin to stretch the hand up behind the back as much as possible, and then do a reverse rope and pulley stretch, beginning ~8 to 10 weeks postoperatively. Typically, restoration of internal rotation lags behind the restoration of the other ranges of motion.

REHABILITATION AFTER ARTHROSCOPIC ANTERIOR INSTABILITY REPAIR

1. Weeks 1 through 4: The patient wears a sling full time and is encouraged to externally rotate the arm only to 0° (the straight-ahead position).
2. After 4 weeks: The sling is discontinued and the patient begins overhead stretching using a rope and pulley.

3. After 6 weeks: The patient begins passive external rotation stretching with a goal of having one half the amount of external rotation that is present on the opposite (normal) side by 12 weeks postoperative. Thera-Band strengthening is also begun after 6 weeks, using the same four pack exercise protocol as described in the section above on rotator cuff rehabilitation.
4. After 3 months: The patient can begin working out with weights in the gym.
5. After 6 months: The patient is released to full activities, including contact sports.

In the event of significant bone deficiency in which a Latarjet procedure is performed, we tend to go a bit slower on mobilization to allow full healing of the coracoid bone graft. Therefore, after the Latarjet procedure, we keep the patient in a sling for 6 weeks, allowing external

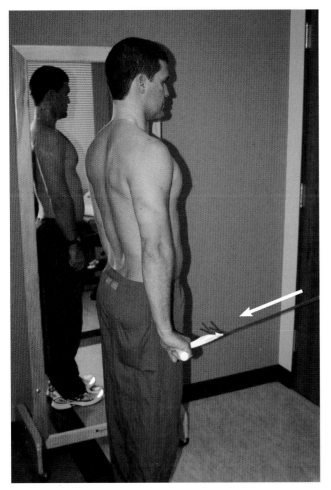

Figure 11-8 The low row is performed with the patient pulling posteriorly (shoulder extension and retraction) with the elbow locked in full extension. This exercise strengthens scapular retractors, particularly the serratus anterior.

rotation only to 0°. At the end of 6 weeks, the patient begins overhead stretching and external rotation stretching. Strengthening is delayed until 3 months postoperative, to allow secure healing of the bone graft as well as full healing of the upper subscapularis tendon (because the upper half of the subscapularis tendon is taken down from its insertion for exposure during the Latarjet procedure). At 4 months postoperative, the patient can begin working out in the gym, and at 6 months postoperative, full unrestricted activities are allowed, assuming that the bone graft is consolidated.

REHABILITATION AFTER ARTHROSCOPIC POSTERIOR INSTABILITY REPAIR

The sequence of rehabilitation efforts after arthroscopic posterior instability repair is essentially analogous to

that for anterior instability repair. The patient is kept in a sling for 4 weeks. During that time, the patient is allowed passive external rotation, as tolerated, but no passive internal rotation. The pillow splint is placed with the large bolster of the pillow anteriorly to keep the arm at approximately 10° of internal rotation, which is closer to the neutral position than we allow during the first 4 weeks after anterior instability repairs. At 4 weeks postoperative, the sling is discontinued and overhead stretching is begun along with external rotation stretching. Specific internal rotation stretching is not done. We simply allow the patient to gradually regain internal rotation as the overall shoulder rehabilitation progresses. At 3 months postoperative, the patient can begin working out in the gym, being careful to avoid the "hands-together" bench press. With the hands located further apart on the bar during the bench press, the force transmission to the shoulder is more perpendicular to the glenoid, protecting the repair. At 6 months postoperative, the patient can return to full unrestricted activities, including contact sports.

REHABILITATION AFTER ARTHROSCOPIC SLAP REPAIR

After SLAP repair, the patient wears a sling for 4 weeks. During that 4-week period, the patient is urged to perform external rotation stretches as far as possible, trying to match the external rotation between the operated arm and the unoperated arm by the end of 4 weeks. Sleeper stretches

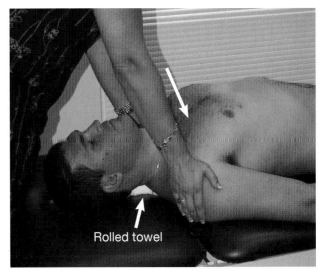

Rolled towel

Figure 11-9 Pectoralis minor stretch. A rolled towel is placed between the shoulder blades. Then, a posteriorly directed force is applied to the anterior aspect of both shoulders at once to stretch the pectoralis minor.

(four sets of ten) are performed twice a day (Fig. 11-5). After 4 weeks, the sling is discontinued. At that point, the patient begins overhead stretching and continues with passive external rotation stretching. At 6 weeks postoperatively, Thera-Band strengthening is begun using the same four-pack program as described above under rotator cuff rehabilitation. In most cases, however, resisted contraction of the biceps at 6 weeks postoperatively will still be somewhat painful because of repair of the SLAP lesion at the biceps root. If the patient experiences pain with resisted forward flexion of the arm 6 weeks postoperatively, we delay the biceps curl until 8 weeks postoperatively. At 8 weeks, closed-chain scapular control exercises are also begun (Fig. 11-6) as is open-chain scapular strengthening (Fig. 11-7). The low row (Fig. 11-8) is particularly good for strengthening scapular retractors.

At 3 months postoperatively, the patient can begin working out with strengthening in the gym. Baseball players can begin to lob a baseball and initiate some slow throwing motions, gradually progressing to an interval throwing program beginning at 4 months postoperatively (Tables 11-1 and 11-2). Baseball players usually need to include pectoralis minor stretches as a part of their regimen (Fig. 11-9). At 7 months postoperatively, the patient can return to full unrestricted activities, including all overhead sports activities.

TABLE 11-1
PHASE I INTERVAL THROWING PROGRAM

45' Phase

Step 1
A: Warm-up throwing
B: 45' (25 throws)
C: Rest 15 minutes
D: Warm-up throwing
E: 45' (25 throws)

Step 2
A: Warm-up throwing
B: 45' (25 throws)
C: Rest 10 minutes
D: Warm-up throwing
E: 45' (25 throws)
F: Rest 10 minutes
G: Warm-up throwing
H: 45' (25 throws)

60' Phase

Step 3
A: Warm-up throwing
B: 60' (25 throws)
C: Rest 15 minutes
D: Warm-up throwing
E: 60' (25 throws)

Step 4
A: Warm-up throwing
B: 60' (25 throws)
C: Rest 10 minutes
D: Warm-up throwing
E: 60' (25 throws)
F: Rest 10 minutes
G: Warm-up throwing
H: 60' (25 throws)

90' Phase

Step 5
A: Warm-up throwing
B: 90' (25 throws)

C: Rest 15 minutes
D: Warm-up throwing
E: 90' (25 throws)

Step 6
A: Warm-up throwing
B: 90' (25 throws)
C: Rest 10 minutes
D: Warm-up throwing
E: 90' (25 throws)
F: Rest 10 minutes
G: Warm-up throwing
H: 90' (25 throws)

120' Phase

Step 7
A: Warm-up throwing
B: 120' (25 throws)
C: Rest 15 minutes
D: Warm-up throwing
E: 120' (25 throws)

Step 8
A: Warm-up throwing
B: 120' (25 throws)
C: Rest 10 minutes
D: Warm-up throwing
E: 120' (25 throws)
F: Rest 10 minutes
G: Warm-up throwing
H: 120' (25 throws)

150' Phase

Step 9
A: Warm-up throwing
B: 150' (25 throws)
C: Rest 15 minutes
D: Warm-up throwing
E: 150' (25 throws)

Step 10
A: Warm-up throwing
B: 150' (25 throws)
C: Rest 10 minutes
D: Warm-up throwing
E: 150' (25 throws)
F: Rest 10 minutes
G: Warm-up throwing
H: 150' (25 throws)

180' Phase

Step 11
A: Warm-up throwing
B: 180' (25 throws)
C: Rest 15 minutes
D: Warm-up throwing
E: 180' (25 throws)

Step 12
A: Warm-up throwing
B: 180' (25 throws)
C: Rest 10 minutes
D: Warm-up throwing
E: 180' (25 throws)
F: Rest 10 minutes
G: Warm-up throwing
H: 180' (25 throws)

Step 13
A: Warm-up throwing
B: 180' (25 throws)
C: Rest 15 minutes
D: Warm-up throwing
E: 180' (25 throws)

Step 14
Begin throwing off the mound or return to respective position.

Each phase is titled according to the distance (in feet) that the athlete is to throw. Throwing program should be performed every other day, unless otherwise specified by physician or rehabilitation specialist. Advance to next step when able to throw the specified number of throws without pain.

TABLE 11-2
PHASE II: INTERVAL THROWING PROGRAM STARTING OFF THE MOUND

STAGE ONE: FASTBALL ONLY

Step 1	Interval throwing 15 throws off mound 50%
Step 2	Interval throwing 30 throws off mound 50%
Step 3	Interval throwing 45 throws off mound 50%
Step 4	Interval throwing 60 throws off mound 50%
Step 5	Interval throwing 30 throws off mound 50%
Step 6	30 throws off mound 75% 45 throws off mound 50%
Step 7	45 throws off mound 75% 15 throws off mound 50%
Step 8	60 throws off mound 75%

STAGE TWO: FASTBALL ONLY

Step 9	45 throws off mound 75% 15 throws in batting practice
Step 10	45 throws off mound 75% 30 throws in batting practice
Step 11	45 throws off mound 75% 45 throws in batting practice

STAGE THREE

Step 12	30 throws off mound 75% warm-up 15 throws off mound 50% BREAKING BALLS 45–60 throws in batting practice (fastball only)
Step 13	30 throws off mound 75% 30 breaking balls 75% 30 throws in batting practice
Step 14	30 throws off mound 75% 60–90 throws in batting practice 25% breaking balls
Step 15	SIMULATED GAME: PROGRESSING BY 15 THROWS PER WORK-OUT.

All throwing off the mound should be done in the presence of a pitching coach to stress proper throwing mechanics.

If the patient has had multiple structures repaired (e.g., combined rotator cuff and SLAP repairs), we tailor our rehabilitation program toward the repaired tissues that require the longest period of immobilization for healing. For example, with a combined SLAP repair and rotator cuff repair, we would not begin strengthening until 12 weeks postoperatively to allow for complete healing of the rotator cuff.

REFERENCES

1. Gerber C. Histologic findings in the healing rotator cuff repair. Presented at the Nice Shoulder Course. Nice, France, May 10, 2004.

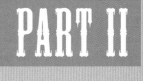

PART II

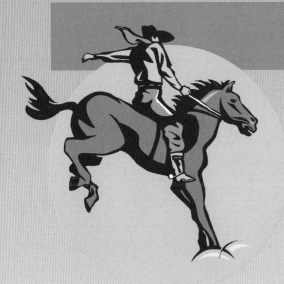

PLAYIN' WITH FIRE

A Cowboy's Guide to
Cookin' (Workin' Smooth), Smokin'
(Workin' Fast), and Brandin' (Leavin' Your Mark)

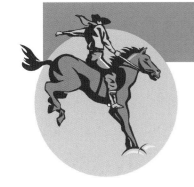

12

Operating Room Set-up

- An overhead perspective of the operating room crystallizes all the elements of our OR set-up (Fig. 12-1).
- The patient, in the lateral decubitus position, is held with a vacuum bean-bag. A Star Sleeve Balanced Suspension System (Arthrex, Inc.; Naples, FL) is used to position the arm. The patient is administered general anesthesia with endotracheal intubation.
- People

  The surgeon stands behind the patient's shoulder. The first assistant is also posterior to the patient, behind the patient's head. The anesthesiologist is at the head of the table. The primary surgical technician stands behind the surgeon, working from Mayo stand #1 and the back instrument table. The second surgical technician, standing in front of the patient, opposite the surgeon, has the following duties:

1. Provides supplemental traction and rotation of the arm, as needed.

2. Manages the cables and suction tubes from the shaver, burr, and electrocautery systems, all of which are positioned on Mayo stand #2.
3. Assists with turbulence control by digitally plugging rapid efflux of fluid from portal sites.

- Tables and stands
  - Mayo stand #1, which contains the most commonly used instruments
  - The back instrument table, which contains all the other procedure-specific instruments
  - Mayo stand #2, which contains the shaver, burr, and electrocautery probes
- Instrument arrays
  - The Tower, which contains the camera box, cautery generator, shaver or burr console, and video monitor
  - A second monitor stand
  - The arthroscopy pump
  - The anesthesia stand

OR SET UP

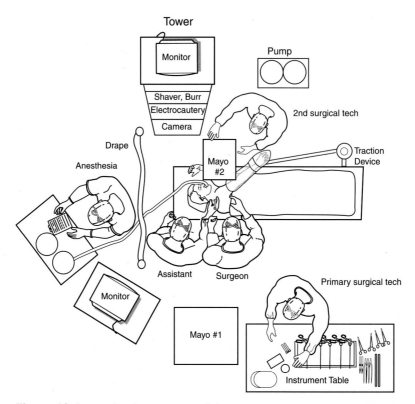

Figure 12-1 Overhead perspective of the operating room set-up used by the authors for shoulder arthroscopy.

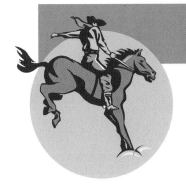

13

Instability

13A

Arthroscopic Bankart Repair

- Assess the Bankart lesion initially from a posterior viewing portal, and check for a superior labrum anterior and posterior (SLAP) lesion.

- Establish an anterosuperolateral portal at the junction of the upper rotator interval with the anterior border of the supraspinatus tendon. It should be placed so that it provides a 45° angle of approach to the superior glenoid rim for easy repair of associated SLAP lesions. This portal will be the primary viewing portal during the arthroscopic Bankart repair.

- Now, assess the Bankart lesion from the anterosuperolateral portal. This portal provides the best view of the anterior glenoid and anterior labrum (Fig. 13A-1).

- Determine the percentage of bone loss by direct measurement with a calibrated probe (see Part I, Chapter 4, for the technique of determining bone loss). If the inferior glenoid has lost no more than 25% of its width, and if no significant engaging Hill-Sachs lesion is present, the patient is considered a good candidate for arthroscopic Bankart repair.

- Dissect the capsulolabral sleeve from the anterior glenoid neck with an arthroscopic elevator until the subscapularis muscle is clearly visible in the cleft deep to the capsule (Fig. 13A-2). If the subscapularis is not visible in the cleft, then the capsule is not adequately mobilized.

- Lightly "dust" the anterior glenoid with a shaver or burr to create a bleeding bone surface. Do not actually resect any glenoid bone.

- Prepare a 2- to 3-mm strip of bleeding bone on the anterior edge of the glenoid face by using a curette to remove a strip of articular cartilage (Fig. 13A-3). This provides a good bleeding surface for capsulolabral healing (Fig. 13A-4).

- Visualize the angle of approach to the 5 o'clock position on the glenoid through the anterior portal. If the angle is too "steep" (i.e., too oblique to the glenoid to obtain good purchase in bone), then a 5 o'clock portal must be used (Fig. 13A-5).

- Create the 5 o'clock portal ~15 mm below the upper border of subscapularis (Fig. 13A-6), using a 3-mm Spear guide to place the suture anchors (BioFASTak or BioSutureTak; Arthrex, Inc.; Naples, FL). Use this guide to place both the 5 o'clock and 4 o'clock anchors onto the prepared anterior glenoid "bone strip."

- Use the standard anterior portal to place the 3 o'clock anchor.

- Pass the sutures from the 5 o'clock anchor. We prefer using a Bankart Viper suture passer (Arthrex) through the anterior portal for antegrade passage (Fig. 13A-7). This allows the suture to be passed through the capsule distal to the anchor, accomplishing a distal-to-proximal shift when the sutures are tied.

- Once the sutures from the 5 o'clock anchor have been passed, tie them before passing the sutures from the next anchor (i.e., tie as you go) (Fig. 13A-8).

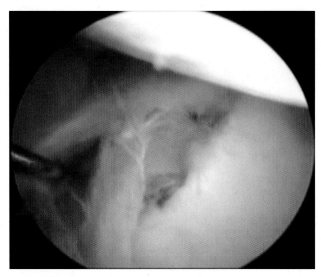

Figure 13A-1   Right shoulder, anterosuperolateral viewing portal. The Bankart lesion and anterior glenoid are clearly visualized through this portal.

- For passing the sutures from the 4 o'clock and 3 o'clock anchors, a 45° BirdBeak (Arthrex) suture passer is used for retrograde suture passage, accomplishing a distal-to-proximal shift of the capsule (Fig. 13A-9).

- The goal is to create an anterior "bumper" of capsulolabral tissue (Fig. 13A-10) and to have the humeral head centered on the glenoid (Fig. 13A-11).

TRICKS AND TIPS

- If a concomitant SLAP lesion is present, place the anchors and pass the sutures for the SLAP repair before addressing the Bankart lesion because the supralabral recess tends to

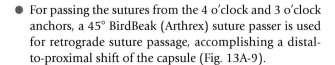

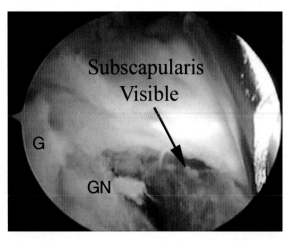

Figure 13A-2   Right shoulder, posterior viewing portal, 70° arthroscope. After dissecting the capsulolabral sleeve from the anterior glenoid neck, the subscapularis muscle is clearly seen in the cleft, deep to the capsule. G, glenoid; GN, anterior glenoid neck.

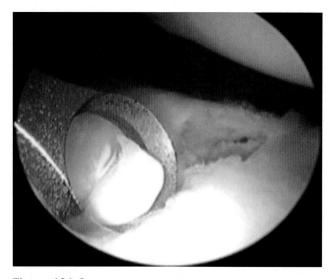

Figure 13A-3   A curette is used to remove a strip of articular cartilage along the anterior glenoid rim.

swell early, obscuring vision. Do not, however, tie the SLAP sutures until after the Bankart repair because SLAP repair will tighten the shoulder sufficiently to compromise the space for working on the Bankart lesion.

- In cases of a "triple labral lesion" consisting of a Bankart lesion, a posterior Bankart lesion, and a SLAP lesion, the order of repair should be as follows:

  1. Place SLAP anchors and pass SLAP sutures, but do not tie them.
  2. Repair Bankart lesion (all steps).
  3. Repair posterior Bankart lesion (all steps).
  4. Tie SLAP sutures.

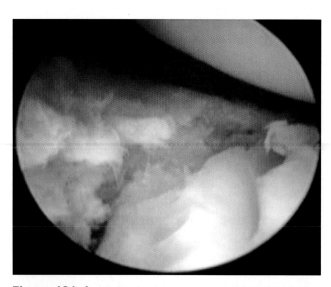

Figure 13A-4   Right shoulder, anterosuperolateral viewing portal. Removal of the articular cartilage strip along the anterior glenoid rim leaves a strip of bleeding bone to which the capsule will be apposed by the repair.

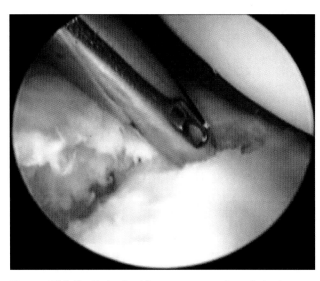

Figure 13A-5 Right shoulder, anterosuperolateral viewing portal. This angle of approach to the 5 o'clock anchor position is too "steep", so a 5 o'clock portal must be created.

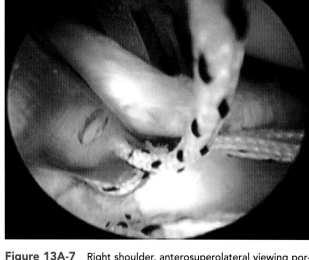

Figure 13A-7 Right shoulder, anterosuperolateral viewing portal. A Bankart Viper (Arthrex, Inc.; Naples, FL) suture passer is used for antegrade suture placement distal to the anchor to achieve a distal-to-proximal capsular shift.

- Many chronic cases of anterior instability will have an anterior labral periosteal sleeve avulsion (ALPSA lesion) in which the capsulolabral tissue has healed in a medialized position on the anterior glenoid neck. In such cases, an arthroscopic elevator must dissect the capsule from the glenoid widely, so that the subscapularis muscle is clearly visible in the cleft deep to the capsule. This wide mobilization frees the capsule to the extent that it "floats" up to the level of the glenoid surface for a tension-free repair.

- Some surgeons have advocated placing the anchors for a Bankart repair onto the glenoid face, 2- to 4-mm onto the articular surface. We have modified this approach by

preparing a 2- to 3-mm strip of bleeding bone at the anterior rim of the glenoid. In this way, when the anchors are placed 2- to 3-mm onto the face of the glenoid, they will appose the capsule against a bleeding bone surface (rather than an articular cartilage surface) for better healing.

- In creating the 5 o'clock portal, use a spinal needle to localize placement, entering the joint ~15 mm below the upper border of the subscapularis tendon. Because this portal will be used only for anchor placement (at 5 o'clock and 4 o'clock), a large cannula is not needed. We use a 3-mm Spear guide (Arthrex, Inc.; Naples, FL),

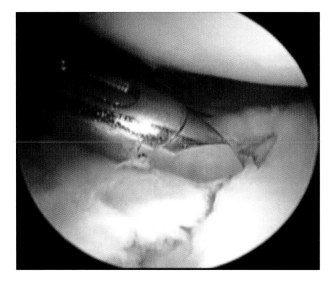

Figure 13A-6 Right shoulder, anterosuperolateral viewing portal. The Spear guide (Arthrex, Inc.; Naples, FL), and trochar are entering the joint through the subscapularis tendon ~15 mm below its superior margin.

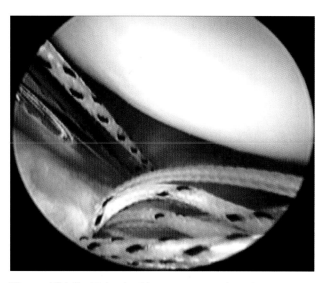

Figure 13A-8 Right shoulder, anterosuperolateral viewing portal. Sutures from each anchor should be sequentially tied "as you go." We prefer static knots tied with a Surgeon's Sixth Finger (Arthrex, Inc.; Naples, FL) knot pusher.

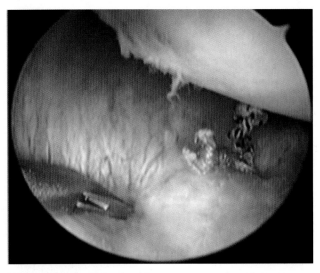

Figure 13A-9 Right shoulder, anterosuperolateral portal. A 45° BirdBeak (Arthrex, Inc.; Naples, FL) suture passer accomplishes retrograde passage of sutures from the 4 o'clock and 3 o'clock anchors.

through which we place the anchors. Suture passage and knot-tying are carried out through the standard anterior portal. Once the spinal needle has appropriately determined the proper angle of approach for the 5 o'clock portal, with two hands, we bimanually "walk" the Spear guide with its sharp trochar alongside the needle, through the subscapularis, and into the joint. A twisting, boring action is most effective in advancing the Spear and trochar in a controlled manner without plunging into the joint (or elsewhere).

● The overriding goals in an arthroscopic Bankart repair are:

1. Accomplish a distal-to-proximal capsular shift by passing the sutures distal to the anchor.

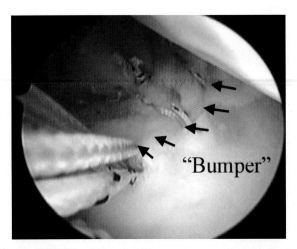

Figure 13A-10 Right shoulder, anterosuperolateral viewing portal. The repair has created an anteroinferior "bumper" of capsulolabral tissue.

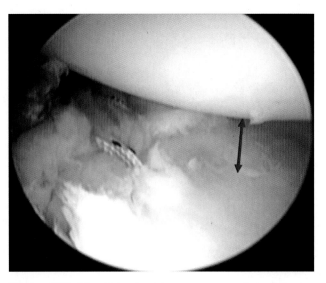

Figure 13A-11 Right shoulder, anterosuperolateral viewing portal. After Bankart repair, the humeral head is now centered on the glenoid.

2. Achieve a "bumper effect" anteriorly with capsulolabral repair.
3. Achieve centralization of the humeral head on the glenoid.

13B
Arthroscopic Latarjet Procedure

● A video of this procedure is provided on the DVD to complete the overview on arthroscopic instability repairs and to show the breadth of surgery that is possible by arthroscopic means.

TRICKS AND TIPS

● Do not try this at home. Stick with the open Latarjet procedure for now. But . . . stay tuned.

13C
Arthroscopic Treatment of Multidirectional Instability

● Arthroscopic inspection reveals patulous capsular recesses with no labral detachment (Fig. 13C-1).

● Establish a posterolateral portal, using a spinal needle as a guide to assure a good angle of approach to the

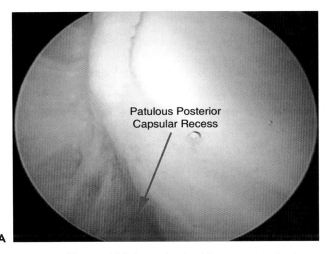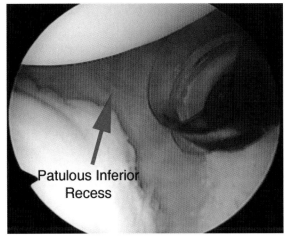

A

B

Figure 13C-1 Right shoulder, posterior viewing portal. This shoulder has a patulous posterior recess. (Fig. 13C-1A). From an anterosuperolateral viewing portal (Fig. 13C-1B), one can see a patulous inferior recess.

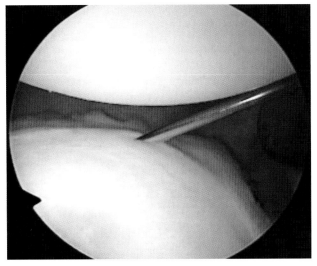

Figure 13C-2 Right shoulder, anterosuperolateral viewing portal. A spinal needle is used as a guide to assure the proper angle of approach for placement of a posterolateral portal. This angle will assure optimal placement of suture anchors into the glenoid.

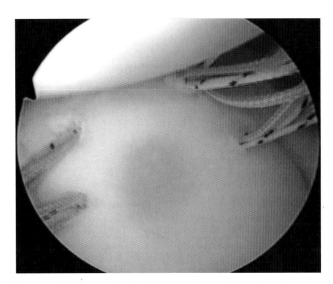

Figure 13C-4 Right shoulder, anterosuperolateral viewing portal. Four double-loaded suture anchors have been placed in the glenoid in preparation for passage of plication sutures.

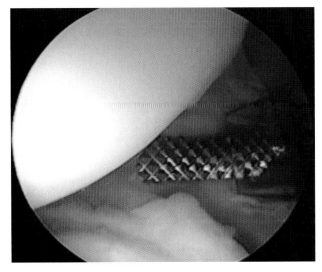

Figure 13C-3 Right shoulder, anterosuperolateral viewing portal. An arthroscopic rasp is used to lightly abrade the capsule in the axillary recess.

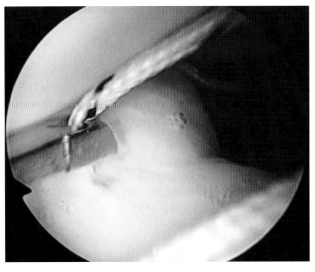

Figure 13C-5 Right shoulder, anterosuperolateral viewing portal. A 45° BirdBeak suture passer introduced through the posterior portal is used to pass plication sutures through the posteroinferior capsule.

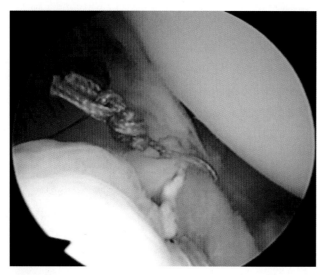

Figure 13C-6   Right shoulder, posterior viewing portal. The rotator interval has been closed by passing a free FiberWire suture to appose the superior glenohumeral ligament to the middle glenohumeral ligament.

posterior and posteroinferior glenoid for anchor placement (Fig. 13C-2).

● Use an arthroscopic rasp to lightly abrade the capsule before capsular plication (Fig. 13C-3).

● Place double-loaded anchors (BioSutureTak; Arthrex, Inc.; Naples, FL) at the glenoid rim to provide firm fixation points for capsular plication (Fig. 13C-4).

● Use a 45° BirdBeak suture passer (Arthrex) through the posterior portal to pass plication sutures (Fig. 13C-5).

● Tie sutures sequentially as suture pairs from a given anchor are passed.

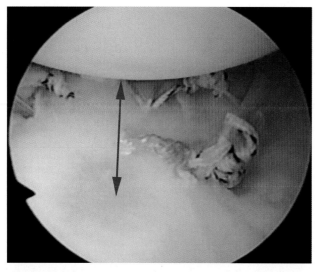

Figure 13C-7   Right shoulder, anterosuperolateral viewing portal. Final result after capsular plication. The humeral head is centered on the glenoid, and the patulous recesses have been eliminated.

● Close the rotator interval by suturing the superior glenohumeral ligament to the middle glenohumeral ligament (Fig. 13C-6).

● The final result is assessed (Fig. 13C-7).

TRICKS AND TIPS

● In patients with multidirectional instability, the labrum is often deficient with poor quality tissue, so we prefer to place suture anchors in the glenoid rim to provide stable fixation points for plication.

● The inferior recess must be plicated, so it is essential to have an anchor near 6 o'clock for that purpose. This anchor is most easily and accurately placed through a posterolateral working portal.

● The posterior portal should enter the joint in the posteroinferior quadrant to provide the best angle of approach for a 45° BirdBeak to plicate the inferior recess.

● A hand-off technique may be helpful in suture passage.

13D
Nonengaging Hill-Sachs Lesion

● By definition, a nonengaging Hill-Sachs lesion is one that does **not** engage the anterior border of the glenoid when the shoulder is in a position of overhead athletic function (combination of 90° abduction and 90° external rotation).

● On the other hand, an engaging Hill-Sachs lesion engages the anterior border of the glenoid in the position of combined abduction of 90° and external rotation of 90° (90-90 positions). Obviously, every Hill-Sachs lesion will engage in some position, but our definition of nonengaging refers to the 90-90 position of overhead athletic function.

● To determine if a Hill-Sachs lesion is engaging or not, place the arthroscope intra-articularly. Then, remove the arm from its balanced suspension and take the shoulder up to 90° abduction combined with 90° of external rotation. Observe the angle that the Hill-Sachs lesion makes with the anterior glenoid (Fig. 13D-1). If the plane of the Hill-Sachs defect diagonally crosses the anterior border of the glenoid, this is a nonengaging Hill-Sachs lesion (Fig. 13D-1).

● With the arm at the side (combined adduction and external rotation), the same Hill-Sachs lesion will engage the anterior glenoid (Fig. 13D-2), but by our definition this is a nonengaging lesion.

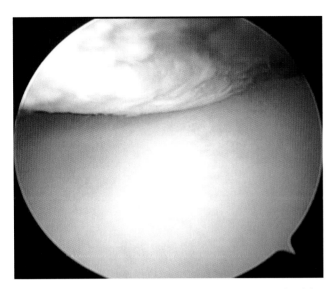

Figure 13D-1 Posterior viewing portal, right shoulder. Nonengaging Hill-Sachs lesion. With the shoulder positioned in 90° abduction and 90° external rotation, this nonengaging lesion crosses the anterior glenoid border at a diagonal angle.

TRICKS AND TIPS

● Our data have shown that a shoulder with an isolated nonengaging Hill-Sachs lesion will do well with an arthroscopic Bankart repair. If an associated inverted-pear glenoid is seen, an arthroscopic repair must not be done because of the very high failure rate. In such a case with a nonengaging Hill-Sachs lesion in association with an inverted-pear glenoid, we recommend an open Latarjet reconstruction.

Open Latarjet Reconstruction

● Perform arthroscopic evaluation, looking for an inverted-pear glenoid (Fig. 13E-1), an engaging Hill-Sachs lesion (Fig. 13E-2), and the presence of any associated pathology (e.g., a superior labrum anterior and posterior [SLAP] lesion) that may need to be addressed arthroscopically before proceeding to the open Latarjet reconstruction (Fig. 13E-3).

● After arthroscopy, place the patient in a modified beach chair position and again prepare and re-drape the shoulder.

● Make a deltopectoral incision.

● Identify the conjoined tendon and follow it proximally to the tip of the coracoid. At that point, identify the *pectoralis minor* attachment insertion into the medial aspect of the distal coracoid (Fig. 13E-4).

● Detach the *pectoralis minor* insertion from the medial coracoid with a pencil-tipped electrocautery probe (Fig. 13E-5).

● Detach the coracoacromial ligament from the lateral coracoid with electrocautery. With a periosteal elevator, clear the soft tissue circumferentially around the coracoid, which is now free of all soft tissue attachments (except for the conjoined tendon) from its tip to its base, where the coracoclavicular ligaments attach (Fig. 13E-6).

● Use an oscillating saw with a 70° angle blade to osteotomize the coracoid just anterior to the coracoclavicular

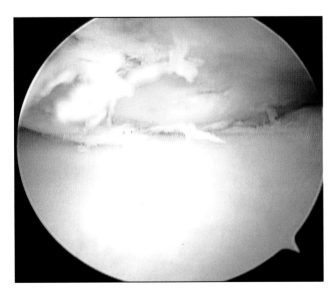

Figure 13D-2 Posterior viewing portal, right shoulder. With the shoulder at the side, combined with 80° of external rotation, the Hill-Sachs lesion engages the anterior glenoid rim. This is still defined as a nonengaging Hill-Sachs lesion.

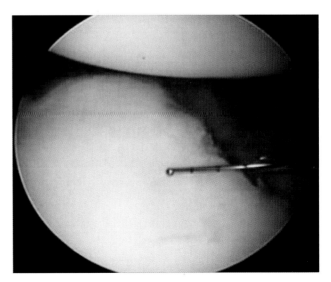

Figure 13E-1 Left shoulder, anterosuperolateral viewing portal. Glenoid bone loss has resulted in the typical inverted-pear glenoid configuration.

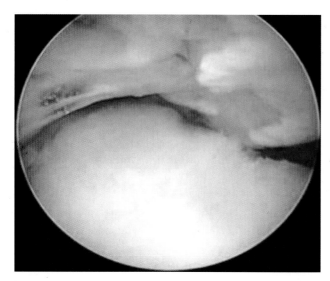

Figure 13E-2 Left shoulder, anterosuperolateral viewing portal. With the shoulder in 90° abduction and full external rotation, the humeral Hill-Sachs lesion engages the anterior rim of the glenoid.

ligaments (Fig. 13E-7). This will usually provide a coracoid bone graft 2.5- to 3-cm in length.

● Detach the upper half of the subscapularis distally and dissect it free from the underlying capsule. Then, develop the plane between the capsule and the lower half of the subscapularis tendon.

● Dissect an inverted L-shaped capsular flap, with the transverse limb of the inverted L at the level of the upper subscapularis tendon and the vertical limb of the L located 1 cm medial to the glenoid rim. Carry this flap down to the 6 o'clock position. A Fukuda ring retractor on the humeral head facilitates this dissection.

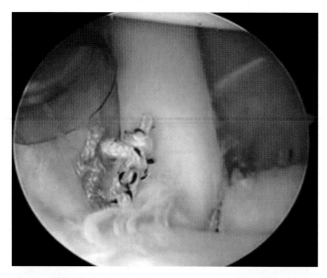

Figure 13E-3 Left shoulder, posterior viewing portal. A superior labrum anterior and posterior (SLAP) lesion has been repaired arthroscopically before proceeding with the open Latarjet reconstruction.

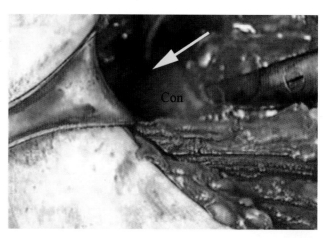

Figure 13E-4 Left shoulder. The conjoined tendon (Con) attaches to the coracoid tip adjacent to the *pectoralis minor* insertion at the medial aspect of the coracoid (*arrow*).

● The medial side of the coracoid graft is the side that will be placed against the glenoid. Prepare this medial side of the coracoid by freshening its surface with an oscillating saw (Fig. 13E-8).

● Then, with a burr, freshen the anterior glenoid neck to a bleeding base of bone.

● Place three BioSutureTak (Arthrex, Inc.; Naples, FL) anchors in the anteroinferior rim of the native glenoid.

● Position the coracoid graft as an extension of the glenoid articular arc, provisionally holding it in place with two K-wires (Fig. 13E-9).

● Secure the graft with two 4.5-mm cannulated screws (Fig. 13E-10).

● Test the security of the construct.

● Repair the capsule with the sutures from the anchors in the glenoid. This repair ensures that the coracoid bone graft is extracapsular (Fig. 13E-10).

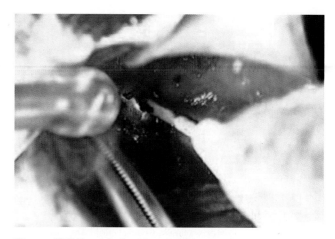

Figure 13E-5 Left shoulder. An electrocautery blade is used to detach the *pectoralis minor* insertion at the medial tip of the coracoid.

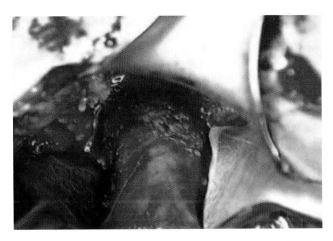

Figure 13E-6 Left shoulder. After medial and lateral soft tissue attachments have been removed, the skeletonized coracoid with its attached conjoined tendon is well-visualized.

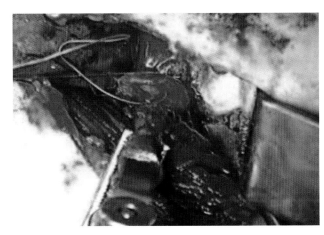

Figure 13E-8 Left shoulder. The medial side of the coracoid graft is freshened to a bleeding base by means of a straight saw blade. The medial surface of the coracoid graft will be placed against the anterior glenoid neck and secured with two screws.

- Repair the upper subscapularis repaired to its anatomic position.

TRICKS AND TIPS

- It is important to perform arthroscopy before the Latarjet reconstruction so as not to miss concomitant pathology. We have arthroscopically repaired SLAP lesions in 20% of our open Latarjet cases before opening the shoulder.

- An oscillating saw with a 70° angle blade greatly simplifies the osteotomy of the coracoid. Care must always be taken to have the end of the saw blade against bone when the saw is activated to avoid neurovascular injury.

- The "best fit" of the coracoid graft is always a "90° twist" in which the medial side of the coracoid is placed against the anterior glenoid neck.

- The coracoid graft should be placed so that it becomes an extension of the glenoid articular arc. There should not be a step-off medially or laterally at the glenoid–graft interface. The graft is *not* intended to act as a bone block.

- The two major stabilizing effects of the graft are:
  1. Elongation of the glenoid articular arc
  2. The sling effect of the conjoint tendon

- If a massive engaging Hill-Sachs lesion is present in association with an inverted pear glenoid, the Latarjet procedure simultaneously addresses the humeral bone defect by virtue of the fact that it lengthens the glenoid articular arc so much that the humerus cannot ever externally rotate far enough to engage the Hill-Sachs lesion. For that reason, we have never had to use a bone graft for a humeral Hill-Sachs lesion, no matter how large, since we began doing the Latarjet reconstruction for instability with bone deficiency.

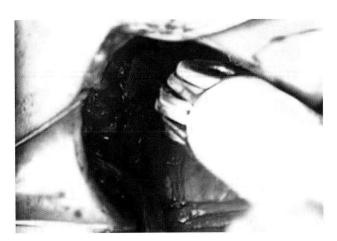

Figure 13E-7 Left shoulder. This surgical photo shows that the coracoid can be well-visualized to its base, as the 70° angle saw begins the coracoid osteotomy.

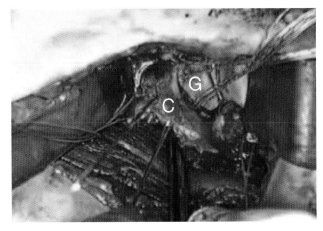

Figure 13E-9 Provisional fixation of the coracoid graft is accomplished with two K-wires. G, glenoid; C, coracoid graft.

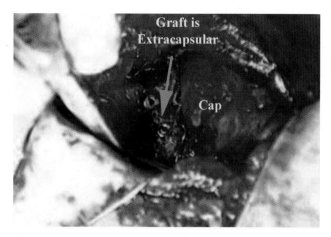

Figure 13E-10 Left shoulder. The capsule has been repaired to the native glenoid, and the coracoid graft is now extracapsular. Cap, repaired anterior capsule.

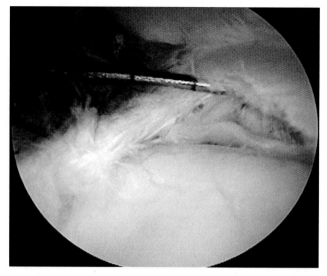

Figure 13F-1 Left shoulder, posterior viewing portal. This arthroscopic photo shows a superior labrum anterior and posterior (SLAP) lesion.

- The coracoid graft should be secured with two 4.5-mm screws, one being 34 mm long (the lower screw) and the other being 36 mm long (the upper screw). These are virtually always the correct length.

- After the coracoid graft has been secured by screws, but before the capsule is repaired, the surgeon should try to manually dislocate the shoulder. We routinely do this, and we have never been able to dislocate the shoulder, even without an intact repaired capsule. This demonstrates the extreme mechanical stability of this construct.

- The capsule is repaired to anchors in the native glenoid, so that the coracoid bone graft is extracapsular. In this way, the humeral head is protected from any abrasion that might result from contact with the coracoid.

- Prepare the posterior glenoid bone bed using a power shaver and ring curettes.

- Place posterior suture anchors.

- Pass the sutures through the posterior glenoid labrum using a 22° or 45° BirdBeak (Arthrex, Inc.; Naples, FL) suture passer through a posterior working portal (Fig. 13F-4).

- Tie the posterior sutures (Fig. 13F-5).

- Tie the SLAP sutures after completing repair of the posterior Bankart lesion.

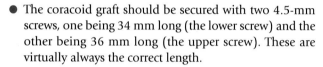

Posterior Bankart and SLAP Repair

- Arthroscopic evaluation reveals a superior labrum anterior and posterior (SLAP) lesion (Fig. 13F-1) as well as a posterior Bankart lesion (Fig. 13F-2).

- Prepare the glenoid bone bed for repair of the SLAP and Bankart lesions.

- Place suture anchors for the SLAP repair and pass, but do not tie, the sutures.

- Now, repair the posterior Bankart lesion.

- Establish a posterolateral working portal at an appropriate angle of approach for placement of suture anchors (Fig. 13F-3).

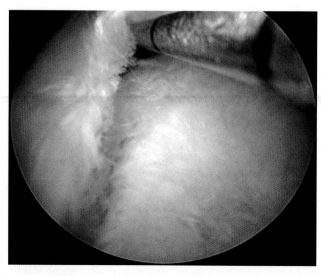

Figure 13F-2 Left shoulder, anterosuperolateral viewing portal. A posterior Bankart lesion is clearly demonstrated.

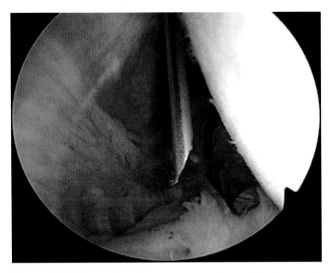

Figure 13F-3   Left shoulder, anterosuperolateral viewing portal. A spinal needle is used to determine the proper angle of approach for a posterolateral working portal.

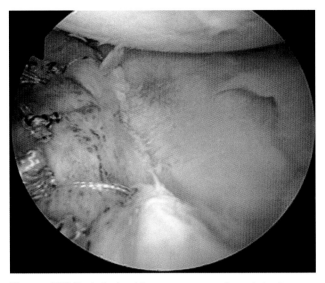

Figure 13F-5   Left shoulder, posterosuperolateral viewing portal. View of completed posterior Bankart lesion repair.

TRICKS AND TIPS

- Place the SLAP anchors and pass the SLAP sutures (but do not tie them) before repairing the posterior Bankart lesion. Suture passage in the supralabral sulcus is much easier early in the case, before onset of swelling in that area.

- Although the SLAP sutures are passed early, they should not be tied until after the posterior Bankart repair has been completed. The reason for this is that a SLAP repair will tighten the joint somewhat, making the posterior Bankart repair (especially the posteroinferior portion) more difficult. This same principle applies to combined SLAP and anterior Bankart repairs.

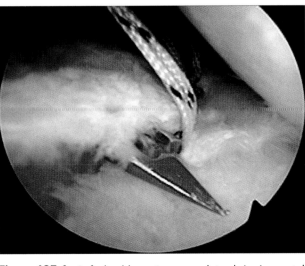

Figure 13F-4   Left shoulder, anterosuperolateral viewing portal. A 45° BirdBeak (Arthrex, Inc.; Naples, FL) suture passer is used through a posterior portal to pass sutures through the posterior labrum.

- We have frequently seen combined SLAP and posterior Bankart lesions as a consequence of weight-lifting, specifically during the bench press. The other category of patient in which we commonly see this combination of pathology is the offensive lineman in football, who repetitively uses his arms to push off in front, sustaining posteriorly directed forces.

13G

Repair of a Bony Bankart Lesion

- Arthroscopic inspection reveals a separate anterior–inferior bone fragment (Fig. 13G-1). Evaluate the posterior humerus to see if an engaging or nonengaging Hill-Sachs lesion is present (Fig. 13G-2).

- Introduce a calibrated probe through the posterior portal to quantify the percentage of bone loss (Fig. 13G-3). In chronic lesions, the fragment can become compressed with repeated dislocations, so direct measurement of the diameter of the fragment itself may underestimate the degree of actual bone loss on the glenoid side (see Part I, Chapter 4 and Chapter 7 for discussion on the specific techniques and calculations for quantifying bone loss).

- Prepare the glenoid by using an arthroscopic elevator to dissect the plane between the fragment and the main glenoid (Fig.13G-4). Clean and prepare to a bleeding base the two apposing bone surfaces (glenoid and fragment).

- Create a 5 o'clock portal for anchor placement. With a spinal needle, locate the entry point for a proper angle of

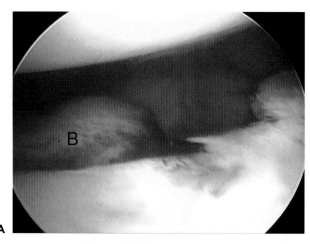
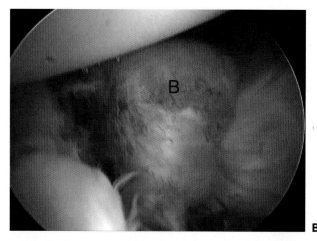

A

B

Figure 13G-1 The bony Bankart fragment in this left shoulder can be visualized through a posterior viewing portal (**A**) or an anterosuperolateral portal (**B**). B, bony Bankart fragment.

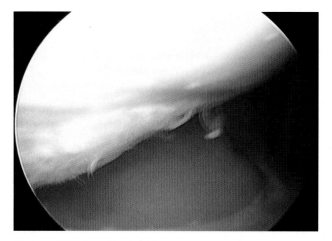

Figure 13G-2 Left shoulder, posterior viewing portal. This arthroscopic photo shows a small nonengaging Hill-Sachs lesion.

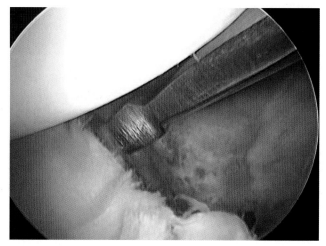

Figure 13G-4 Left shoulder, anterosuperolateral viewing portal. An arthroscopic elevator is used to locate and develop the plane between the glenoid and the bone fragment.

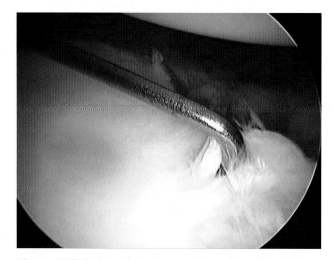

Figure 13G-3 Left shoulder, anterosuperolateral viewing portal. A calibrated probe introduced through a posterior portal can be used to quantify the bone loss as a percentage of the inferior glenoid diameter.

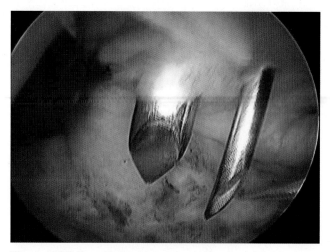

Figure 13G-5 Left shoulder, anterosuperolateral viewing portal. The trocar tip of the Spear guide penetrates the capsule adjacent to the spinal needle that was used to localize the entry point for the 5 o'clock portal.

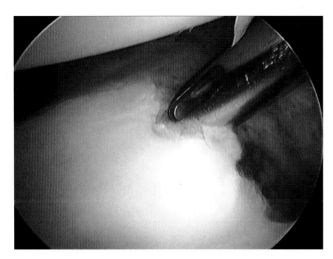

Figure 13G-6   Left shoulder, anterosuperolateral viewing portal. The Spear guide in this photo provides a perfect angle of approach (by means of a 5 o'clock portal) for placing the lowermost suture anchor firmly into bone.

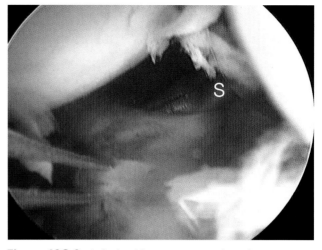

Figure 13G-8   Left shoulder, anterosuperolateral viewing portal. A Sidewinder (Arthrex, Inc.; Naples, FL) suture passer (*S*) is introduced through the anterior portal in preparation for suture passage through the bone fragment.

approach, and then walk down the BioSutureTak Spear guide (Arthrex, Inc.; Naples, FL) adjacent to the needle so that it penetrates the capsule next to the needle (Fig. 13G-5). A twisting, boring motion to the Spear guide aids in its passage through the tough subscapularis tendon. This guide will then provide an excellent angle of approach for passing the two lower anchors (Fig. 13G-6).

- With a Bankart Viper (Arthrex) suture passer, pass the lowermost sutures (below the bone fragment) with an antegrade approach, distal to the lowest anchor (Fig. 13G-7).

- With a Sidewinder (Arthrex) suture passer (Fig. 13G-8), pass sutures through the bone fragment by pushing its sharp tips through the bone (S, Sidewinder suture

passer). Then, with a hand-off technique, pass the suture (Fig. 13G-9).

- Sequentially, tie the sutures from distal to proximal (Fig. 13G-10).

- At the conclusion of the repair, the humeral head is centered over the bare spot of the glenoid (Fig. 13G-11).

TRICKS AND TIPS

- If an overhead athlete has a bony Bankart lesion in the dominant shoulder, the surgeon should make every effort to obtain bone union of the Bankart fragment to the glenoid. This is the only way to preserve motion *and*

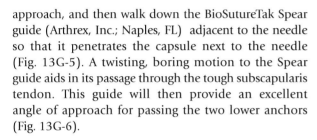

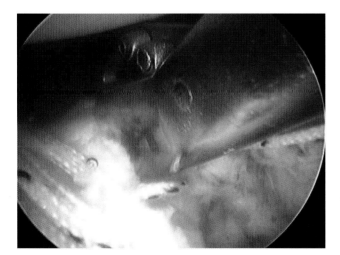

Figure 13G-7   Left shoulder, anterosuperolateral viewing portal. A Bankart Viper (Arthrex, Inc.; Naples, FL) suture passer is used to place a suture distal to the lowermost anchor.

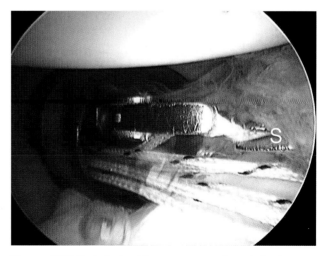

Figure 13G-9   Left shoulder, anterosuperolateral viewing portal. The Sidewinder (Arthrex, Inc.; Naples, FL) suture passer's tips (*S*) have been passed through the bone fragment, where they will accept a suture from a suture retriever by a "hand-off" technique.

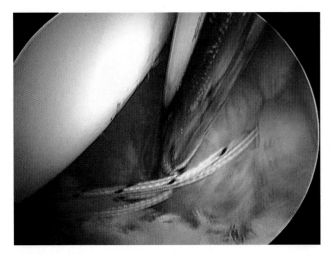

Figure 13G-10   Left shoulder, anterosuperolateral viewing portal. Knots are sequentially tied with the Surgeon's Sixth Finger (Arthrex, Inc.; Naples, FL) knot pusher, beginning with the distal-most sutures.

restore stability at the extremes of motion required in throwing. If a Latarjet procedure is done in the dominant shoulder of a baseball player, he will not regain enough external rotation to be able to throw effectively, although his shoulder will be stable and functional for other activities.

● In the case of a bony Bankart lesion, we have found that a 5 o'clock portal is always necessary for placement of the most inferior anchor. With glenoid bone loss, the angle of approach to the 5 o'clock or 7 o'clock position on the glenoid through a standard anterior portal is too oblique to predictably gain purchase in the bone with a glenoid suture anchor.

● The 5 o'clock portal is used *only* for placement of suture anchors. Suture passage and knot-tying are performed through a standard anterior portal.

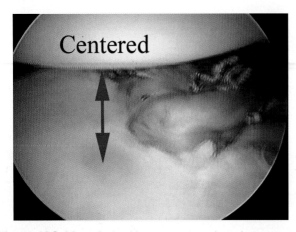

Figure 13G-11   Left shoulder, anterosuperolateral viewing portal. Final result, in which the humeral head is centered exactly over the glenoid bare spot.

● The 45° Sidewinder (Arthrex) suture passer is ideal for passing sutures through the bone fragment because it has sharp tips that can be used to bore through the bone. Once the tips have been passed through the bone, they are opened slightly to accept a suture "hand-off" from a suture retriever placed through the posterior portal; this is done while viewing from the anterosuperolateral portal.

13H

Repair of Reverse Humeral Avulsion of Glenohumeral Ligament (RHAGL) Lesion

● We have seen a few cases wherein a small posterior Bankart lesion and a large reverse HAGL lesion are found. In such cases, first repair the posterior Bankart lesion with suture anchors to provide a firm fixation point on one side of the unstable sheet of posterior capsule.

● Recognize the reverse HAGL lesion as a posterior capsular defect, which has been avulsed from the humerus, in which the underlying muscle is visible through the defect (Fig. 13H-1). Once the reverse HAGL lesion has been identified, create a posterolateral portal through the defect. G, glenoid; H, humerus.

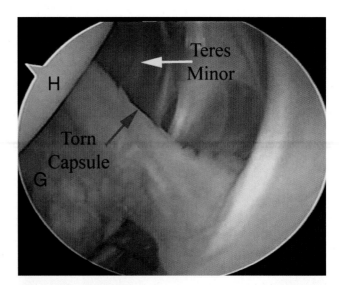

Figure 13H-1   Right shoulder, anterosuperolateral viewing portal. The reverse humeral avulsion of glenohumeral ligaments RHAGL lesion is clearly visible as a capsular rent above the posterior cannula in this arthroscopic photo, and muscle is seen deep to the capsular defect.

- Using a grasper, determine if the detached capsule is reducible to its bone bed on the posterior aspect of the proximal humerus (Fig. 13H-2).

- Prepare the bone bed on the posterior aspect of the humeral head, using a curette, (Fig. 13H-3) and then place a suture anchor (Fig. 13H-4).

- Pass capsular sutures by antegrade (Fig. 13H-5) or retrograde techniques through the posterolateral portal.

- Then withdraw the posterolateral cannula barely past the capsule, and blindly tie the capsular sutures within the cannula to complete the repair.

TRICKS AND TIPS

- An accessory posterolateral cannula, which is inserted through the center of the reverse HAGL lesion, is essential for suture passage.

- The angle for suture anchor insertion for a reverse HAGL repair is not as severe as for a HAGL repair (the "killer angle"), but the suture passage and knot-tying have a high degree of difficulty in this confined and relatively inaccessible space.

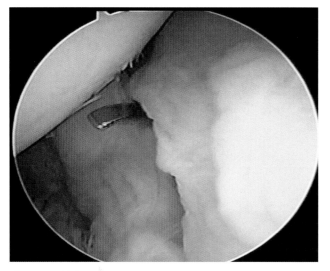

Figure 13H-2 Right shoulder, anterosuperolateral viewing portal. A grasper is used to reduce the edge of the capsule to assess its reparability.

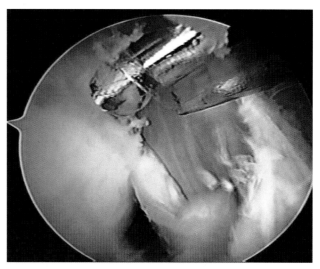

Figure 13H-4 Right shoulder, anterosuperolateral viewing portal. A BioCorkscrew (Arthrex, Inc.; Naples, FL) suture anchor is placed in the prepared bone bed in the proximal humerus.

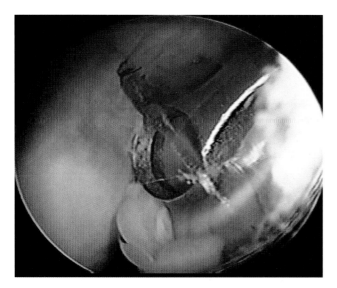

Figure 13H-3 Right shoulder, anterosuperolateral viewing portal. A curette introduced through a posterolateral portal is used to prepare the bone bed of the humerus.

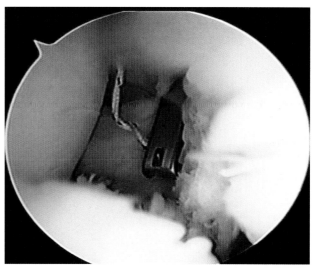

Figure 13H-5 Right shoulder, anterosuperolateral viewing portal. Capsular sutures from the anchor are placed with a Viper (Arthrex, Inc.; Naples, FL) suture passer.

13I

Repair of Triple Labral Lesion

- A triple labral lesion is one that has a combination of three labral lesions: (a) superior labrum anterior and posterior (SLAP) lesion; (b) Bankart lesion; and (c) posterior Bankart lesion.

- The case shown here has a Type III SLAP lesion (Fig. 13I-1). The bucket-handle segment is excised, but the Type II component of the SLAP lesion will also require repair.

- A posterior Bankart lesion is present (Fig. 13I-2) as well as an anterior Bankart lesion (Fig. 13I-3).

- Also, significant inferior labral pathology with labral detachment is seen all along the axillary pouch (Fig. 13I-4).

- Begin the repair by preparing the glenoid bone bed, leaving a horseshoe-shaped labral lesion around the inferior glenoid (Fig. 13I-5) in addition to the SLAP lesion.

- Place the SLAP anchors and pass their sutures through the superior labrum (Fig. 13I-6), but do not tie them until after all the other sutures (anterior and posterior) have been tied.

- Place a posteroinferior anchor through a posterolateral portal (Fig. 13I-7), and an anteroinferior anchor through a 5 o'clock portal (Fig. 13I-8).

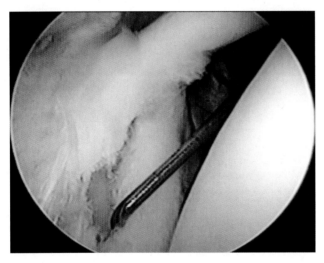

Figure 13I-1 Right shoulder, posterior viewing portal. This arthroscopic photo shows a Type III superior labrum anterior and posterior (SLAP) lesion with a bucket-handle segment.

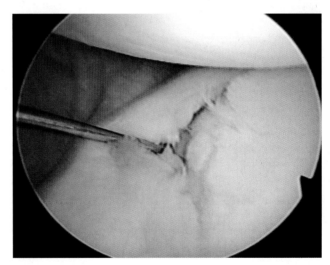

Figure 13I-3 Right shoulder, anterosuperolateral viewing portal. Anterior Bankart lesion is seen in this view.

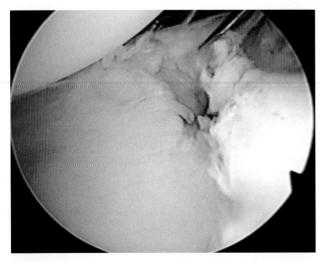

Figure 13I-2 Right shoulder, anterosuperolateral viewing portal. Posterior Bankart lesion is present.

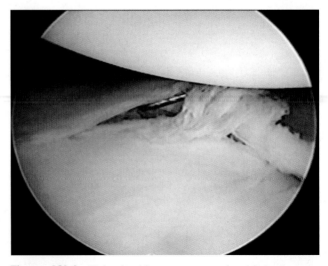

Figure 13I-4 Right shoulder, anterosuperolateral viewing portal. The inferior labral lesion connects the anterior and posterior Bankart lesions.

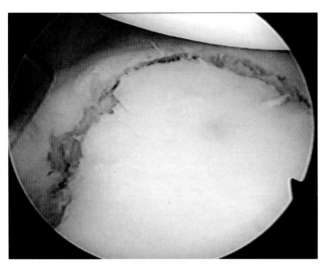

Figure 13I-5 Right shoulder, anterosuperolateral viewing portal. After glenoid preparation, the horseshoe shape of this extensive inferior labral lesion is apparent.

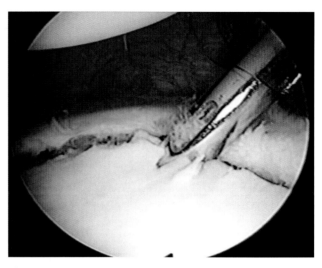

Figure 13I-7 Right shoulder, anterosuperolateral viewing portal. A posteroinferior anchor is placed through the posterolateral portal.

- The easiest way to pass the anteroinferior sutures distally below the anchor is with an antegrade technique using a Bankart Viper (Arthrex, Inc.; Naples, FL) suture passer (Fig. 13I-9), whereas the posteroinferior sutures are most easily passed retrograde by a 45° BirdBeak (Arthrex) suture passer through the posterior portal (Fig. 13I-10). Tie the sutures from the inferior anchors, then sequentially place additional anchors and pass and tie the sutures.

- After tying all the anterior and posterior sutures, tie the previously-passed SLAP lesion sutures.

- After all sutures have been tied, the humeral head should be centered over the glenoid bare spot (Fig. 13I-11).

TRICKS AND TIPS

- If a Type III SLAP lesion is encountered, as in this case, it is important to realize that a Type II component always accompanies this lesion, with disruption of the superior labrum from the glenoid bone bed. For that reason, simple excision of the bucket-handle segment is not

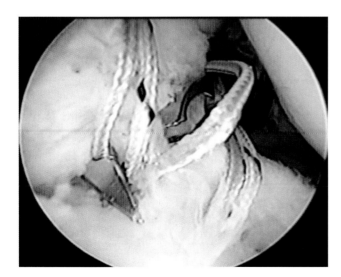

Figure 13I-6 Right shoulder, posterior viewing portal. A BirdBeak (Arthrex, Inc.; Naples, FL) suture passer is used to pass sutures through the superior labrum. These will be tied last (after all other sutures have been tied) to achieve repair of the superior labrum anterior and posterior (SLAP) lesion.

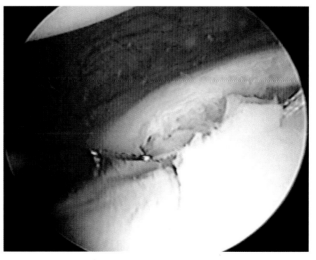

Figure 13I-8 Right shoulder, anterosuperolateral viewing portal. An anteroinferior anchor is placed through a 5 o'clock portal.

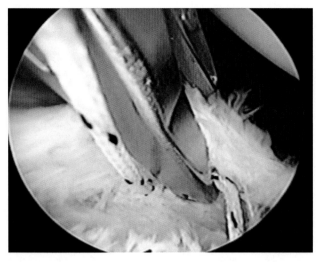

Figure 13I-9 Right shoulder, anterosuperolateral viewing portal. A Bankart Viper (Arthrex, Inc.; Naples, FL) suture passer is used to place sutures distal to the 5 o'clock anchor using an antegrade technique.

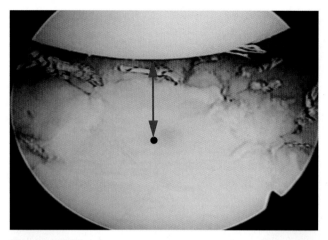

Figure 13I-11 Right shoulder, anterosuperolateral viewing portal. At the conclusion of the triple labral repair, the humeral head is centered over the glenoid bare spot.

enough, but it must be combined with repair of the Type II component.

● If the posterolateral portal is placed somewhat low (at the same level as our usual low posterior portal, which enters the joint in the posteroinferior quadrant), then a very low anchor placement (at 6 o'clock or 6:30 position) is possible.

● Penetration of the capsule at the 6 o'clock position is necessary to achieve a proximal shift of the posteroinferior capsule. This can easily be done at 6 o'clock with a

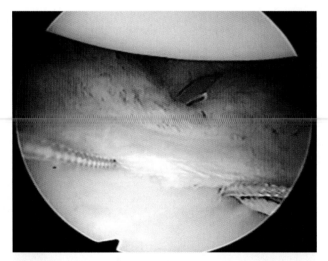

Figure 13I-10 Right shoulder, anterosuperolateral viewing portal. A 45° BirdBeak (Arthrex, Inc.; Naples, FL) suture passer through a posterior working portal easily achieves retrograde suture passage through the capsule at the 6 o'clock and 7 o'clock positions.

45° BirdBeak suture passer introduced through a low posterior portal. (see Fig. 13I-10).

13J

Arthroscopic Repair of Humeral Avulsion of Glenohumeral Ligament (HAGL) Lesion

● From a posterior viewing portal, the lateral edge of the anterior capsule can be seen to be retracted medially, and subscapularis muscle fibers can be seen anterolateral to the retracted edge of the capsule (Fig. 13J-1).

● Establish an anterior portal and a 5 o'clock portal (Fig. 13J-2).

● Prepare the bone bed on the humerus through the 5 o'clock portal.

● Insert anchors into the bone bed on the humerus through the 5 o'clock portal. The angle of approach is so steep (oblique) that portal placement must be perfect to obtain satisfactory purchase in bone. We call this the "killer angle" (Fig. 13J-3).

● If space permits, we prefer to place two suture anchors into the proximal humerus.

● Pass sutures in antegrade fashion through the capsular margin by means of instruments inserted through the anterior portal.

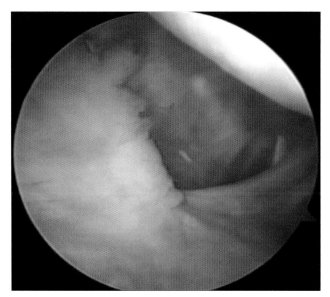

Figure 13J-1 Right shoulder, posterior viewing portal. The lateral edge of the avulsed anterior capsule is visible, with muscle fibers of the subscapularis deep to the capsular margin.

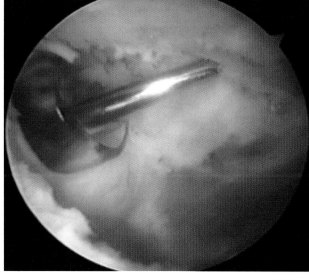

Figure 13J-3 Right shoulder, anterosuperolateral viewing portal. Even with optimal placement of the 5 o'clock portal, the "killer angle" is very obliquely oriented to the surface of the bone bed in the proximal humerus.

- We prefer to tie the sutures with a Surgeon's Sixth Finger (Arthrex, Inc.; Naples, FL) knot pusher. As the sutures are tied, the space closes down and visualization can become very difficult.

- At the completion of the repair, the capsular attachment to the humerus is restored, and the underlying subscapularis muscle belly is no longer visible (Fig. 13J-4).

TRICKS AND TIPS

- A spinal needle is used to direct placement of the 5 o'clock portal. It must be placed far laterally, entering the joint near the humeral bone bed, and must be at or below the midpoint of the subscapularis to "hit" the bone bed at an angle that will allow purchase of the anchor in bone.

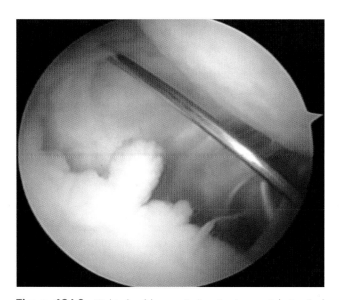

Figure 13J-2 Right shoulder, posterior viewing portal. A spinal needle is used to choose an appropriate angle of approach for the 5 o'clock portal, which will allow firm suture anchor fixation into the proximal humerus.

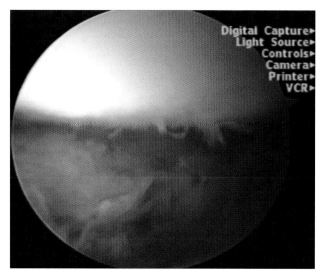

Figure 13J-4 Right shoulder, posterior viewing portal. Completed repair of the capsule. The subscapularis muscle is no longer visible. (Compare to pre-repair appearance in Fig. 13J-1).

14

SLAP Repair

- Evaluate superior labrum with a hook probe.

- An anterior superior labrum anterior and posterior (SLAP) lesion will have a displaceable biceps root (Fig. 14-1) in which no continuity exists of soft tissue attachment from the biceps root to the superior glenoid. In essence, the biceps root has no bone attachment.

- A posterior SLAP lesion will have a positive peel-back test (Fig. 14-2).

- Combined anterior–posterior SLAP lesions will have both a displaceable biceps root and a positive peel-back test.

- An anterosuperolateral portal is established as a working portal for anchor placement, suture passing, and knot-tying.

- The superior glenoid neck is prepared down to a bleeding base of bone before anchor placement.

- Through the anterosuperolateral portal, insert a suture anchor directly below the biceps root (Fig. 14-3).

- If a more posterosuperior anchor is additionally required, place it through a posterolateral portal (Port of Wilmington), which is located 1 cm lateral and 1 cm anterior to the posterolateral corner of the acromion (Figs. 14-4 and 14-5).

- Using a 45° BirdBeak (Arthrex, Inc.; Naples, FL) suture passer, pass sutures through the anterosuperolateral portal to penetrate through the superior and posterosuperior labrum (Fig. 14-6).

- If the superior glenohumeral ligament attachment is disrupted anterior to the biceps root, perform a suture anchor repair of that ligament (Fig. 14-7).

- Sequentially tie the sutures from anterior to posterior.

- The most important suture for neutralizing peel-back forces is the one just posterior to the biceps root (Fig. 14-8).

TRICKS AND TIPS

- The superior and posterosuperior labra are best visualized in panoramic fashion if the viewing portal is a low posterior portal, entering the joint in the posteroinferior quadrant.

- In creating the anterosuperolateral portal, use a spinal needle initially to choose the proper entry point and angle of approach. When viewing through a posterior portal, a soft-tissue "ridge" should been seen directly above the biceps tendon. This ridge marks the junction of the thicker supraspinatus tendon with the thinner rotator interval tissue. The portal should enter just anterior to this ridge, through the rotator interval tissue, in order not to damage the supraspinatus tendon. Furthermore, the angle of approach to the superior glenoid rim should be a 45° angle for optimal anchor placement.

- In preparing the glenoid neck, all soft tissue should be removed down to a bleeding base of bone. Ring curettes are useful to precisely remove the thick articular cartilage at the corner of the glenoid. When the shaver is used, it is more effective to run it on forward or reverse (depending on whether the surgery is being performed on a left or right shoulder) rather than the oscillate mode. Furthermore, working portals must be changed, depending on which part of the glenoid neck is being prepared. For the superior glenoid neck (underneath the biceps

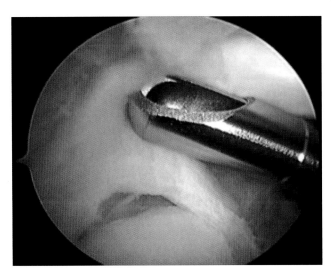

Figure 14-1 Right shoulder, posterior viewing portal. A shaver blade is used to pull the biceps root away from the superior glenoid bone bed, demonstrating a displaceable biceps root.

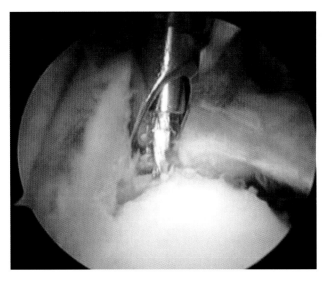

Figure 14-3 A suture anchor is inserted directly beneath the biceps root.

root as well as posterior to it), an anterior working portal is used for bone preparation. To prepare the bone anterior to the biceps root, an anterosuperolateral working portal should be used.

- If the SLAP lesion extends anterior to the biceps root, the superior glenohumeral ligament (SGHL) has been disrupted and must be repaired to bone with a suture anchor.

- Doubly loaded anchors give greater security of fixation and we preferentially use them (BioSutureTak or BioFASTak [Arthrex]).

- We prefer to use simple sutures rather than mattress sutures because they are more effective at resisting peel-back forces.

- For placement of posterosuperior anchors, the anterosuperolateral portal is usually not satisfactory because of the very oblique angle of approach it provides to that portion of the glenoid rim. The Port of Wilmington portal provides a much more direct angle for secure anchor placement.

- We use the Port of Wilmington for anchor placement only, so that we can use a small (3-mm) Spear guide (Arthrex, Inc.; Naples, FL) rather than a larger diameter cannula. This small diameter puncture is preferable because this portal penetrates the rotator cuff very close to the musculotendinous junction of the infraspinatus tendon.

- Using the 45° BirdBeak through an anterosuperolateral portal provides the perfect angle for penetrating the superior and posterosuperior labrum for suture passage.

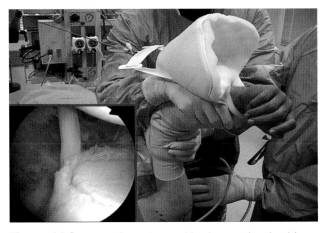

Figure 14-2 To perform the peel-back test, the shoulder is brought into 90° abduction and 90° external rotation. If the biceps root is not firmly anchored to bone, the biceps superior labral complex will peel back medially over the edge of the glenoid (*inset*), demonstrating a positive peel-back test.

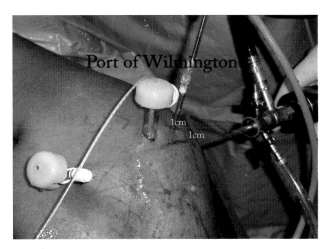

Figure 14-4 External view of a right shoulder showing the entry point for the Port of Wilmington portal.

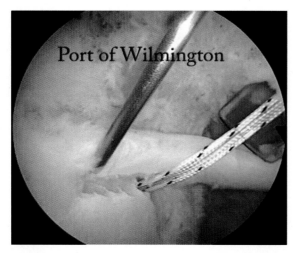

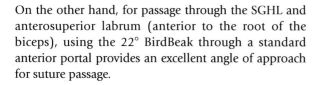

Figure 14-5 Intra-articular arthroscopic view of a right shoulder through a posterior viewing portal. This view demonstrates the excellent angle of approach afforded by the Port of Wilmington portal for anchor placement.

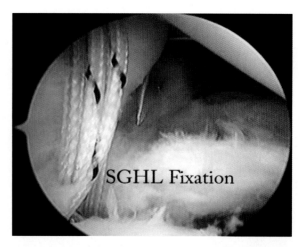

Figure 14-7 A suture anchor repair of the superior gleno-humeral ligament (SGHL) and anterosuperior labrum is performed when the superior labrum anterior and posterior (SLAP) lesion extends anterior to the biceps root.

On the other hand, for passage through the SGHL and anterosuperior labrum (anterior to the root of the biceps), using the 22° BirdBeak through a standard anterior portal provides an excellent angle of approach for suture passage.

- The single most effective suture at resisting peel-back forces is the one just posterior to the root of the biceps. We call this the "money stitch" for SLAP repair because of its critical biomechanical role in the durability of the repair.

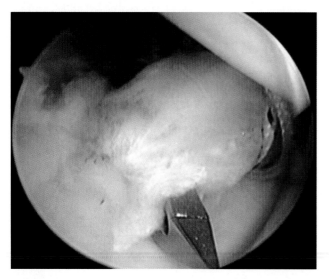

Figure 14-6 A 45° BirdBeak (Arthrex, Inc.; Naples, FL) suture passer is used through the anterosuperolateral portal for suture passage.

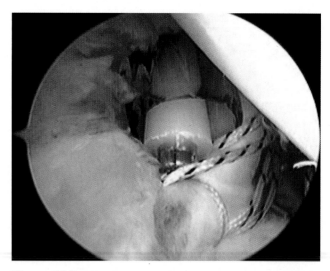

Figure 14-8 The "money stitch" just posterior to the biceps root is the most effective suture for resisting peelback forces.

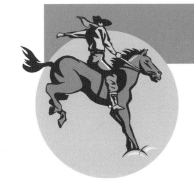

Subacromial Procedures (Non-cuff)

15A

Arthroscopic Acromioplasty

- We prefer, initially, to place the arthroscope in the part of the subacromial space that has the largest volume of open bursal space. The bursa occupies the anterior half of the subacromial space, and the largest part of that bursal space is beneath the anterolateral corner of the acromion, which is where we direct the tip of our scope.

- While viewing from a posterior portal, use a spinal needle to choose the proper lateral portal placement, underneath the anterior half of the acromion and parallel to it.

- Introduce a power shaver through a lateral portal and perform a bursectomy in the anterior half of the subacromial space. Identify the acromion, the coracoacromial ligament, and the rotator cuff (Fig. 15A-1).

- Divide the internal deltoid fascia longitudinally with an electrocautery probe from the portal site to the lateral acromial border, then distally past the edge of the greater tuberosity to expose the lateral gutter (Fig. 15A-2).

- Use an electrocautery probe to remove the soft tissues from the undersurface of the acromion as well as from the distal clavicle. Excise the coracoacromial (CA) ligament.

- While viewing from posteriorly, perform a "provisional" anterior acromioplasty by introducing a motorized burr through a lateral portal. This simply provides a bleeding bone surface at the anterior acromion, which is a useful landmark to aim for when the final acromioplasty is done by a cutting-block technique.

- Next, while viewing through a lateral portal, bring a power shaver in through a posterior portal to remove the fibrofatty soft tissues from the posterior aspect of the subacromial space.

- Identify the dome, or highest point, of the acromion. Typically, a "hump" of bone will be seen between the dome of the acromion and the bleeding surface of the provisional acromioplasty (Fig. 15A-3). Remove this hump of bone during the cutting-block portion of the procedure to create a flat undersurface to the acromion (Fig. 15A-4).

- Next, switch the scope to the posterior viewing portal, and perform the final refinement of the acromioplasty, if necessary. If the acromion has a lateral downslope, perform a lateral bevel on the acromion with a high-speed burr to diminish any lateral impingement (Fig. 15A-5).

TRICKS AND TIPS

- The portion of the subacromial space that has the greatest volume is directly beneath the anterolateral corner of the acromion. To maximize the chance of placing the scope in an actual "space," it is important to aim the scope from the posterior portal toward the anterolateral tip of the acromion. Even if that space is compromised, a trick will allow the surgeon to enter it every time. In

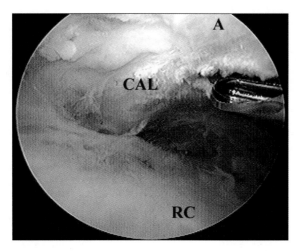

Figure 15A-1   Right shoulder, posterior viewing portal. The acromion *(A)*, coracoacromial ligament *(CAL)*, and rotator cuff *(RC)* are easily identifiable.

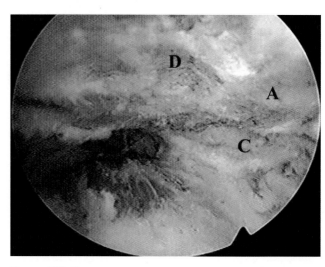

Figure15A-3   Right shoulder, lateral viewing portal. The hump of bone between the dome of the acromion *(D)* and the provisional acromioplasty at the anterior acromion *(A)* must be removed during the cutting-block procedure. C, distal clavicle.

pushing the scope toward a point beneath the anterolateral tip of the acromion, intentionally push the scope beyond the subacromial space and into the deltoid muscle. Then, with the scope and camera in place, slowly withdraw the arthroscopic sheath. At first, only the deltoid muscle will be seen. A slight "give" or "pop" will be felt as the scope withdraws past the deltoid fascia, and then will appear a clear view of whatever space exists.

● There are three reasons to incise the internal deltoid fascia with an electrocautery probe through the lateral portal. The first reason is that it provides an easy way to locate the lateral border of the acromion (as the cautery probe divides the fascia proximally). The second reason is for visualization. Dividing the internal deltoid fascia distally into the lateral gutter provides a clear view of the greater tuberosity and the lateral-most portions of the rotator cuff. The third reason is for freedom of movement for instruments introduced through the lateral working portal. Releasing the fascia allows the surgeon much greater freedom to move the arthroscopic instruments without being bound and restricted by noncompliant muscle fascia.

● Clear the undersurface of the distal clavicle to detect any distal clavicular osteophytes that may need to be coplaned.

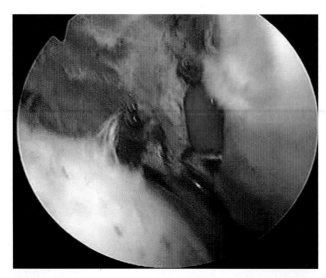

Figure 15A-2   Right shoulder, posterior viewing portal. The internal deltoid fascia is incised distally by an electrocautery probe to expose the lateral gutter.

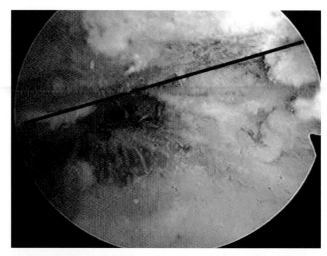

Figure 15A-4   Right shoulder, lateral viewing portal. At the conclusion of the cutting-block procedure, the undersurface of the acromion should be flat, as indicated by the *solid black line.*

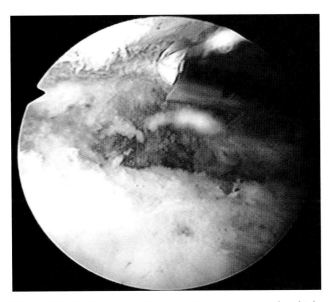

Figure15A-5   Right shoulder, posterior viewing portal. A high-speed burr has been introduced through a lateral portal to create a lateral bevel to the acromion.

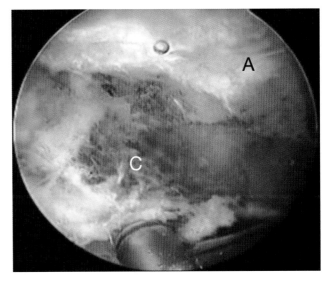

Figure 15B-2   Right shoulder, posterior viewing portal, 30° arthroscope. A provisional resection of 1 cm of the inferior aspect of the distal clavicle has been done. C, distal clavicle; A, acromion.

15B

Arthroscopic Distal Clavicle Excision

- Perform a subacromial bursectomy along with excision of the medial fibrofatty tissue around the distal clavicle and the scapular spine.

- Expose the scapular spine (Fig. 15B-1). This is located posterior to the acromioclavicular (AC) joint and is sur-rounded by dense fibrofatty tissue that must be removed. The scapular spine resembles the keel of a boat, and it marks the border between supraspinatus and infraspinatus muscles.

- Refine the acromioplasty, as indicated.

- Expose the AC joint, using instrumentation through an anterior working portal.

- Make a provisional resection of the inferior aspect of the distal clavicle (Fig. 15B-2), using a power burr through an anterior portal.

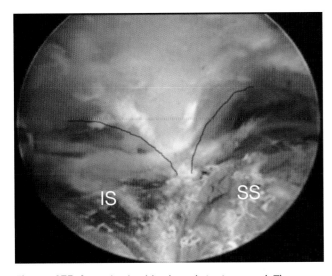

Figure 15B-1   Right shoulder, lateral viewing portal. The scapular spine has been exposed. Note the keel shape of scapular spine and its location between the muscle bellies of supraspinatus (SS) and infraspinatus (IS).

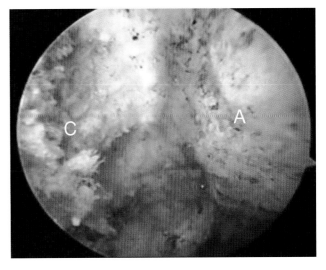

Figure 15B-3   Right shoulder, posterior viewing portal, 70° arthroscope. Note: The superior portion of the distal clavicle can be seen in its entirety all the way to the acromioclavicular (AC) joint. C, distal clavicle; A, acromion.

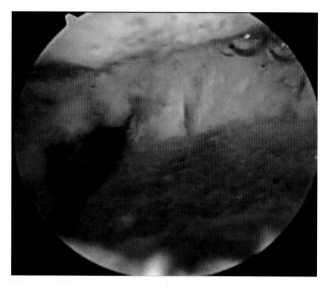

Figure 15B-4 Right shoulder, posterior viewing portal, 70° arthroscope. Final result after resection, leaving a 1-cm space at the acromioclavicular (AC) joint.

- After the provisional resection, insert a 70° arthroscope through a posterior portal for a better view of the superior AC joint (Fig. 15B-3).

- Complete the resection. The endpoint is to create a 1-cm space at the AC joint (Fig. 15B-4).

TRICKS AND TIPS

- The best view of the AC joint is through a posterior viewing portal in which the scope passes directly against the lateral aspect of the scapular spine. The dense fibrofatty tissue surrounding the scapular spine and the distal clavicle must be removed, however, to be able to visualize the AC joint from this approach.

- The scapular spine is easily identified by locating the medial acromion just posterior to the AC joint, then following the bony arch posteromedially as it dives inferiorly between the muscle bellies of supraspinatus and infraspinatus tendons (Fig. 15B-1). After débriding the overlying fibrofatty tissue, the scapular spine has a shape that is like the keel of a boat.

- We prefer to excise the distal clavicle with a high-speed burr introduced through an anterior working portal. We use the same skin puncture used for an intra-articular anterior portal, which is an outside-in portal that enters the joint over the lateral half of the subscapularis tendon. If that portal is established for the intra-articular portion of the arthroscopy, the same skin puncture can be used for the distal clavicle excision. In doing this, we have found that the angle of approach to the AC joint is

virtually always exactly on target in the plane of the AC joint for precise excision of the distal clavicle.

- Although some surgeons try to preserve all the AC ligaments except the inferiorly-located ones, we believe that the posterior and anterior AC ligaments must be excised for adequate bone resection, so we routinely excise them. We have not seen any adverse effects as a result of excising the anterior and posterior ligaments. We believe, however, that it is important to preserve the superior ligaments.

- We believe that it is essential to use a 70° arthroscope when excising the superior portion of the distal clavicle. Many AC joints are angled up to 45° from inferomedial to superolateral, and the only way to completely visualize the entire distal clavicle without excising some of the medial acromion (which we never do) is to use a 70° arthroscope.

- A 1-cm resection of the distal clavicle is always sufficient to prevent abutment of the distal clavicle against the medial acromion when the arm is taken across the body into horizontal adduction. In fact, we have done this maneuver intraoperatively while viewing the AC joint arthroscopically in >100 patients, and we have never observed AC abutment after resection of 1 cm of bone from the distal clavicle.

15C

Coplaning of Distal Clavicle

- While viewing through a lateral viewing portal, clear the scapular spine of fibrofatty tissue (Fig. 15C-1). This will permit later placement of the arthroscope sufficiently

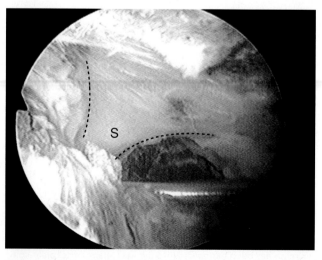

Figure 15C-1 Scapular spine (S) (dotted lines) of a left shoulder, as viewed from a lateral portal, has been cleared of fibrofatty tissue.

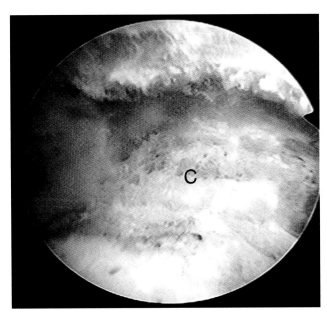

Figure 15C-2   Distal clavicle after coplaning, demonstrating a lateral bevel to the undersurface of the distal clavicle. C, distal clavicle.

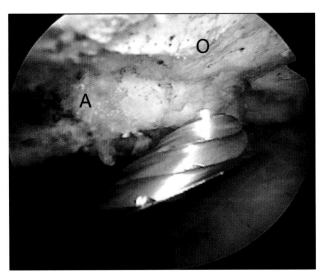

Figure 15D-1   Right shoulder, lateral viewing portal. "Refining acromioplasty," in which the body of the acromion is flattened by a cutting-block technique before excising the os acromiale. A, acromial body; O, os acromiale.

medial (through a posterior viewing portal) for excellent visualization of the distal clavicle.

- After the acromioplasty has been completed, clear all soft tissue from the undersurface of the distal clavicle while viewing through a posterior portal.

- Coplaning of the distal clavicle (Fig. 15C-2) is achieved by alternately viewing through a posterior portal while using a burr through a lateral portal, then viewing through a lateral portal while using a burr through an anterior portal.

- Usually a hook of bone projects downward at the anterior border of the body of the acromion. Remove that hook by a cutting-block technique, while viewing through a lateral portal (Fig. 15D-1), before excising the os acromiale. We term this portion of the procedure a "refining acromioplasty."

- Coplane the undersurface of the clavicle, if necessary, to remove inferiorly projecting osteophytes.

- Next, excise the os (mesoacromion) with a high-speed burr while viewing from posteriorly. As the excision progresses, the 30° arthroscope must be switched to a 70° arthroscope to see around the cleft and be able to

TRICKS AND TIPS

- Clearing the scapular spine of fibrofatty tissue will greatly enhance visualization of the acromioclavicular joint with the arthroscope placed through a posterior portal.

15D

Os Acromiale Excision

- A mesoacromion is the type of os acromiale whose posterior border lies in line with the posterior border of the clavicle. The mesoacromion is usually mobile to palpation.

- In the case of a symptomatic mesoacromion, we prefer to remove the mobile fragment.

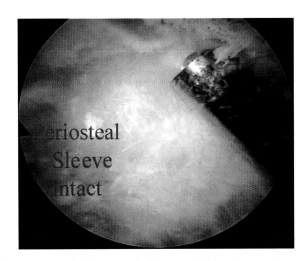

Figure 15D-2   Posterior viewing portal, right shoulder. In excising the os acromiale, the periosteal sleeve is preserved.

fully excise all the bone. Preserve the periosteal sleeve so as not to disrupt deltoid and trapezial muscle attachments (Fig. 15D-2).

TRICKS AND TIPS

● In our experience, preacromion and mesoacromion types of os acromiale can be completely excised without creating any functional deficit or cosmetic deformity. We have never seen a nontraumatic meta-acromion, and we doubt its existence as an anatomic variant.

● By preserving the periosteal sleeve that is continuous with the deltotrapezial fascia, we have never had a case of deltoid detachment following excision of an os acromiale.

Stiffness

16A

Capsular Release for Adhesive Capsulitis

● Release rotator interval with electrocautery wand. Excise all rotator interval tissue between the upper subscapularis and the superior glenohumeral ligament (SGHL), being careful to preserve the medial sling of the biceps (Fig. 16A-1).

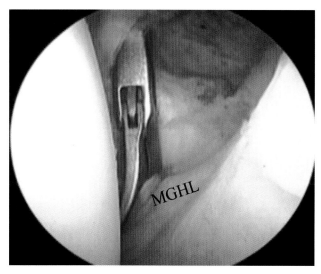

Figure 16A-2 Scissors perform release of middle glenohumeral ligament *(MGHL)*.

● Release the middle glenohumeral ligament (MGHL) (Fig. 16A-2).

● Place the arthroscope anteriorly and perform a posterior capsular release from 1 o'clock to 5 o'clock with a pencil-tip electrode.

● Use the pencil-tipped electrode to make multiple perforations in the capsule of the axillary pouch (Fig. 16A-3).

● Release the anterior capsule inferior glenohumeral ligament (IGHL) using a pencil-tip electrode placed through the posterior portal, with an angle of approach parallel to the joint line (Fig. 16A-4).

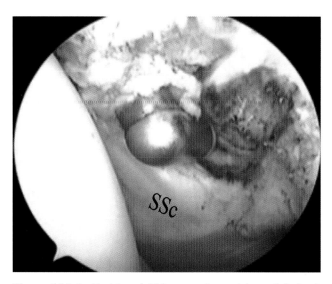

Figure 16A-1 Excision of thick rotator interval tissue (left shoulder, posterior viewing portal). SSc, subscapularis tendon.

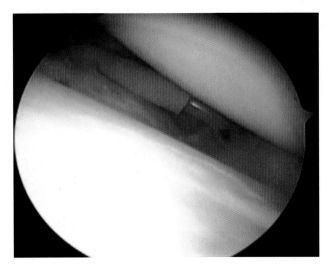

Figure 16A-3 Pencil-tip electrode (introduced through posterior portal) is used to make multiple perforations in the axillary pouch (left shoulder, anterosuperior viewing portal).

- Manipulate the shoulder in order to fully release the "perforated" axillary pouch.

- Reassess arthroscopically.

TRICKS AND TIPS

- Lateral excursion of the subscapularis tendon must be restored by rotator interval release and anterior capsular release.

- Because the posterior portal is created at an angle that is parallel to the face of the glenoid, a pencil-tip electrode

through that portal provides the perfect angle of approach for performing the anterior release of the IGHL.

- Surgically created perforations in the axillary pouch capsule cause sufficient capsular weakening that manipulation will usually release the axillary pouch after all other releases have been completed arthroscopically.

16B

Capsular Release for Postoperative Stiffness after Rotator Cuff Repair

- Assess healing of cuff repair (Fig. 16B-1).

- Release "captured" subscapularis tendon by first creating a window in the rotator interval, then dissect the subscapularis tendon from the coracoid, releasing adhesions that prevent lateral excursion of the tendon with passive external rotation (Fig. 16B-2).

- Perform posterior capsular release with a pencil-tip electrode (OPES electrosurgical system; Arthrex, Inc.; Naples, FL).

- The posterior release should extend from 11 o'clock to 7 o'clock (Fig. 16B-3). Then, use the pencil-tip electrode to perforate the capsule multiple times in the axillary pouch.

- Manipulate the shoulder, which typically releases the axillary pouch in line with the perforations.

- Release any subacromial adhesions.

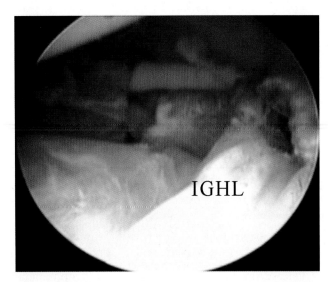

Figure 16A-4 The anteriorly located inferior glenohumeral ligament (IGHL) is released using a pencil-tip electrode introduced through a posterior working portal, parallel to the surface of the glenoid (left shoulder, anterosuperior viewing portal).

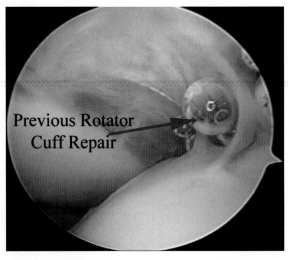

Figure 16B-1 Healed rotator cuff repair (right shoulder, posterior viewing portal).

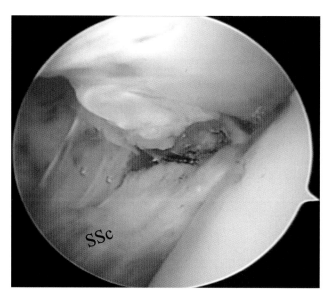

Figure 16B-2 Subscapularis tendon mobilization is begun by releasing the upper subscapularis tendon from rotator interval tissue, taking care to preserve the medial sling of biceps, then excising the rotator interval tissue to create a rotator interval "window," followed by release of any adhesions between the coracoid and subscapularis. SSc, subscapularis tendon. (Right shoulder posterior viewing portal.)

TRICKS AND TIPS

- If external rotation is limited, then the "captured" subscapularis tendon must have its lateral excursion restored by releasing it from surrounding adhesions.

- The posterior capsular release should be done 1-cm from the posterior labrum, extending from 11 o'clock to 7 o'clock.

- Multiple perforations of the capsule in the axillary pouch, using a pencil-tip electrode, usually direct its tearing along those perforations during manipulation.

16C
Manipulation Under Anesthesia

- For adhesive capsulitis and for postoperative stiffness, manipulation is done only after arthroscopic anterior and posterior capsular releases have been performed, along with multiple perforations in the capsule of the axillary pouch. The perforations weaken the axillary pouch so that it can be manipulated into full forward elevation as the capsule fails along the perforations. This provides a more controlled release than manipulation alone.

- After performing arthroscopic releases, remove all instruments and cannulas from the shoulder, and take the arm out of balanced suspension.

- First, externally rotate the shoulder while the arm is at the side. Then, take the arm up into full combined elevation and external rotation while an assistant stabilizes the inferolateral border of the scapula (Fig. 16C-1).

- Next, manipulate the shoulder up into combined elevation and internal rotation while the assistant stabilizes the scapula (Fig. 16C-2).

- Next, manipulate the shoulder into full elevation (Fig. 16C-3), then into horizontal abduction.

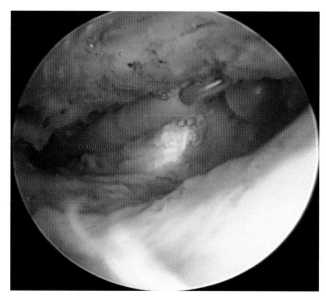

Figure 16B-3 Posterior release with a pencil-tip electrocautery probe. Note: The posterior capsule is too thick (~1 cm) to accomplish a release by shoulder manipulation alone. (Right shoulder anterior viewing portal.)

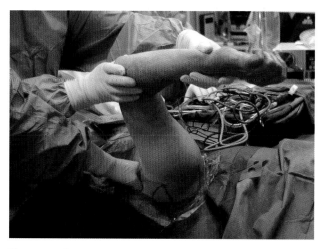

Figure 16C-1 The surgeon manipulates the shoulder into combined elevation and external rotation while the assistant stabilizes the scapula.

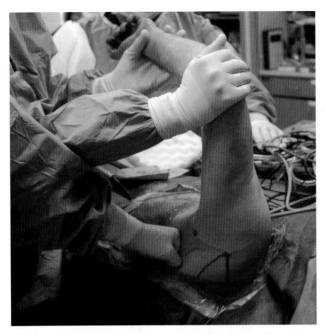

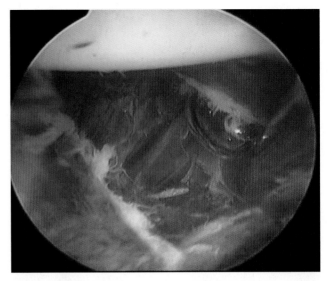

Figure 16C-4 Intra-articular view after manipulation shows that the capsule in the axillary recess has been disrupted a few millimeters from the labrum, where the perforations had been made. (Right shoulder, anterosuperolateral viewing portal.)

Figure 16C-2 The shoulder is manipulated into combined elevation and internal rotation while the scapula is stabilized.

- Finally, with the shoulder held at 90° abduction, sequentially rotate it into maximal internal and external rotation.

- Reinsert the arthroscope intra-articularly to assess the adequacy of the release (Fig. 16C-4).

TRICKS AND TIPS

- An arthroscopic-assisted manipulation provides a more controlled release of the capsule than a standard manipulation, reducing the chance of fracture and inadvertent tissue avulsion from overly aggressive manipulation.

- The only part of the capsule that is not released (not even with multiple perforations) is the superior capsule (between 11 o'clock and 1 o'clock).

- Stabilization of the scapula concentrates the forces of manipulation at the glenohumeral joint for maximal effectiveness.

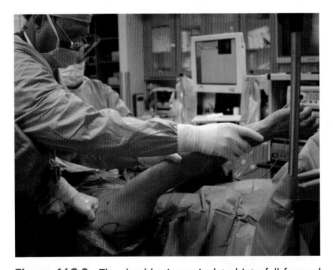

Figure 16C-3 The shoulder is manipulated into full forward elevation.

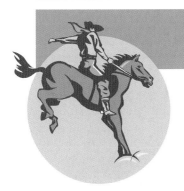

Rotator Cuff

17A

Completion of a PASTA Lesion to a Full-Thickness Cuff Tear

- We recommend converting a partial articular surface tendon avulsion (PASTA) lesion to a full-thickness cuff tear when only a thin tenuous layer of lateral cuff tissue is available (Fig. 17A-1).

- In this case, excise the poor-quality lateral cuff tissue with electrocautery and shaver and prepare the bone bed.

- Repair the lesion using a double-row technique (Fig. 17A-2)

TRICKS AND TIPS

- The decision to complete the tear is a judgment call. In general, if palpation of the lateral cuff tissue suggests that it is of poor quality and only 1 to 2 mm thick, we recommend completing the tear.

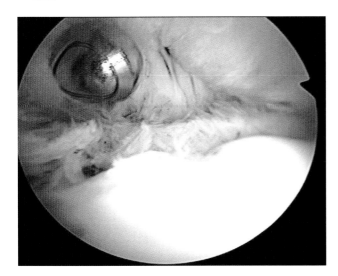

Figure 17A-1 Left shoulder, posterior intra-articular viewing portal. This arthroscopic photo shows that the residual lateral cuff tissue is very thin and of poor quality.

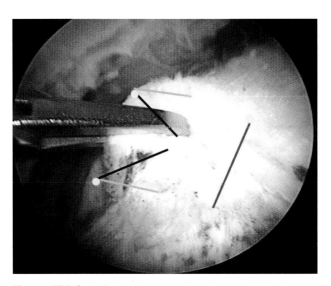

Figure 17A-2 Left shoulder, posterior subacromial viewing portal. A KingFisher tendon grasper (Arthrex, Inc.; Naples, FL) is used to reduce the tear. The superimposed schematic demonstrates the proposed double-row repair.

249

17B

Coracoplasty with Nonretracted Subscapularis Tendon

- Palpate coracoid through rotator interval tissue.

- Make a "window" in the rotator interval.

- Locate the coracoid just anterior to the upper border of the subscapularis tendon; it will be visible through the window in the rotator interval (Fig. 17B-1).

- Identify the coracoid tip, coracoacromial ligament, and conjoint tendon (Fig. 17B-2).

- Remove soft tissues from the coracoid tip with electrocautery and shaver.

- Perform the coracoplasty with a high-speed burr introduced through an anterosuperolateral portal in a plane that is anterior to the "comma sign" (Fig. 17B-3).

Figure 17B-2 Right shoulder, posterior viewing portal, 70° arthroscope. The coracoid tip (*CT*), coracoacromial ligament (*CAL*), and conjoint tendon (*Con*) are easily identifiable.

TRICKS AND TIPS

- The coracoid tip is always located just anterior to the upper border of the subscapularis tendon. It is most easily found from a posterior viewing portal with a 30° arthroscope. The coracoplasty itself is more clearly performed and visualized using a 70° arthroscope.

- When making the "window" in the rotator interval, it is important to preserve the medial sling of the biceps (which is the "comma sign") laterally, as well as the superior glenohumeral ligament (SGHL).

- Only after the "window" has been made in the rotator interval should the soft tissues be removed from the coracoid and the coracoplasty performed with instruments that pass anterior to the "comma sign" so that the comma tissue will not be damaged during the coracoplasty.

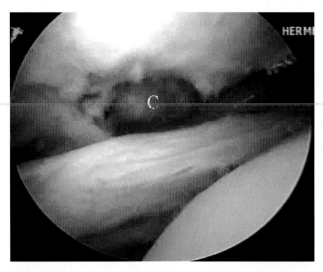

Figure 17B-1 Right shoulder, posterior viewing portal. The coracoid tip (*C*) is easily seen through the window in the rotator interval.

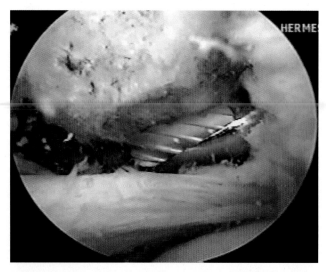

Figure 17B-3 Right shoulder, posterior viewing portal, 70° arthroscope. Coracoplasty being performed by a high-speed burr through an anterosuperolateral portal.

17C

Double-Pulley Technique of Double-Row Repair

- Prepare the bone bed on the greater tuberosity to a bleeding base while viewing through a posterior intra-articular portal.

- Place the scope in the subacromial space and do an arthroscopic subacromial bursectomy, débridement of the rotator cuff tear margin, acromioplasty, and distal clavicle excision (if indicated).

- Place two medial-row suture anchors (BioCorkscrew-FT; Arthrex, Inc.; Naples, FL) adjacent to the articular margin (Fig. 17C-1).

- Pass all four suture limbs from each anchor sequentially through two single points in the rotator cuff, to result in two fixation points in the tendon, with a tendon bridge between them. Pass the sutures using a shuttling technique with a FiberWire SutureLoop (Arthrex, Inc.; Naples, FL) (Fig. 17C-2). Pass the SutureLoop ~15 mm from the free margin of the rotator cuff tear using a long-jaw NeedlePunch or a Scorpion suture passer (Arthrex). Then retrieve the medial sutures through an alternative "holding" portal, because they should not be tied until after tying the lateral row sutures.

- Place the lateral row anchors. If only enough room is available for one lateral anchor, consider adding a third suture to a BioCorkscrew anchor so that it is triple-loaded.

- Pass the lateral sutures ~10 mm from the free margin of the cuff tear. We prefer a Viper suture passer for passing the lateral row sutures.

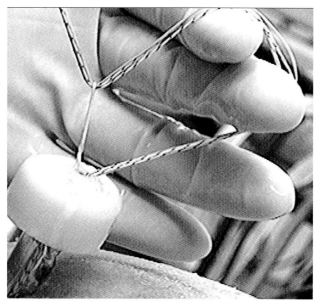

Figure 17C-2 External view showing that the four suture limbs from the anteromedial anchor have been placed through the loop of the SutureSnare (Arthrex, Inc.; Naples, FL) in preparation for shuttling the sutures through the rotator cuff.

- Tie the lateral row sutures as simple sutures. This establishes the muscle tendon length and tension before compressing the cuff broadly over the footprint with the medial row sutures.

- Tie the medial row sutures using a double-pulley technique. For this technique, retrieve a Tigerwire (Arthrex) suture limb from each of the medial anchors through the lateral portal and manually tie it as a six-throw surgeon's knot over a metal rod (Fig. 17C-3). Then, pull the two free ends of Tigerwire to transport the knot over the top of the tendon bridge (Fig. 17C-4). In this maneuver, the eyelets of the two medial anchors serve as pulleys (hence, the term "double-pulley technique") in pulling the knot

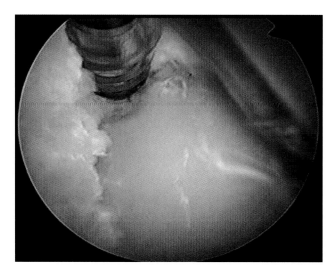

Figure 17C-1 Right shoulder, posterior viewing portal. A BioCorkscrew-FT (Arthrex, Inc.; Naples, FL) suture anchor is being placed adjacent to the articular margin.

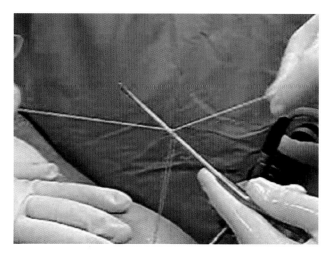

Figure 17C-3 External view showing the surgeon tying a six-throw surgeon's knot over a metal rod. The two suture limbs originate from two different medial anchors.

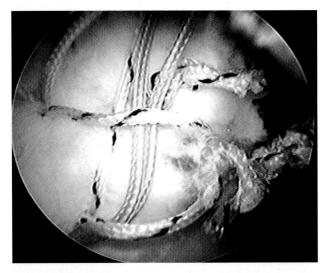

Figure 17C-4 Right shoulder, posterior viewing portal. The externally tied surgeon's knot is transported to a compressive position over the top of the cuff by pulling on the other two suture limbs of the same color from the two medial anchors.

down over the tendon bridge. Then tie the two free TigerWire suture limbs with a Surgeon's Sixth Finger (Arthrex) knot pusher as a static, nonsliding knot. This produces a double mattress suture between the two medial anchors. Repeat this same double-pulley sequence for the blue FiberWire sutures from the two medial anchors to create a second double mattress suture.

- The final subacromial view will show good indentation of the rotator cuff by the sutures (Fig. 17C-5).

- Reinsert the arthroscope intra-articularly to be sure that the rotator cuff is firmly in contact with the bone footprint all the way to the articular margin.

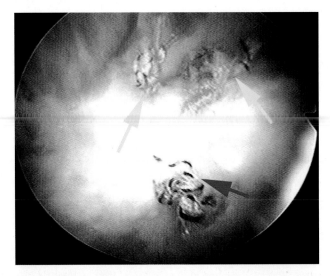

Figure 17C-5 Right shoulder, posterior viewing portal. Final result from the subacromial perspective. Good tissue indentation is seen from the medial sutures (*yellow arrows*) and the lateral suture (*red arrow*).

TRICKS AND TIPS

- In preparing the bone bed, ring curettes are helpful to sharply define the medial border of the footprint at the articular margin.

- In placing the BioCorkscrew-FT anchors, it is not necessary to tap, even in hard bone. We use a conical punch to make a tapered bone socket. The internal hex drive of this anchor allows very large insertional torques with minimal risk of stripping, breaking, or otherwise disrupting the anchor.

- In placing anchors, try to have ~1 cm of intact bone between the anchors. If the footprint is too small to allow insertion of 5.5-mm BioCorkscrew-FT or 5.0-mm BioCorkscrew anchors, the smaller 3.7-mm Corkscrew anchors (Arthrex) can be used.

- In passing the medial row sutures, we prefer suture placement ~2 to 3 mm lateral to the musculotendinous junction.

- Tie lateral sutures first and medial sutures last.

- As an exercise, look inside the joint after tying the lateral row sutures, and see the residual uncovered area of footprint medially. After tying the medial sutures, look inside the joint again to see full footprint restoration.

17D
Double-Row Rotator Cuff Repair

- In cases where the subscapularis tendon is torn as well as the supraspinatus and/or infraspinatus tendon, repair the subscapularis tendon before proceeding to a double-row repair of the supraspinatus and infraspinatus tendons.

- Prepare the bone bed on the greater tuberosity with electrocautery, ring curettes, power shaver, and burr.

- Measure the medial-to-lateral dimension of the rotator cuff footprint.

- Grasp the cuff with a tendon grasper and determine the tear pattern and whether sufficient lateral excursion exists to perform a double-row repair.

- Place the medial row suture anchors (BioCorkscrew-FT; Arthrex, Inc.; Naples, FL) (Fig. 17D-1).

- Place the sutures ~14 or 15 mm from the cuff margin, if sufficient cuff excursion exists, to obtain complete footprint reconstruction (Fig. 17D-2).

- Place the lateral row anchors.

- Pass the lateral row sutures ~10 to 12 mm from the cuff margin.

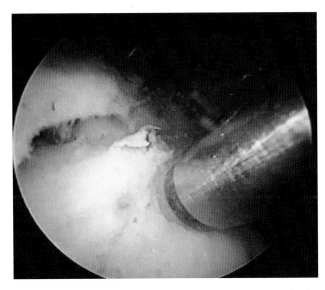

Figure 17D-1 Right shoulder, posterior viewing portal. The medial anchors are placed on the prepared greater tuberosity, directly adjacent to the articular margin.

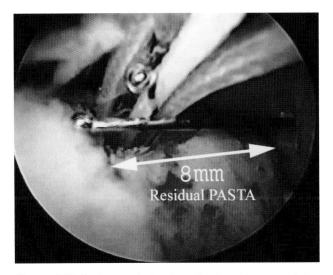

Figure 17D-3 Intra-articular view after lateral row repair has been done. Note: A residual 8-mm partial articular sided tendon avulsion (PASTA) lesion remains because of the uncovered footprint that existed before securing the medial row sutures.

- Tie the lateral sutures as "simple" suture loops.

- Secure the suture limbs of the medial anchors to prepare for completion of medial row repair with "double-pulley" mattress sutures (see Chapter 17C).

- Place the arthroscope intra-articularly and observe any residual uncovered footprint on the bone bed (Fig. 17D-3).

- Tie and secure the medial row sutures, obtaining good tissue indentation (Fig. 17D-4).

- Observe intra-articularly again to be sure that the footprint is completely covered (Fig. 17D-5).

TRICKS AND TIPS

- The quickest way to prepare the bone bed on the greater tuberosity is first, remove the soft tissues with an ablative electrocautery electrode, then lightly burr the bone surface. It is important to stop burring when the charcoal (i.e., the residue from the soft tissue ablation by the electrocautery) has been burred away.

- A well-defined medial border to the bone bed can be created by using a ring curette to sharply remove residual soft tissue all the way to the articular margin.

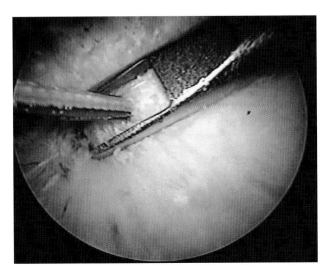

Figure 17D-2 Sutures from the medial anchors are passed ~14 to 15 mm from the cuff margin using a Scorpion (Arthrex) suture passer.

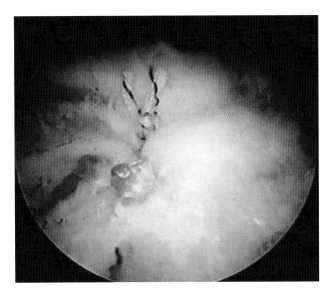

Figure 17D-4 Subacromial view of completed repair showing good tissue indentation by all sutures, indicating good loop security.

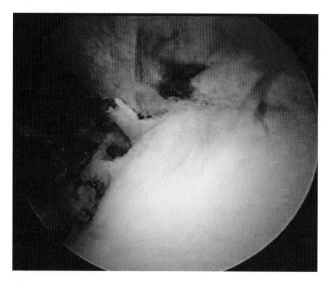

Figure 17D-5 Intra-articular view of completed repair after all medial and lateral sutures have been tied, showing complete coverage of the footprint of the rotator cuff.

- Measuring the medial-to-lateral dimension of the footprint with a calibrated probe provides a good estimate of how far medial from the edge of the cuff the medial row sutures should be placed. The footprint averages ~15 mm in width, but can range between 12 and 21 mm, depending on the size of the person.

- In passing sutures with the Scorpion (Arthrex) device, it is important to recognize that the suture limb being passed should not be under tension, or else the nitinol needle cannot effectively push it through the soft tissues. Excessive tension can inadvertently be applied by friction in the diaphragm of the cannula as the Scorpion is advanced through it. The easiest way to avoid excessive tension is, initially, push the Scorpion medially past the spot at which the suture is to be placed, and then pull it back laterally to the edge of the cuff. This maneuver creates sufficient slack in the suture to allow easy passage with the Scorpion.

- Some cases of double-row repair will present a situation in which the medial portion of the footprint has a longer anterior-to-posterior dimension than the lateral portion of the footprint. Such cases may provide room for two medial anchors, but the narrower lateral footprint may permit only one lateral anchor to be placed. In such cases, lateral fixation can be improved by loading a third suture into a BioCorkscrew anchor (Arthrex) using a nitinol threader, so that three lateral fixation points can be obtained from one anchor. It is easier to thread a third suture through the eyelet of a standard BioCorkscrew anchor rather than a BioCorkscrew-FT, because the eyelet of the standard anchor is located above the profile of the body of the anchor.

- Loop security is best judged by observing tissue indentation below the suture loop. For medial row sutures, the best way to tension the sutures to indent the tissues is by means of a Sixth Finger (Arthrex) knot pusher introduced through an anterosuperolateral portal so that the tip of the knot pusher is oriented down toward the cuff as the knot is tied rather than parallel to the cuff.

17E

L-Shaped Tear Assessment

- Use a KingFisher (Arthrex, Inc.; Naples, FL) tendon grasper to assess the mobility of the tear. When the "corner" of the posterior leaf is properly selected, the L-shape of the tear is obvious as the tendon is inset into the defect (Fig. 17E-1).

- While holding the tendon, envision where anchors need to be placed (Fig. 17E-2).

TRICKS AND TIPS

- The mobility of anterior and posterior leaves of the cuff can be assessed with a tendon grasper. If one leaf has significantly greater anteroposterior (AP) mobility than the other, then the tear is probably an L-shaped or reverse L-shaped tear. The tendon grasper must then be used to grasp different points along the margin of the tear to identify the "corner" of the L-shaped tear.

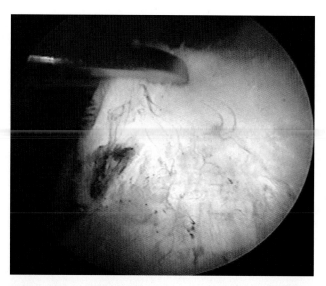

Figure 17E-1 Subacromial view of a left shoulder from a posterior viewing portal. The tendon grasper has properly identified the "corner" of the L-shaped tear, which can be easily inset into the defect.

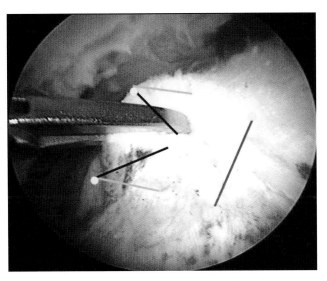

Figure 17E-2 Proposed repair construct (*yellow dots* indicate anchor location). Medial mattress sutures (*red line*) between the medial anchors. Simple sutures (*blue and black lines*) from lateral anchors. Side-to-side sutures also need to be placed between the anterior and posterior leaves of the rotator cuff.

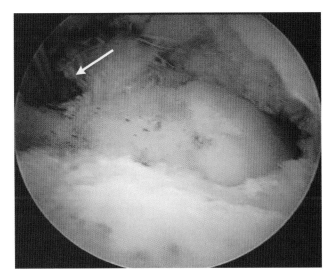

Figure 17F-2 A biceps tenodesis has been performed with a BioTenodesis screw before cuff repair (*arrow*). The sutures from the BioTenodesis construct will later be incorporated into the lateral row repair of the rotator cuff.

Margin Convergence to Bone in a Reverse-L Tear

- The reverse-L tear configuration is one in which the supraspinatus tendon avulses from the bone, and a split occurs between the supraspinatus and infraspinatus tendons.

- Confirm the reverse-L configuration by grasping the anterior leaf at the corner of the L, and observing how it inserts anatomically into the cuff defect (Fig. 17F-1).

- Perform biceps tenodesis, if necessary, before beginning cuff repair. Place the BioTenodesis (Arthrex, Inc.; Naples, FL) screw at the anterolateral aspect of the greater tuberosity (Fig. 17F-2). Later, incorporate the sutures from this construct into the lateral row of the rotator cuff repair.

- For the anteromedial anchor, use a 3.7-mm BioCorkscrew (Arthrex) anchor, due to the limited space available because the 8-mm BioTenodesis screw occupies a significant portion of the anterior part of the greater tuberosity.

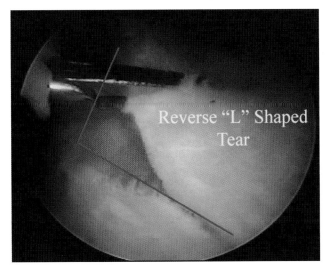

Figure 17F-1 A KingFisher (Arthrex, Inc.; Naples, FL) tendon grasper is used to assess the tear pattern configuration, pulling the "corner" of the L to its anatomic position on the greater tuberosity.

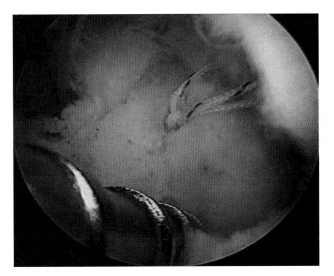

Figure 17F-3 A bone tap prepares a socket for insertion of the posteromedial BioCorkscrew (Arthrex, Inc.; Naples, FL) anchor. The sutures from this anchor will be passed for side-to-side margin convergence to bone repair.

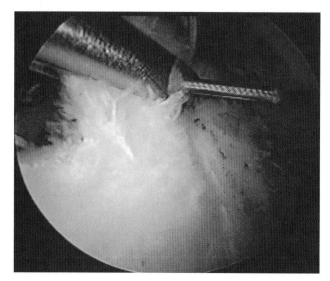

Figure 17F-4 A Scorpion (Arthrex, Inc.; Naples, FL) suture passer is used to pass the sutures antegrade through the posterior border of the supraspinatus tendon.

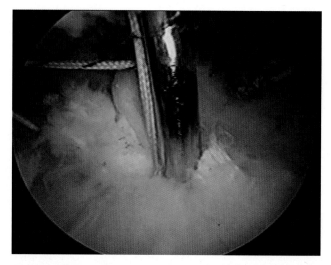

Figure 17F-6 Suture pairs from the posteromedial anchor are tied with the Surgeon's Sixth Finger (Arthrex, Inc.; Naples, FL) knot pusher, achieving margin convergence to bone.

- Pass sutures from the anteromedial anchor with a Scorpion (Arthrex) suture passer for later tying as medial row mattress sutures.

- Place a posteromedial BioCorkscrew anchor (Fig. 17F-3). Pass its sutures in a side-to-side fashion between the anterior and posterior leaves of the cuff to achieve "margin convergence to bone" fixation.

- Pass the anterior limb of each suture pair (from the posteromedial anchor) in antegrade fashion with a Scorpion suture passer through the posterior border of the supraspinatus tendon (Fig. 17F-4).

- Pass the posterior limb of each suture pair in retrograde fashion through the infraspinatus tendon with a BirdBeak (Arthrex) suture passer (Fig. 17F-5).

- Tie the suture pairs with a Surgeon's Sixth Finger (Arthrex) knot pusher (Fig. 17F-6). This technique accomplishes margin convergence between the two leaves of the cuff and anchors the cuff to bone (margin-to-bone-fixation), providing very secure fixation.

- Perform lateral row repair using sutures from the BioTenodesis screw (Arthrex) construct.

- The final construct has restored the anatomic footprint of the rotator cuff (Fig. 17F-7).

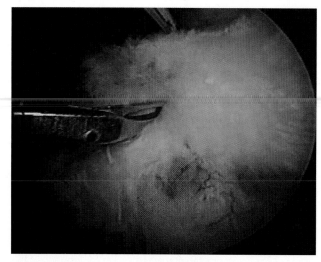

Figure 17F-5 A BirdBeak (Arthrex, Inc.; Naples, FL) suture passer is used for retrograde passage of sutures through the anterior border of the infraspinatus tendon.

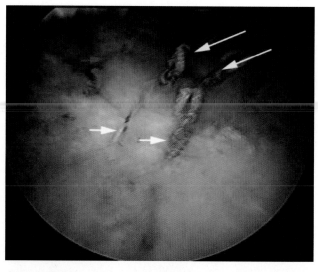

Figure 17F-7 Final construct. Margin convergence to bone repair (*white arrows*); medial mattress sutures (*yellow arrows*); and lateral simple sutures (*red arrow*).

TRICKS AND TIPS

- If limited footprint is available, 3.7-mm BioCorkscrew suture anchors can be used medially.

- Margin convergence to bone has the mechanical strain reduction advantage of margin convergence coupled with strong fixation to bone. This provides a very secure component to the overall fixation construct.

- If a biceps tenodesis is done in addition to the cuff repair, it is important to incorporate the sutures from the BioTenodesis construct into the lateral row of the cuff repair.

- The medial row mattress sutures should be tied after tying the lateral row sutures.

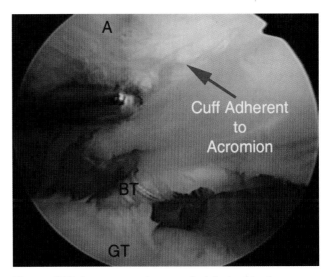

Figure 17G-1 Intra-articular view of a left shoulder from a posterior viewing portal. The glenohumeral joint space is continuous with the subacromial space, and the rotator cuff is adherent to the acromion. A, *acromonial process* (acromion); BT, biceps tendon; GT, greater tuberosity.

17G

Massive Adhesed Rotator Cuff Tear: Repair by Modified Double Interval Slide

- Definition: A modified double interval slide accomplishes a double slide by means of (a) a standard posterior interval slide plus (b) an anterior interval slide in continuity rather than a standard anterior interval slide. The anterior interval slide in continuity is performed when a massive retracted tear includes the subscapularis tendon, and dissection of the adhesed subscapularis from the base of the coracoid also accomplishes release of the coracohumeral ligament (anterior interval slide) without having to cut across the anterior border of the supraspinatus tendon.

- A massive adhesed rotator cuff tear usually results from a failed attempt at repair of a massive cuff tear. Occasionally, a previously unoperated massive tear will also develop dense adhesions.

- The adhesions that form are dense sheets of fibrous tissue that cause the cuff to be adherent to the *acromonial process* (acromion) and deltoid muscle.

- From an intra-articular perspective, the cuff can be seen to be adherent to the acromion, but the lateral margin of cuff tendon is obscured by scar tissue (Fig. 17G-1).

- Develop a plane between the cuff and the acromion while viewing through a lateral portal and working through a posterior portal (Fig. 17G-2). In this way, the cuff is "excavated" from the acromion.

- Identify the fat pad just behind the acromioclavicular (AC) joint (Fig. 17G-3). It is always present, even in multiply operated shoulders, and is a guide to the plane of dissection between the cuff and acromion.

- Dissect the fat plane laterally over the top of the cuff, using a power shaver, until the underlying tissue thins out into a layer of "bursal leader" that extends from the cuff margin to the deltoid fascia (Fig. 17G-4).

- Cut the bursal leaders from the deltoid fascia to free the margins of the rotator cuff.

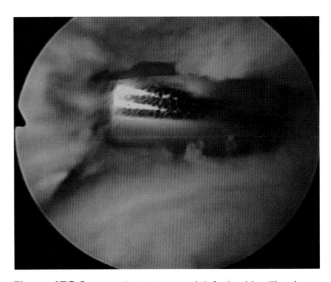

Figure 17G-2 Lateral viewing portal, left shoulder. The shaver has been introduced through a posterior working portal and is developing the plane between the *acromonial process* (acromion) and the rotator cuff. This plane is defined by a fat layer that is being débrided by the shaver.

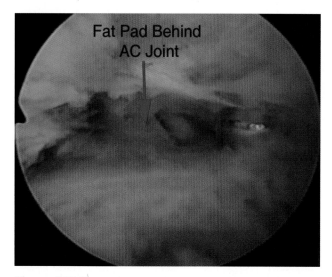

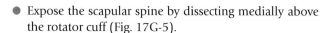

Figure 17G-3 Lateral viewing portal, left shoulder. The fat pad behind the acromioclavicular (*AC*) joint is identified. This fat pad is in the fat plane between the *acromonial process* (acromion) and the rotator cuff.

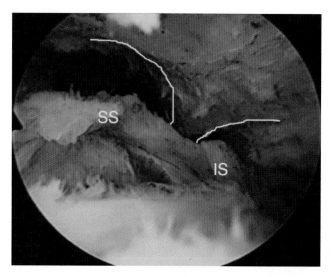

Figure 17G-5 Lateral viewing portal, left shoulder. The keel-shaped scapular spine (*solid line*) defines the border between supraspinatus (*SS*) and infraspinatus (*IS*) muscles.

- Expose the scapular spine by dissecting medially above the rotator cuff (Fig. 17G-5).

- If the subscapularis is torn, dissect, mobilize, and repair it before beginning repair of the rest of the rotator cuff.

- Evaluate the cuff through a lateral viewing portal to determine the location of the supraspinatus and infraspinatus tendons and their relationship to the scapular spine (Fig. 17G-5).

- While viewing through a lateral portal, assess the mobility of the supraspinatus (Fig. 17G-6) and infraspinatus tendons using a KingFisher (Arthrex, Inc.; Naples, FL) tendon grasper.

- Prepare the bone bed of the greater tuberosity to a bleeding surface while viewing through a posterior portal.

- Next, perform a biceps tenodesis, if necessary, using the BioTenodesis (Arthrex) interference screw fixation technique. Do this before performing the posterior interval slide. The sutures from the BioTenodesis construct can later be incorporated into the rotator cuff repair.

- Place two traction sutures, one near the posterior border of the supraspinatus tendon and one near the anterior border of the infraspinatus tendon (Fig. 17G-7).

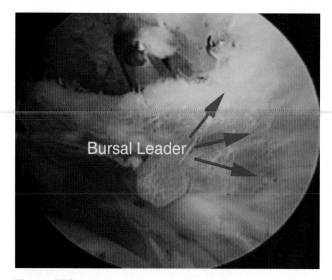

Figure 17G-4 Lateral viewing portal, left shoulder. "Bursal leaders" (*red arrows*) connect the lateral margin of the rotator cuff to the deltoid fascia.

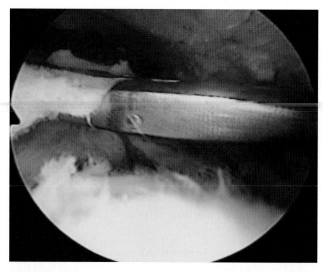

Figure 17G-6 Lateral viewing portal, left shoulder. The mobility of the cuff is assessed by means of a KingFisher (Arthrex, Inc.; Naples, FL) tendon grasper.

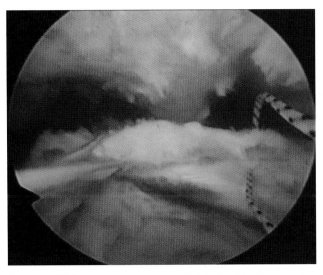

Figure 17G-7 Lateral viewing portal, left shoulder. Two traction sutures have been placed along the cuff tear margin, one near the posterior border of the supraspinatus tendon and the other near the anterior border of the infraspinatus tendon.

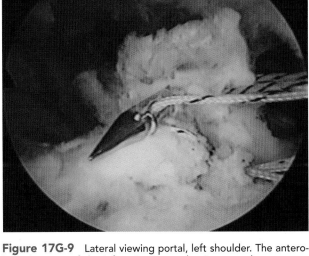

Figure 17G-9 Lateral viewing portal, left shoulder. The antero-lateral corner of the infraspinatus tendon is secured to a suture anchor by retrograde suture passage through the tendon.

- While viewing from a posterolateral portal, introduce an arthroscopic scissor through a lateral working portal. With the scissor, incise the tendon bridge between the two traction sutures and cut in a direction toward the base of the scapular spine (Fig. 17G-8).

- Release the thin capsular tissue between the rotator cuff and the glenoid with an arthroscopic elevator.

- Reassess tear mobility. In most cases, 4 to 5 cm of increased lateral excursion will be noted, providing

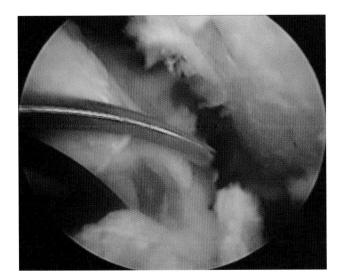

Figure 17G-8 Posterolateral viewing portal, left shoulder. An arthroscopic scissor is used to perform the posterior interval slide, beginning laterally between the two traction sutures and aiming toward the base of the scapular spine as traction is applied.

sufficient tendon length for at least 1 cm of medial-to-lateral footprint coverage.

- Identify the point on the greater tuberosity where the anterolateral corner of the infraspinatus tendon can easily reach and place a suture anchor there to secure the corner. Pass the sutures from the anchor through the infraspinatus tendon in a retrograde fashion (Fig. 17G-9) and tie with a Surgeon's Sixth Finger (Arthrex) knot pusher.

- Secure the posterolateral corner of the supraspinatus tendon to bone with a suture anchor (Fig. 17G-10). Retrograde suture passage through a modified Neviaser portal assures that an adequate bite of soft tissue is captured for a secure repair. Alternatively, a Scorpion (Arthrex) suture passer can capture a 15-mm bite of tendon with antegrade suture passage.

- Tie suture pairs as static, nonsliding knots with a Surgeon's Sixth Finger knot pusher (Fig. 17G-11).

- Secure the residual cuff margins to bone with additional suture anchors, as needed.

- Close the cleft between supraspinatus and infraspinatus tendons with side-to-side sutures.

- Arthroscopically confirm stability of the final construct (Fig. 17G-12).

TRICKS AND TIPS

- In developing the plane between the rotator cuff and the acromion, it is crucial to preserve as much tendon length as possible. To accomplish this, it is important to dissect

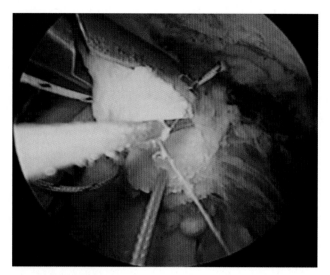

Figure 17G-10 Lateral viewing portal, left shoulder. The supraspinatus tendon is repaired to bone by a suture anchor. Retrograde suture passage through the posterior portion of the supraspinatus tendon is achieved using a Penetrator (Arthrex, Inc.; Naples, FL) suture passer introduced through a modified Neviaser portal.

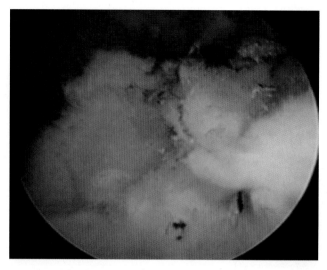

Figure 17G-12 Posterior viewing portal, left shoulder. Final repair. A complete repair has been achieved with adequate single-row footprint coverage.

the soft tissues from the acromion as far lateral as possible. The best way to locate this plane is to view from a lateral portal as a 4.5 mm power shaver is inserted through a posterior portal. The shaver tip is directed so that it "hugs" the undersurface of the acromion as the tip is pushed anteromedially until it strikes the scapular spine. Then the shaver tip can be swept anterolaterally to further excavate the appropriate plane of dissection. As the tip of the shaver advances laterally, it will be seen to tent the soft tissues beneath the lateral acromion. At that point, it can be popped through the last layer of soft tissue so that the shaver tip is now visible through the

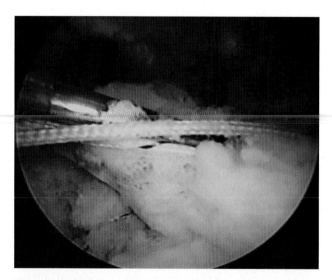

Figure 17G-11 Posterior viewing portal, left shoulder. Surgeon's Sixth Finger (Arthrex, Inc.; Naples, FL) knot pusher is used to tie static, nonsliding knots.

arthroscope. The shaver tip and cautery probe are next used to sufficiently enlarge the lateral opening into this tissue plane so that the arthroscope can be advanced through that opening into the dissection plane. In this way, the rest of the cuff dissection can take place under direct visualization. The inferior aspect of the distal clavicle is cleared of soft tissue, and the fat pad posterior to the AC joint is identified. The portion of the acromion just posterior to the AC joint is cleared of soft tissue and followed posteriorly. This part of the acromion arches downward in a posteromedial direction to become a thick strut of bone that is shaped like the keel of a boat. This keel-shaped structure is the lower portion of the scapular spine (Fig. 17G-5).

● The fat plane between the rotator cuff and the acromion is the desired plane of dissection. This plane is most easily located by initially finding the large fat pad just posterior to the AC joint, which is in the plane of dissection.

● As the dissection of the cuff from the acromion progresses laterally, the soft tissue thins so that it can be difficult to tell where the cuff ends. Remember, the cuff scars to the deltoid fascia by means of thin "bursal leaders." These thin sheets of bursal tissue that insert directly into the deltoid fascia must be divided and débrided back to normal tendon to accurately define the lateral border of the rotator cuff.

● Lateral traction sutures are placed into the posterior aspect of the supraspinatus and the anterior aspect of the infraspinatus for four reasons:

1. They are used as a guide for incising the cuff for the posterior interval slide. The scissor tips begin incising the tendon edge between the two traction sutures as they aim toward the base of the scapular spine.

2. They protect the suprascapular nerve by pulling the tendon edge toward the scissor and away from the nerve as the posterior slide is done.

3. Traction is produced by pulling the two traction sutures in divergent directions, with the anterior suture being pulled in an anterolateral direction and the posterior suture being pulled in a posterolateral direction. In this way, as the tendon is incised for the posterior interval slide, the apex of the tendon incision opens in a V-like fashion so that the portion of the tendon to be incised next is always clearly visible.

4. Once the posterior interval slide has been completed, the two traction sutures allow control of the two separate tendon flaps while sutures are passed through them for tendon-to-bone repair. Without these traction sutures, the tendon flaps would be extremely floppy and difficult to control for suture passage.

- Technical points to help protect the suprascapular nerve during the posterior interval slide are:

1. Cut the tendon margin only when lateral traction is being applied.

2. Lift the scissor blades upward as each scissor cut is made. The suprascapular nerve is located tightly against the glenoid neck at the base of the scapular spine, so lifting the scissor blades will pull them away from the nerve.

3. Stop the posterior interval slide's tendon incision as soon as the tendon margin gives way to a fat pad. This fat pad comprises the perineural fat around the suprascapular nerve. Most of the time, as the last tendon fibers are cut, the two flaps of tissue (supraspinatus and infraspinatus) will suddenly snap apart. This snap is much like the recoil that occurs when a rubber band under tension is cut, and the fat pad at the apex of the cut will immediately be seen. At that point, the posterior interval slide is complete.

- After completing the posterior interval slide, we release the capsular tissue between the rotator cuff and the glenoid with an arthroscopic elevator. The traction sutures are pulled laterally during the capsular release to prevent injury to the suprascapular nerve by the elevator. In our experience, however, this capsular release adds (at most) 2 or 3 mm of additional lateral excursion, and as an isolated release (i.e., without interval slides) it is useless.

- After double interval slide, a double-row repair is seldom possible. This is a salvage situation in which the goal should be to achieve the best possible single-row repair.

- After performing the posterior interval slide, the corners of the two tissue flaps should be secured to bone first to eliminate the floppiness of the tissue.

- Side-to-side sutures between the two tissue flaps (supraspinatus and infraspinatus) are placed after the tendon edges have been secured to bone. The tissues are too floppy to pass side-to-side sutures before tendon-to-bone repair. The side-to-side sutures are essential, however, to help diminish strain at the tendon-to-bone interface by means of the mechanical effect of margin convergence. This mechanical effect provides additional protection to the repair.

- We prefer to tie static, nonsliding knots, using the Surgeon's Sixth Finger knot pusher. This technique provides excellent loop and knot security. In addition, it avoids the "cheese-cutter" effect of suture cutting through tendon as it slides through the often-attenuated soft tissue in these challenging cases. This technique preserves tendon integrity as much as possible. Another advantage to the Surgeon's Sixth Finger knot pusher is that it can be used to manipulate tissue to the desired repair site, removing extrinsic tension at the repair site as the suture is tied.

17H

PASTA Repair: One Anchor Repair

- Arthroscopic inspection reveals a small partial articular surface tendon avulsion (PASTA) lesion that comprises a portion of the supraspinatus tendon footprint (Fig. 17H-1).

- Once the decision has been made to repair a PASTA lesion, move the arthroscope to the subacromial space and perform a complete subacromial bursectomy.

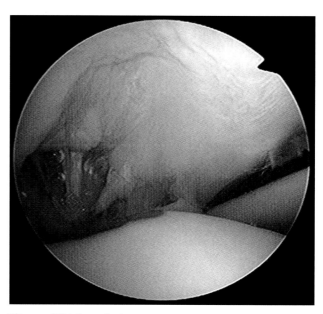

Figure 17H-1 Left shoulder, posterior intra-articular viewing portal. A small partial articular surface tendon avulsion (PASTA) lesion is seen involving a portion of the supraspinatus tendon.

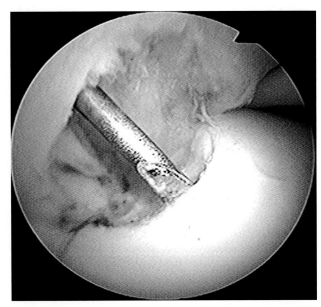

Figure 17H-2 Left shoulder, posterior intra-articular viewing portal. A spinal needle is used to determine the optimal position and angle of approach for transtendon suture anchor placement.

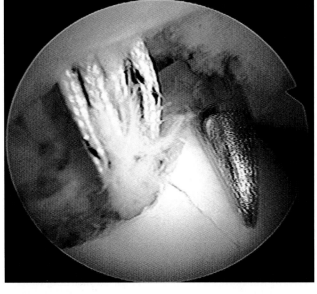

Figure 17H-4 Left shoulder, posterior intra-articular viewing portal. A Penetrator (Arthrex, Inc.; Naples, FL) suture passer has been placed through a separate transtendon puncture and will remove two of the suture limbs.

- Place the arthroscope intra-articularly again and prepare the bone bed to a bleeding base.

- Use a spinal needle as a guide to transtendon suture anchor placement (Fig. 17H-2).

- Make a bone socket for a suture anchor (BioCorkscrew or BioCorkscrew-FT; Arthrex, Inc.; Naples, FL) by a transtendon punch. Then, place the anchor through the

same skin puncture and through the same puncture in rotator cuff tendon (Fig. 17H-3).

- Use a Penetrator (Arthrex) suture passer to pass two suture limbs from the anchor through a separate puncture site in the rotator cuff (Fig. 17H-4). This allows a suture bridge (between the two sets of sutures) to be apposed to the bone bed when the sutures are tied.

- Tie the sutures subacromially.

- The final result is confirmed by good tissue indentation by the sutures from the subacromial perspective (Fig. 17H-5A) and good restoration of the rotator cuff footprint on the intra-articular view (Fig. 17H-5B).

TRICKS AND TIPS

- The subacromial bursa must be thoroughly excised before anchor insertion so that the sutures can be easily located subacromially without having to shave around them. Shaving around the sutures might cut or damage them.

- When tying the knots, the best angle of approach for the knot pusher is through a superolateral portal adjacent to the *acromonial process* (acromion). From this angle, it is easy to hold a tight suture loop with the Surgeon's Sixth Finger (Arthrex) knot pusher while advancing sequential half-hitches.

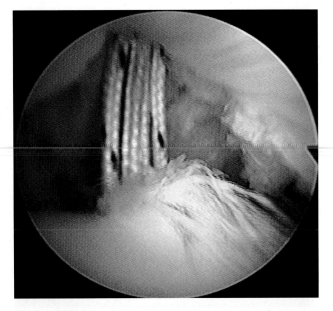

Figure 17H-3 Left shoulder, posterior intra-articular viewing portal. A transtendon suture anchor has been placed.

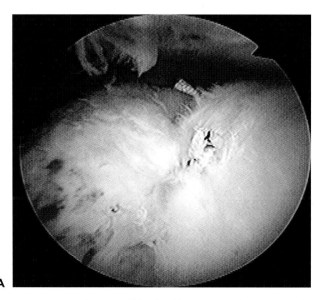

A

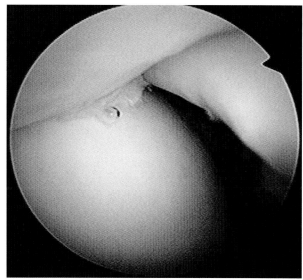

B

Figure 17H-5 Final result. The subacromial view **(A)** shows good tissue indentation by the sutures. The intra-articular view **(B)** shows good restoration of the rotator cuff footprint all the way out to the articular margin.

17I

Repair of a Partial (Upper) Subscapularis Tendon Tear

● Evaluate the upper subscapularis tendon.

● Before making a standard anterior portal, create an anterosuperolateral portal at a 5° to 10° angle of approach toward the lesser tuberosity bone bed (Fig. 17I-1). This is the primary working portal for upper subscapularis repair.

● Evaluate the relationship of the biceps tendon to the subscapularis tendon while using a 70° arthroscope through a posterior portal, producing an "aerial" view. On this view, the biceps should normally not be located posterior to the plane of the subscapularis. If it is even partially posterior to the place of the subscapularis (Fig. 17I-2), then a tear of the upper subscapularis tendon is present, allowing the biceps tendon to sublux medially and posteriorly behind the upper subscapularis tendon.

● Next, address the biceps tendon, either by definitive tenotomy or by tenotomy and application of a whip-

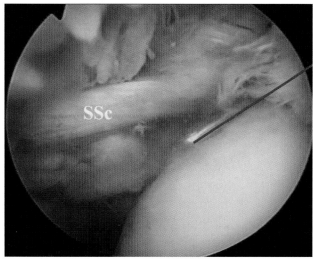

Figure 17I-1 Right shoulder, posterior viewing portal. Use a spinal needle to determine the proper angle of approach for the anterosuperolateral portal. SSc, subscapularis tendon.

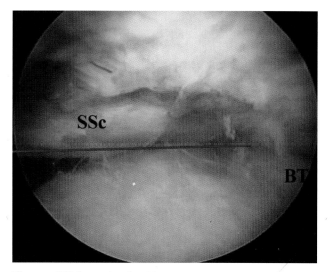

Figure 17I-2 Right shoulder, posterior viewing portal, 70° arthroscope. The biceps tendon (*BT*) is situated posterior to the plane of the subscapularis (*SSc*) tendon (*solid line*), indicating a tear of the upper subscapularis associated with posteromedial subluxation of the biceps tendon.

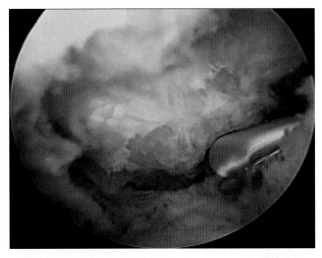

Figure 17I-3 Right shoulder, posterior viewing portal, 70° arthroscope. Coracoplasty is performed with a high-speed burr to create a 7-mm space between the coracoid tip and the subscapularis tendon.

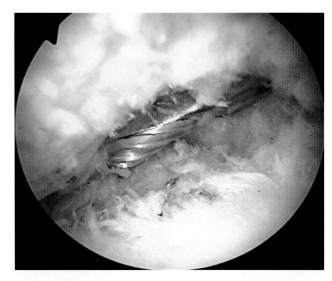

Figure 17I-4 Right shoulder, posterior viewing portal, 70° arthroscope. The bone bed on the lesser tuberosity is prepared with a high-speed burr.

stitch in preparation for tenodesis. Getting the biceps tendon out of the way greatly improves visualization for subscapularis tendon repair.

● Make a window in the rotator interval to expose the tip of the coracoid.

● Perform a coracoplasty with a high-speed burr through an anterosuperolateral working portal to create a 7-mm space between the reconfigured coracoid tip and the anterior plane of the subscapularis tendon (Fig. 17I-3). This space will serve to protect the subscapularis tendon repair from abrasion by the coracoid.

● Prepare the bone bed for subscapularis tendon repair on the lesser tuberosity, first outlining the proposed bone bed with an electrocautery probe, then "burring off the charcoal" to a bleeding bone base. Use a curette to further define the precise margins of the bone footprint (Fig. 17I-4).

● Place a single BioCorkscrew-FT (Arthrex, Inc.; Naples, FL) suture anchor at the anterolateral aspect of the bone footprint on the lesser tuberosity. The portal for anchor placement is an accessory anterior portal (chosen by spinal needle for the proper angle of approach) in which it is usually necessary to place the hand very close

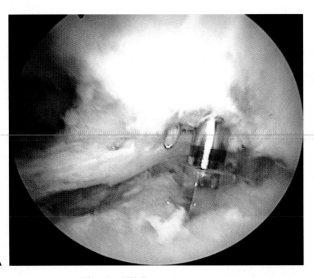
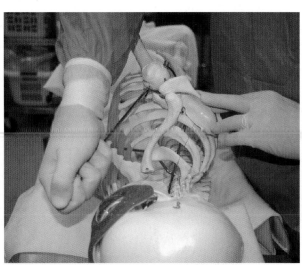

Figure 17I-5 A: A suture anchor is placed at the superior aspect of the lesser tuberosity. **B:** In placing the anchor for repair of the upper subscapularis tendon, the surgeon's hand must come very close to the patient's face. This unusual position is necessary because of the retroversion of the proximal humerus.

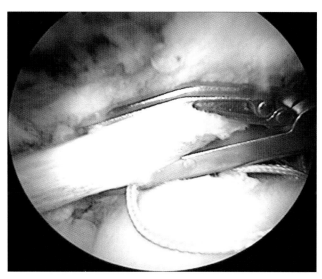

Figure 17I-6   Right shoulder, posterior viewing portal. A Viper (Arthrex, Inc.; Naples, FL) suture passer is used to pass sutures through the upper border of the subscapularis tendon.

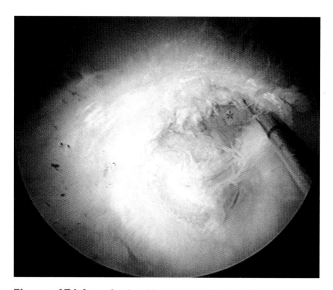

Figure 17J-1   Left shoulder, posterolateral viewing portal. Palpation of the cuff tear reveals an intact medial wall of capsule with some intact overlying cuff fibers.

to the patient's face to achieve the proper angle of approach (Fig. 17I-5).

- Pass sutures antegrade with a Viper (Arthrex) suture passer over the superolateral edge of the subscapularis (Fig. 17I-6). This position for suture placement provides a nice rolled edge from the tendon to bone. Furthermore, the adjacent "comma sign" tissue, whose fibers are at right angles to the subscapularis tendon fibers, helps to prevent lateral cut-through of the sutures.

- Knots are tied with the Surgeon's Sixth Finger (Arthrex) knot pusher.

TRICKS AND TIPS

- When making the window in the rotator interval and identifying the coracoid tip, it is important to use the 30° arthroscope so as not to inadvertently stray inferior to the coracoid. After identifying the coracoid tip, the rest of the case (coracoplasty and subscapularis repair) is best visualized while using a 70° arthroscope through a posterior viewing portal.

- The anterosuperolateral portal is virtually parallel to the plane of the subscapularis tendon. As such, it provides the perfect angle of approach for performing the coracoplasty, bone bed preparation, suture passing, and knot-tying.

- Suture passage through the upper part of the subscapularis tendon is most easily performed with an antegrade passer (e.g., the Viper). Retrograde passage is very difficult because the coracoid is in the way.

17J

Repair of Bursal Sided Rotator Cuff Tear

- Palpate the cuff defect with a probe, confirming an intact medial wall of cuff or capsule (Fig. 17J-1).

- Prepare the bone bed with a combination of ring curette, electrocautery, and motorized burr.

- Use 3.7-mm BioCorkscrew (Arthrex, Inc.; Naples, FL) suture anchors. Using smaller anchors permits double-row fixation over this small footprint.

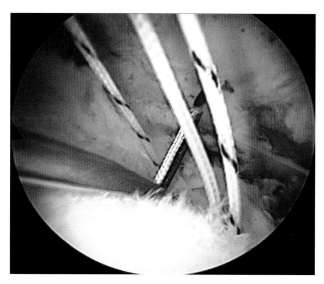

Figure 17J-2   Medial-row sutures are passed with a Scorpion (Arthrex, Inc.; Naples, FL) suture passer.

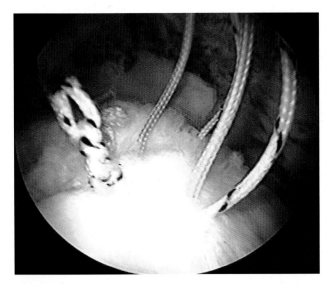

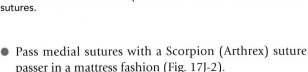

Figure 17J-3 Lateral sutures have been tied as simple sutures. Medial sutures have been placed and will be tied as mattress sutures.

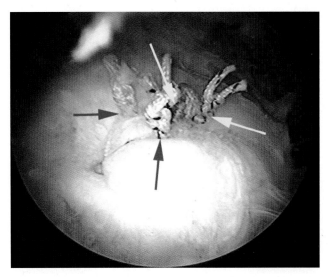

Figure 17J-4 Final double-row repair: (*red arrows*) lateral row sutures and (*yellow arrows*) medial row sutures.

- Pass medial sutures with a Scorpion (Arthrex) suture passer in a mattress fashion (Fig. 17J-2).

- Pass lateral sutures with a Scorpion or Viper (Arthrex) suture passer, so that they can be tied as simple sutures.

- Tie lateral sutures first (simple sutures) to "set" the length of the repair construct. Then, tie medial suture pairs as mattress sutures (Figs. 17J-3 and Fig. 17J-4).

TRICKS AND TIPS

- Small suture anchors (3.7-mm BioCorkscrew anchors) allow double-row fixation on a small bone footprint.

- It is important to tie lateral sutures first (simple sutures), and then tie medial suture pairs (mattress sutures).

17K

Repair of Complete Subscapularis Tendon Tear

- Evaluate long head of biceps tendon for tenotomy versus tenodesis procedure. If tenodesis is to be done, place half-racking sutures, then whipstitch after tenotomy. Either way, pull the tenotomized biceps out of the way to provide better visualization of the subscapularis tendon.

- Identify the "comma sign," the comma-shaped arc of tissue at the superolateral border of the subscapularis tendon, which is the remnant of the avulsed medial sling of the biceps (Fig. 17K-1).

- Identify the coracoacromial ligament, which will lead the way to the coracoid tip, where it inserts.

- Place a traction suture at the junction of the comma sign with the upper subscapularis tendon. We prefer antegrade suture passage with a Viper (Arthrex, Inc.; Naples, FL) suture passer.

- While pulling laterally on the traction suture, make a "window" in the rotator interval, preserving the comma tissue laterally. Use a shaver and electrocautery probe alternately to make the window.

- The coracoid will become visible through the window just anterior to the upper border of the subscapularis.

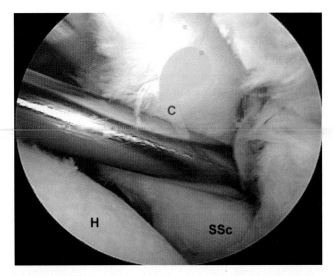

Figure 17K-1 Left shoulder, posterior viewing portal. The comma sign (*C*) is the remnant of the avulsed medial sling of the biceps, which is located at the superolateral border of the subscapularis tendon. C, comma sign; H, humeral head; SSc, subscapularis tendon.

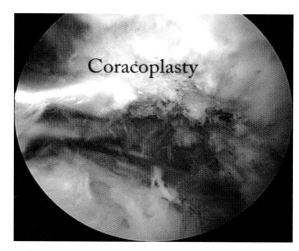

Figure 17K-2 Coracoplasty is performed by a burr introduced through an anterosuperolateral portal.

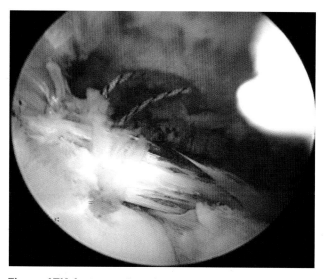

Figure 17K-4 Sutures from the upper anchor invert the supero-lateral corner of the subscapularis tendon repair, while the intact comma tissue provides a buttress to resist lateral cut-out of the sutures.

- Perform a coracoplasty (Fig. 17K-2) using a burr intro-duced through the anterosuperolateral portal. The cora-coplasty should create a 7- to 8-mm space between the re-configured coracoid and the anterior plane of the subscapularis tendon. This space will protect the sub-scapularis repair from abrasion.

- Perform a three-sided release of the subscapularis ten-don as follows:

  1. Skeletonize the posterolateral coracoid from its tip to the coracoid neck for anterior release. This releases adhesions between the coracoid and the anterosupe-rior subscapularis.

  2. Achieve superior release (Fig. 17K-3) by viewing through the rotator interval window with a 70° arthroscope while applying lateral traction to the

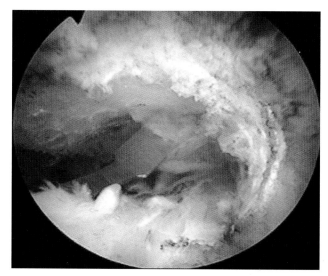

Figure 17K-3 Superior release of the subscapularis tendon is achieved by using a 30° elevator to release adhesions to the cora-coid neck and coracoid base, while viewing through a 70° arthro-scope.

subscapularis tendon. Clear the base of the coracoid of soft tissue. Then, with a 30° elevator disrupt the adhesions between the superior aspect of the sub-scapularis tendon and the inferolateral corner of the coracoid neck and coracoid base.

  3. Perform posterior release using a 15° elevator in the interval between the posterior subscapularis and the anterior glenoid neck.

- Prepare the lesser tuberosity bone bed with electro-cautery, shaver, curettes, and burr.

- Place the inferior anchor, then pass sutures (antegrade with Viper), and tie sutures before placing the upper anchor.

- Place the upper anchor.

- Pass sutures from the upper anchor antegrade with a Viper suture passer at the junction of the upper border of the subscapularis tendon with the comma arc area. This inverts the upper tendon margin toward the bone bed, and the laterally-placed comma tissue helps to resist suture cut-out (Fig. 17K-4).

TRICKS AND TIPS

- An anterosuperolateral portal, just off the anterolateral tip of the acromial process (acromion), provides an ideal angle of approach for (a) coracoplasty, (b) prepa-ration of the lesser tuberosity bone bed, and (c) ante-grade suture passage through the subscapularis tendon.

- Identifying the "comma" is the key to locating a retracted subscapularis tendon.

- The coracoid is located anterior to the upper border of subscapularis tendon. It is most easily located by viewing with a 30° arthroscope through a window made through the rotator interval.

● Once the coracoid is located, it is important to skeletonize its posterolateral aspect by "getting on bone and staying there." The posterolateral aspect of the coracoid is its safe side, because no neurovascular structures are adjacent to that side of the coracoid.

● The superior release of the subscapularis tendon must be done while viewing through a 70° arthroscope, and using a 30° elevator to release adhesions. This portion of the subscapularis tendon release will gain the most lateral excursion for a captured subscapularis tendon.

● Be sure to use one anchor for every linear centimeter of superior-to-inferior detachment of the subscapularis tendon.

● Double-row fixation of a retracted subscapularis tendon is seldom possible.

● If insufficient lateral excursion exists of the subscapularis tendon for tension-free repair, the footprint can be medialized 5 to 7 mm without adversely affecting the functional result.

● After subscapularis tendon repair, the intact comma tissue can be incorporated into the repair of the remainder of the cuff tear (supraspinatus and infraspinatus tendons).

17L
Repair of Interstitial Rotator Cuff Tear

● Suspect an interstitial tear based on the appearance on preoperative magnetic resonance imaging (MRI) of a

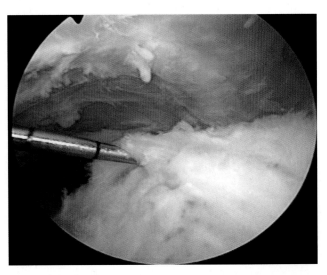

Figure 17L-2   Left shoulder, posterior subacromial viewing portal. A hook probe has penetrated the outer layer of the cuff and has entered the interstitial defect.

linear longitudinal high signal within the supraspinatus tendon. In addition, a capsular "dimple" within the rotator crescent suggests a possible tear (Fig. 17L-1).

● The "bubble sign" (see Chapter 17O) in this case was negative, probably because the injected fluid escaped into the joint by way of the capsular "dimple."

● Use an arthroscopic probe in the subacromial space to detect (by palpation) relative motion between layers of the interstitial cuff tear. Then use the probe to penetrate into the interstitial defect (Fig. 17L-2).

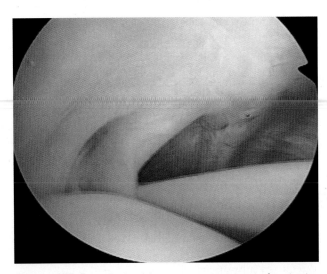

Figure 17L-1   Left shoulder, posterior intra-articular viewing portal. A capsular "dimple" within the rotator crescent is suggestive of an interstitial cuff tear that communicates with the joint.

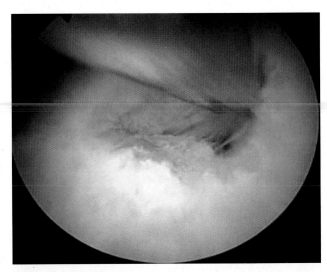

Figure 17L-3   Left shoulder, posterior subacromial viewing portal. A power shaver is used to débride the poor-quality tissue surrounding the defect.

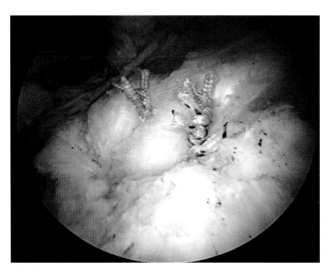

Figure 17L-4 Left shoulder, posterior subacromial viewing portal. Completed double-row repair.

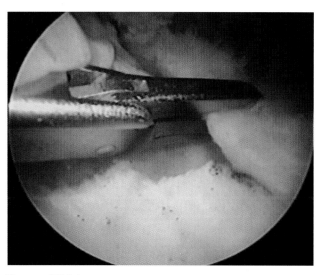

Figure 17M-1 A KingFisher (Arthrex, Inc.; Naples, FL) tendon grasper is used to manipulate the leaves of the cuff tear to assess tear pattern and tear mobility.

- Débride the poor-quality tendon surrounding the defect (Fig. 17L-3) to complete the tear.
- Perform a double-row repair using standard techniques (Fig. 17L-4).

TRICKS AND TIPS

- Palpation by a probe over the interstitial tear will provide the tactile sensation of relative motion between two layers of the rotator cuff. If that palpatory sensation is present, the hook probe can easily penetrate the outer layer of cuff, at which point it falls into the interstitial defect.

17M
Reverse L-Shaped Tear: Evaluation and Repair

- Assess tear pattern configuration and tear mobility using a KingFisher (Arthrex, Inc.; Naples, FL) tendon grasper (Fig. 17M-1).
- While holding the tear margin reduced, envision proposed positions for anchor insertion and suture configuration for an optimized repair (Fig. 17M-2).

TRICKS AND TIPS

- For the side-to-side portion of the repair, margin convergence to bone provides an extremely strong element to the repair construct.

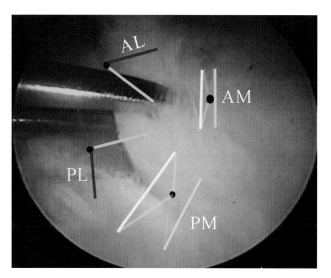

Figure 17M-2 The optimal repair construct is planned while holding the tear margin reduced. The anteromedial anchor (*AM*) will provide two mattress sutures. The posteromedial anchor (*PM*) will provide two margin convergence to bone sutures. The anterolateral (*AL*) and posterolateral (*PL*) anchors will each provide two simple sutures.

17N
Small Bursal-Surface Crescent Tear with Single Lateral Row Fixation

- This is the simplest tear pattern to repair.
- Prepare the bone bed to a bleeding base (Fig. 17N-1).
- Place a single anchor at the lateral aspect of the prepared bone bed.

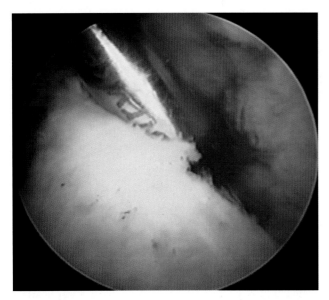

Figure 17N-1   Left shoulder, posterior viewing portal. Preparation of the bone bed on the greater tuberosity.

- Use a Viper (Arthrex, Inc.; Naples, FL) suture passer for antegrade passage of sutures to create two simple sutures as the repair construct (Fig. 17N-2).

- Tie static simple knots.

- The final repair is anatomic (Fig. 17N-3).

TRICKS AND TIPS

- This is a very straightforward procedure and all pertinent information is included in the directions above.

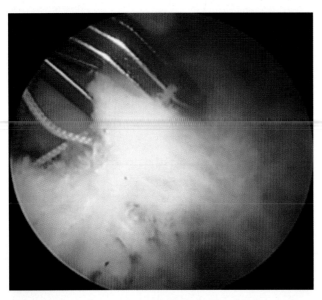

Figure 17N-2   A Viper (Arthrex, Inc.; Naples, FL) suture passer accomplishes antegrade passage of sutures from the anchor.

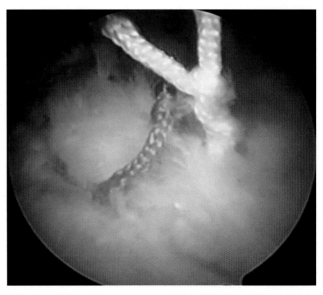

Figure 17N-3   Left shoulder, posterior viewing portal. Final repair construct composed of two simple sutures.

17O

The "Bubble" Sign: A Method of Detecting an Interstitial Rotator Cuff Tear

- While viewing through a posterior subacromial portal, introduce a spinal needle from a lateral position at a 45° angle of approach to the rotator cuff (Fig. 17O-1).

- Based on the preoperative magnetic resonance imaging (MRI), insert the needle into the area of suspected interstitial tear (Fig. 17O-2). Usually, a subtle "give" will be

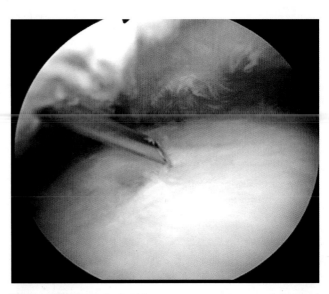

Figure 17O-1   Left shoulder, posterior viewing portal. A spinal needle is introduced at a 45° angle to the rotator cuff.

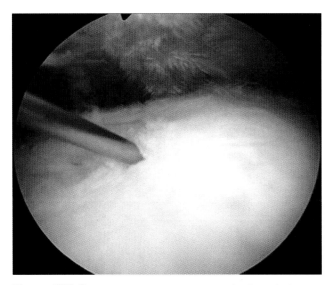

Figure 17O-2 The needle is inserted partially through the tendon in the area of suspected interstitial tear.

felt as the interstitial soft tissue plane is entered if, in fact, an interstitial tear is present.

● Have a syringe with 3 mL of saline connected to the spinal needle and attempt to rapidly inject 1 or 2 mL of fluid. If the needle tip is in a normal densely packed rotator cuff tendon, it is not possible to push any fluid from the syringe into the tendon. If the needle tip is in an interstitial defect, 1 to 2 mL of fluid should be easily injected into the cuff defect (depending on its size), and then a firm resistance will be felt to any further injection of fluid once the defect has been filled. As the cuff defect fills with fluid, it forms a dome-shaped "bubble" (Fig. 17O-3). Sequentially aspirate the defect with the syringe

(deflating the bubble) and re-inject the defect (to reconfirm the bubble sign).

TRICKS AND TIPS

● This is a very straightforward procedure and all pertinent information is included in the directions above.

17P
The "Triple Double" Technique of Rotator Cuff Footprint Reconstruction

● This is a useful technique for providing extremely secure double-row fixation in large and massive (but mobile) crescent-shaped rotator cuff tears.

● After preparing the bone bed, place two medial row suture anchors (BioCorkscrew-FT; Arthrex, Inc.; Naples, FL) adjacent to the articular margin (Fig. 17P-1).

● Pass the four suture limbs from each anchor through a single point in the rotator cuff ~15 mm from the free edge of the tendon. This passage is accomplished by a shuttling technique using a SutureLoop (Arthrex), suture with a loop on the end through which other sutures are passed and shuttled.

● Pass the SutureLoop (Arthrex) through the cuff 15 mm from the free edge using a NeedlePunch or Scorpion (Arthrex) (Fig. 17P-2). Pull the loop of the snare through

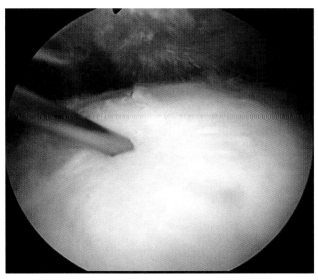

Figure 17O-3 A dome-shaped bubble has formed with injection of fluid into the cuff, indicating that the tear is an interstitial tear that is completely contained within the rotator cuff.

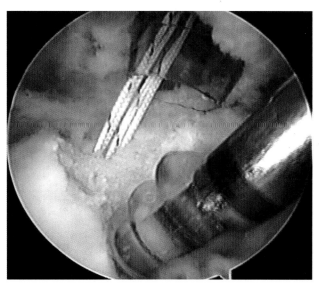

Figure 17P-1 Right shoulder, posterior viewing portal. Two medial row suture anchors (BioCorkscrew-FT; Arthrex, Inc.; Naples, FL) are placed adjacent to the articular margin.

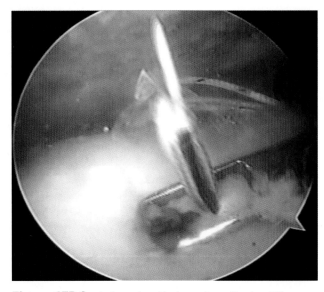

Figure 17P-2 A Scorpion (Arthrex, Inc.; Naples FL) suture passer is used to pass the free end of the SutureLoop (Arthrex) through the rotator cuff.

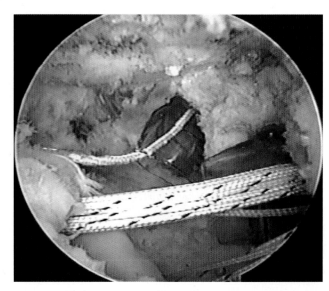

Figure 17P-4 Right shoulder, posterior viewing portal. The SutureLoop (Arthrex, Inc.; Naples, FL) is seen shuttling the four limbs from the suture anchor through the rotator cuff.

a lateral portal along with the four suture limbs from one of the anchors. Thread the ends of the suture limbs through the loop in the SutureLoop (Fig. 17P-3).

- Retrieve the free end of the SutureLoop through the anterior portal. Then, pull on the free end, which pulls the entire SutureLoop through the cuff, shuttling the anchor sutures with it (Fig. 17P-4).

- Next, shuttle (through a separate puncture in the rotator cuff) the sutures of the posteromedial anchor.

- Next, place two lateral row anchors (BioCorkscrew-FT [Arthrex]).

- Then, secure one pair of suture limbs from the antero-medial anchor to the same color suture limbs of the posteromedial anchor using a double mattress configu-

ration that is achieved by means of the "double-pulley" technique. For this technique, initially tie a suture limb from one anchor to a suture limb of the other anchor by exteriorizing the sutures outside the body and then tie them over a rod (Fig. 17P-5).

- Then, pull the other two "free" suture limbs from those same two pairs of sutures in a to-and-fro fashion, pulling the knot down over the top of the cuff at the medial part of the footprint. Tie these two suture limbs securely as a static, nonsliding knot using the Surgeon's Sixth Finger (Arthrex) knot pusher (Fig. 17P-6). This technique is called the "double-pulley" technique because the eyelets of two suture anchors are used like pulleys to bring the knots down onto the cuff.

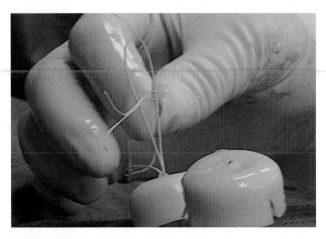

Figure 17P-3 The four suture ends from one of the medial anchors are loaded through the loop of the SutureLoop (Arthrex, Inc.; Naples, FL).

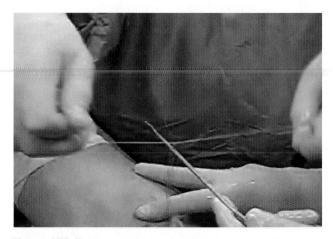

Figure 17P-5 A six-throw surgeon's knot is manually tied over a rod before transporting it inside the shoulder by pulling on the opposite ends of the suture pairs.

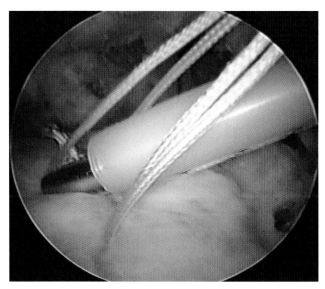

Figure 17P-6 Right shoulder, posterior viewing portal. The Surgeon's Sixth Finger (Arthrex, Inc.; Naples, FL) knot pusher is used to tie a static, nonsliding knot to complete the double-pulley construct.

- After tying the double-mattress suture on the medial row, two sets of suture pairs (one from each medial anchor) remain to be used later in separate diagonal double-pulley constructs, with the lateral row anchors to optimize footprint compression by means of a criss-cross configuration.

- Next, pass a single suture from each lateral anchor 10 to 12 mm from the cuff margin with the Viper (Arthrex) or Scorpion suture passer. Tie these two sutures as simple sutures, which will hold the edge of the cuff down to the bone (Fig. 17P-7).

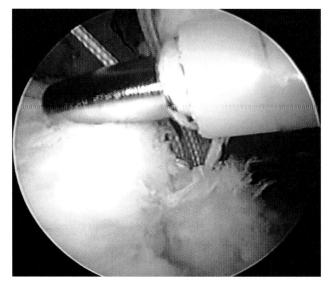

Figure 17P-7 Right shoulder, posterior viewing portal. One suture from each of the lateral anchors is tied as a simple suture.

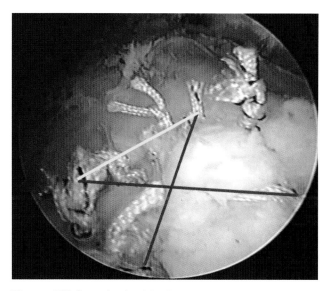

Figure 17P-8 Right shoulder, lateral viewing portal. The criss-cross sutures (*red lines*) and the medial mattress sutures (*yellow line*) provide excellent footprint contact.

- At this point, there remains one suture pair in each of the four anchors (total of four suture pairs) not tied. Tie these as diagonal mattress sutures using the double-pulley technique for each diagonal set of sutures. The two diagonal pairs cross each other to form a criss-cross pattern (Fig. 17P-8).

TRICKS AND TIPS

- In shuttling sutures through the cuff with a SutureLoop, it is important initially to maintain a grip on the proximal portions of the sutures as the SutureSnare begins to pull the distal (free) ends of the sutures into the shoulder. In this way, a redundancy is created in the proximal part of the sutures such that the loop of the SutureSnare "leads" the sutures through the cuff. If the SutureSnare is simply pulled through without creating the redundancy in the proximal portion of the sutures, the loop will pull all the way to the eyelet of the anchor before the suture limbs begin to pull through the cuff. When this happens, the suture limbs will bind between the eyelet and the cuff, and it will be very difficult, if not impossible, to pull them through the cuff.

- Diagonal criss-cross sutures create a very extensive contact pattern between the cuff and the bone.

- In performing the double-pulley technique, it is important to realize that once the first knot has been pulled down against the cuff, the suture will no longer slide through the soft tissues, and a sliding knot is not an option. We prefer to tie the second knot of the double-pulley construct as a static, nonsliding knot using a Surgeon's Sixth Finger knot pusher.

17Q

The Roller-Wringer Phenomenon

- The roller-wringer phenomenon refers to the mechanism by which the tip of the coracoid contributes to subscapularis tendon tears, particularly partial undersurface tears near its insertion to its lesser tuberosity.

- The coracoid tip is consistently located just anterior to the upper border of the subscapularis tendon. If the subcoracoid space is compromised, the coracoid tip will actually indent the subscapularis tendon, particularly with combined forward flexion and external rotation of the shoulder. Indentation of the subscapularis tendon creates high tensile forces on the posterior aspect of the subscapularis tendon, producing partial articular surface failure from bone and linear longitudinal tears near the insertion of the tendon (see Part I, Chapter 5: *The Tough Stuff*, section on subscapularis tears).

- An identified partial tear of the upper subscapularis tendon suggests coracoid impingement. The coracoid can be identified through the rotator interval tissue as a posteriorly directed bulge at the upper border of the subscapularis tendon (Fig. 17Q-1).

TRICKS AND TIPS

- The coracoid is easily identified as a "moving bulge" that can be seen through the rotator interval tissue at the top of the subscapularis tendon as the shoulder is internally and externally rotated.

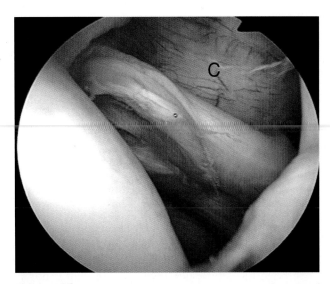

Figure 17Q-1 Left shoulder, posterior viewing portal. A partial subscapularis tendon tear near its insertion should alert the surgeon to probable coracoid impingement. C, capsular indentation from coracoid tip.

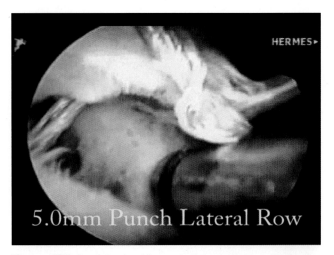

Figure 17R-1 Right shoulder, posterior viewing portal. A 5-mm bone socket is created in the lateral portion of the greater tuberosity.

17R

The "Shoestring" Technique of Knotless Lateral Row Fixation

- Knotless lateral row fixation is a technique that provides a fast, secure lateral fixation that can be done after standard medial row fixation has already been performed. It is particularly useful for reverse-L tears.

- This technique uses the concept of an interference fit of a 5.5-mm BioTenodesis (Arthrex, Inc.; Naples, FL) screw against 3-mm FiberTape (Arthrex) instead of knots.

- The FiberTape has a thin leading end of #2 FiberWire (Arthrex), which allows it to be passed through the rotator cuff with standard suture-passing instruments. In the

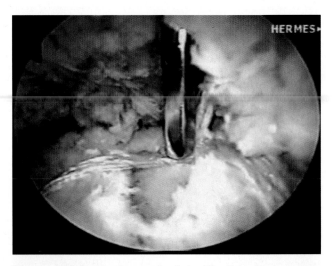

Figure 17R-2 The free ends of the FiberTape (Arthrex, Inc.; Naples, FL) have been loaded through a loop of suture at the tip of the BioTenodesis (Arthrex) inserter.

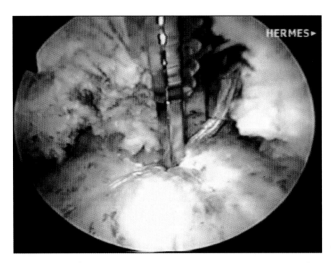

Figure 17R-3   The tip of the BioTenodesis (Arthrex, Inc.; Naples, FL) inserter pushes the FiberTape (Arthrex) to the base of the prepared bone socket.

case of a reverse-L tear, the FiberTape is woven across the tear like a shoestring.

● With a 5-mm BioCorkscrew (Arthrex) punch, create a slightly undersized bone socket for the 5.5-mm BioTenodesis screw on the lateral aspect of the greater tuberosity (Fig. 17R-1).

● Thread a loop of #2 FiberWire through the cannulation of the BioTenodesis driver. Then pass the two ends of the FiberTape through the loop at the tip of the inserter and tighten the loop around the FiberTape (Fig. 17R-2). In this way, the tip of the inserter can be used to manipulate the FiberTape into the prepared bone socket.

● With the BioTenodesis driver, push the FiberTape to the base of the prepared bone socket (Fig. 17R-3). Before inserting the screw, tension the FiberTape appropriately

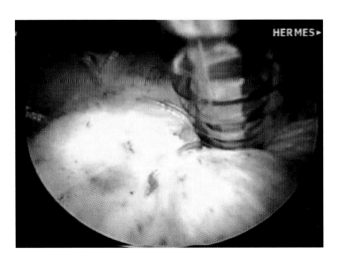

Figure 17R-4   Insertion of BioTenodesis (Arthrex, Inc.; Naples, FL) screw.

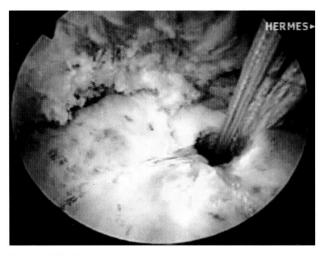

Figure 17R-5   Final construct of a knotless lateral row fixation.

to draw the tendon margins to the edge of the bone socket.

● Then insert the BioTenodesis screw (Fig. 17R-4) while holding appropriate tension on the FiberTape.

● Indentation of the tendon by the FiberTape indicates good loop security (Fig. 17R-5).

TRICKS AND TIPS

● Inserting the BioTenodesis screw through an accessory superolateral portal (adjacent to the acromion) while bringing the free ends of the FiberTape out a standard lateral portal after they have been passed through the loop in the BioTenodesis inserter allows greater control during tensioning of the FiberTape.

17S

Tuberoplasty: Arthroscopic Treatment of Greater Tuberosity Malunion

● Perform intra-articular evaluation. If the subscapularis tendon is torn, repair it before proceeding to the tuberoplasty.

● Because fracture lines can extend intra-articularly, smooth any step-offs in the articular surface with a shaver or burr.

● Place needles to mark the posterior extent of the proposed tuberoplasty (Fig. 17S-1).

● Use a pencil-tipped cautery probe to take down the superior portion of the rotator cuff, which overlies the prominent malunion of the greater tuberosity (Fig. 17S-2).

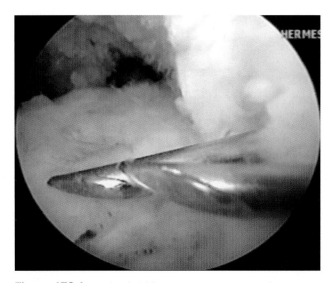

Figure 17S-1 Right shoulder, posterior intra-articular viewing portal. Needles are placed to mark the posterior extent of the superior aspect of the greater tuberosity. This will mark the posterior limit of the rotator cuff that is to be taken down for the tuberoplasty.

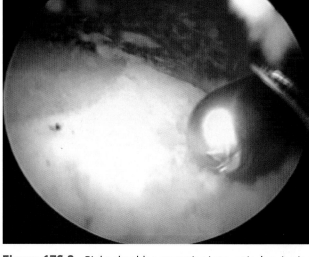

Figure 17S-3 Right shoulder, posterior intra-articular viewing portal. A high-speed burr introduced through a lateral portal reduces the prominent greater tuberosity until it is at or below the level of the articular margin of the humerus.

● Gradually reduce the size of the prominent malunited greater tuberosity by sculpting it down with a high-speed burr through a lateral working portal (Fig. 17S-3).

● In this case, a malunited intra-articular fragment caused a mechanical block to external rotation and had to be sculpted down to the same level as the adjacent articular surface by means of a high-speed burr (Fig. 17S-4).

● The final contour is a continuation of the normal humeral head convexity (Fig. 17S-5).

● After completion of the tuberoplasty, repair the rotator cuff by standard double row suture anchor fixation (Fig. 17S-6).

TRICKS AND TIPS

● It is better to take the greater tuberosity down to a lower level than to leave it with a profile that is too high. It is

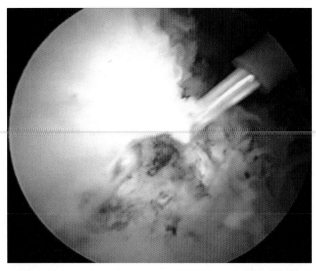

Figure 17S-2 Right shoulder, posterior subacromial viewing portal. A pencil-tip electrocautery (OPES electrosurgical system; Arthrex, Inc.; Naples, FL) is used to take down the superior portion of the rotator cuff that overlies the prominent malunited greater tuberosity.

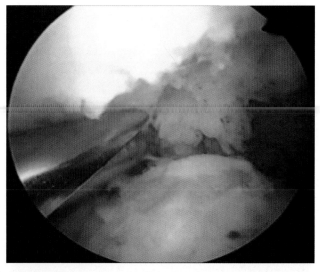

Figure 17S-4 Right shoulder, lateral viewing portal, 70° arthroscope. The malunited posterior step-off is sculpted by a burr introduced through a posterior portal.

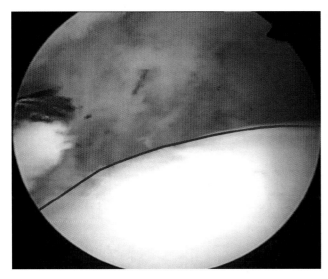

Figure 17S-5 After sculpting, the articular surface of the humerus has a smooth convexity (*solid line*).

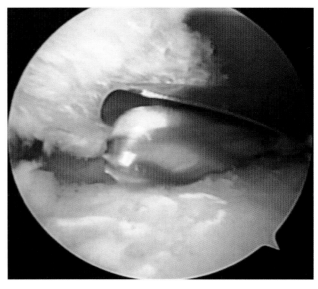

Figure 17T-1 Right shoulder, posterior intra-articular viewing portal. A burr is used to lightly abrade the bone bed of the greater tuberosity in preparation for cuff repair.

best to take it down to the level of the articular margin or even slightly lower (1 or 2 mm) than the articular margin.

● Intra-articular step-offs must be specifically looked for and corrected, because many fractures of the greater tuberosity extend into the posterior articular surface. If this occurs, the step-off will cause a mechanical block to external rotation, which will (by means of the coupled effect of external rotation on forward elevation) limit forward elevation.

● Cuff repair should be done by double-row techniques.

17T

Margin Convergence to Bone: Double-Row Repair of a Small U-Shaped Tear

● Evaluate the cuff tear from an intra-articular perspective initially.

● While viewing intra-articularly, prepare the bone bed on the greater tuberosity of the humerus (Fig. 17T-1).

● Place a medial anchor adjacent to the articular margin (Fig. 17T-2).

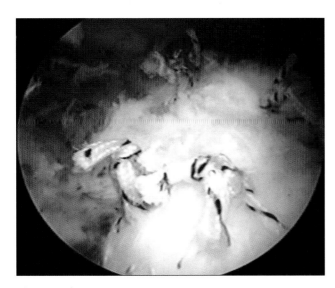

Figure 17S-6 Right shoulder, posterior viewing portal. The rotator cuff has been repaired by a double-row suture anchor technique.

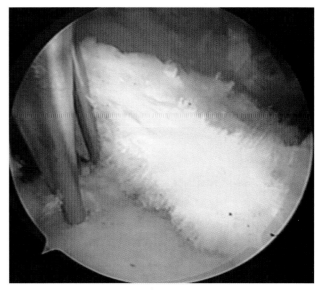

Figure 17T-2 Right shoulder, lateral subacromial viewing portal. A medial suture anchor is placed adjacent to the articular margin.

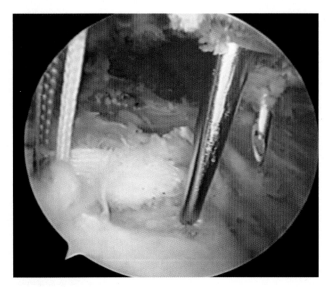

Figure 17T-3   Right shoulder, posterior viewing portal. A lateral anchor is placed.

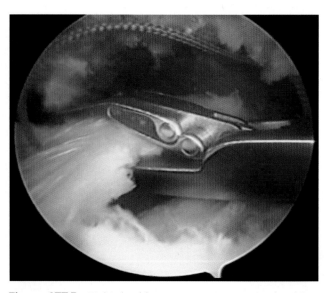

Figure 17T-5   Right shoulder, posterior viewing portal. A Viper (Arthrex, Inc.; Naples, FL) suture passer is used for antegrade suture passage through the anterior leaf of the cuff.

- Place a lateral anchor on the lateral aspect of the greater tuberosity (Fig. 17T-3).

- Pass sutures through the posterior leaf of the cuff in retrograde fashion with a Penetrator (Arthrex, Inc.; Naples, FL) suture passer (Fig. 17T-4).

- Pass sutures through the anterior leaf with an antegrade Viper (Arthrex) suture passer (Fig. 17T-5).

- Tie suture pairs, beginning with the medial sutures and progressing to the lateral sutures.

- Complete margin convergence to bone construct (Fig. 17T-6).

TRICKS AND TIPS

- In passing sutures retrograde through the posterior leaf of the cuff, it is useful to think that one is "lining up the putt" by choosing an entry point through the cuff that will line up the Penetrator directly toward the suture that is to be retrieved.

- In tying sutures, the most medial suture pairs should be tied first. This medial-to-lateral progression of margin convergence sequentially decreases the strain at the new "converged margin" of the cuff.

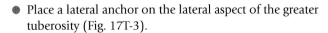

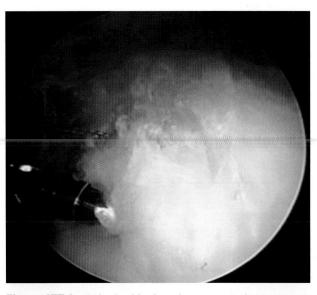

Figure 17T-4   Right shoulder, lateral viewing portal. A Penetrator (Arthrex, Inc; Naples, FL) suture passer is used to "line up the putt" for retrograde suture passage through the posterior leaf of the rotator cuff.

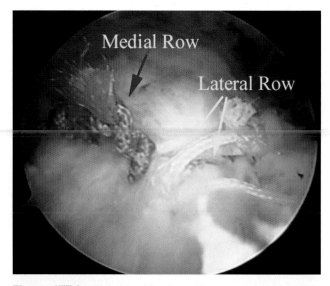

Figure 17T-6   Right shoulder, lateral viewing portal. Final construct. *Red arrows* denote the medial row sutures and *yellow arrows* indicate the lateral sutures that have accomplished margin convergence to bone.

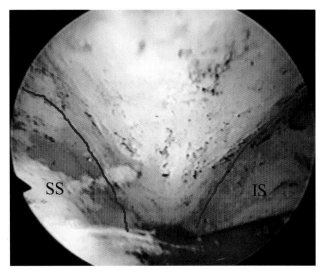

Figure 17U-2 Lateral view of the OPES (Arthrex, Inc.; Naples, FL) device inserted through the posterior portal to clean off the spine of the scapula. This structure appears much like the keel of a boat (*red line*). All tissue anterior to the spine is the supraspinatus (*SS*) and all tissue posterior is the infraspinatus (*IS*).

17U

Double Interval Slide Technique

- Massive rotator cuff tears are frequently (almost always) associated with partial or complete tears of the sub-scapularis tendon. In this situation, first repair the sub-scapularis tendon as outlined in Chapters 4 and 5 of this textbook.

- Once the subscapularis is appropriately repaired, follow the "comma" tissue to the anterior border of the supraspinatus tendon (Fig. 17U-1).

- Before attempting a mobilization procedure, perform a complete subacromial bursectomy. Extend this bursectomy all the way medially to the scapula spine (Fig. 17U-2).

- When completely cleared of all soft tissue, the scapula spine looks much like the keel of a boat.

- Proceed posteriorly with the bursectomy, being careful to differentiate bursal tissue from true cuff tissue (Fig. 17U-3) because bursal repairs tend to perform poorly.

- Next, use a cuff grasper to try to gauge the degree of cuff mobility (Fig. 17U-4). When assessing mobility, pull in multiple directions—medial to lateral, anterior to posterior, and posterior to anterior. Based on this mobility the tear pattern can be recognized.

- Once the anterior, medial, and posterior extent of the tear is exposed, place one or two traction sutures in the

supraspinatus and infraspinatus tendons, using either the Scorpion (Arthrex, Inc.; Naples, FL) or Viper (Arthrex) suture passer (Fig. 17U-5).

- If the cuff feels tight anterior to the supraspinatus tendon and if it feels like the comma tissue is inhibiting lateral excursion of the supraspinatus, then use an arthroscopic scissor to incise the tissue anterior to the supraspinatus tendon, including its attachment with the comma tissue (Fig. 17U-6). Use the scissor to release the tissue all the way to the base of the coracoid. The proper trajectory is

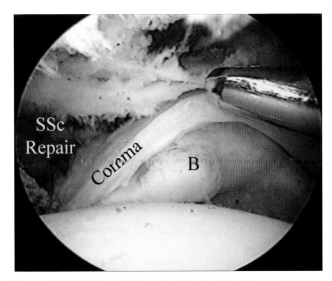

Figure 17U-1 Lateral view of a left shoulder after repair of the subscapularis tendon. The sutures from the subscapularis repair can be seen and the tissue running from the repaired subscapularis superiorly is the "comma" tissue. This comma tissue will lead the surgeon to the anterior edge of the supraspinatus tendon. The shaver is pointing to the supraspinatus tendon. SSc, subscapularis tendon; B, bursal tissue.

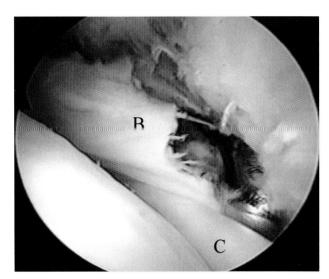

Figure 17U-3 Lateral portal viewing posteriorly. The shaver is removing the bursal tissue (*B*) overlying the intact rotator cuff tissue (*C*). The bursal tissue is noted to insert into the deltoid fascia, whereas the cuff tissue inserts onto the tuberosity.

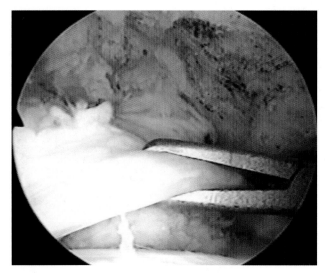

Figure 17U-4 The arthroscopic cuff grasper is used to determine cuff mobility. The tissue is pulled in multiple directions to gain a sense of where the tissue is tight and where releases need to be performed.

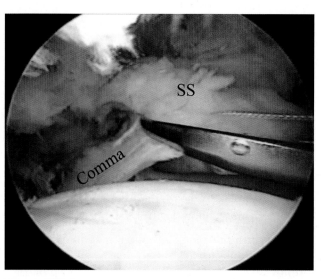

Figure 17U-6 Arthroscopic scissor used to perform the anterior interval slide. The tissue anterior to the supraspinatus (*SS*) tendon is cut. The scissor should be directed over the anterior biceps root and toward the base of the coracoid. The anterior interval slide separates the comma tissue from the SS tendon.

achieved by aiming directly anteromedial to the root of the biceps tendon (the anterior interval slide).

● Next, re-insert the cuff grasper and reassess cuff mobility.

● If increased lateral excursion is still required, then use the arthroscopic scissor to incise the tissue between the supraspinatus and infraspinatus tendons (posterior interval slide) while pulling laterally on the traction sutures that were previously placed in these two tendons. This release should proceed toward the spine of

the scapula (Fig. 17U-7) until the fat pad of the suprascapular nerve is reached. This nerve travels at the base of the scapula spine. Traction sutures on the cuff will help prevent injury to the suprascapular nerve.

● Once the anterior and posterior interval slides are completed, repair the rotator cuff (Fig. 17U-8). If a complete repair still cannot be achieved, make every effort to advance the infraspinatus tendon superiorly to optimize the rotator cuff force couples.

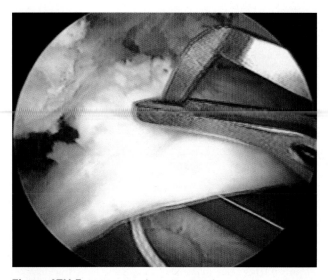

Figure 17U-5 A Viper (Arthrex, Inc.; Naples, FL) suture passer is used to place a traction suture into the anterior aspect of the supraspinatus tendon.

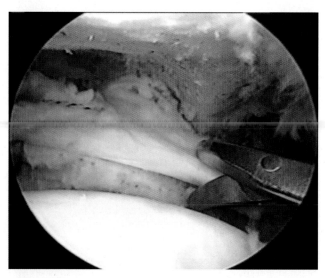

Figure 17U-7 While pulling the traction sutures laterally, the arthroscopic scissor is placed between the supraspinatus and infraspinatus tendons and aimed toward the scapula spine. This is the posterior interval slide.

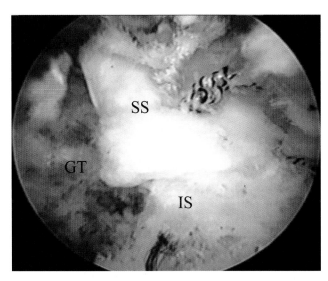

Figure 17U-8 After a double interval slide is completed, sufficient cuff mobility remains to allow for a complete repair of the rotator cuff. SS, supraspinatas; IS, infraspinatus; GT, greater tuberosity.

TIPS AND TRICKS

- Some surgeons may find it difficult to differentiate cuff tissue from bursal tissue during the subacromial bursectomy. One helpful "trick" is to follow the tissue to its distal attachment. If the tissue has attachments to the deltoid fascia, then it is bursal tissue and not cuff tissue. This tissue should be removed.

- Assessment of cuff mobility is one of the most critical aspects in all rotator cuff repairs. Not all cuffs should simply be repaired from medial to lateral! If the cuff demonstrates increased posterior to anterior mobility, it may be an L-shaped tear; if increased anterior to posterior mobility, it may be a reverse L-shaped tear; and if the anterior to posterior mobility is approximately equal and much greater than the medial to lateral mobility, it may be a U-shaped tear and margin convergence can be effective. Previous sections of this book concentrate on understanding tear patterns. We cannot overemphasize the importance of this skill.

- Typically, an anterior interval slide provides between 1 to 2 cm of increased lateral excursion of the supraspinatus tendon.

- To protect the suprascapular nerve during the posterior interval slide, we use two important techniques. First, we pull laterally on the traction sutures, thereby pulling the tissue away from the nerve. Secondly, we lift up on the arthroscopic scissor before each cut. We also watch for the medial fat pad while we are performing the posterior interval slide. This fat pad signifies that we are getting close to the suprascapular nerve and it is time to stop.

- The posterior interval slide can often provide 4 to 5 cm of increased lateral excursion. It is particularly effective for freeing the infraspinatus tendon.

- We described the anterior interval slide in this section, but we typically attempt to perform the anterior interval slide in continuity (see Chapter 17Y) if possible. The primary difference between the two techniques is that the anterior interval slide in continuity preserves the comma tissue. This is usually stout tissue and can often be incorporated into the rotator cuff repair.

17V

Routine Margin Convergence Technique

- Once a complete bursectomy has been performed, assess the mobility of the rotator cuff tear with the arthroscopic cuff grasper.

- Tears that exhibit more posterior to anterior and anterior to posterior mobility (as compared with medial to lateral mobility) are typically U-shaped tears (Fig. 17V-1). These tears are often amenable to margin convergence techniques.

- Multiple methods exist to perform margin convergence. The "hand-off" technique is described here.

- Load a suture at its midpoint onto a Penetrator (Arthrex, Inc.; Naples, FL) suture passer. While visualizing from a lateral viewing portal, insert the Penetrator through the posterior portal to pierce the posterior cuff tissue.

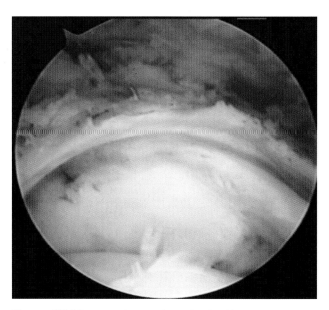

Figure 17V-1 Lateral view of a right shoulder with a massive rotator cuff tear.

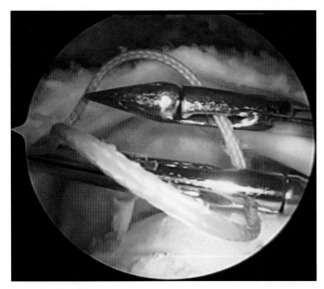

Figure 17V-2 Lateral view demonstrates two Penetrator (Arthrex, Inc.; Naples, FL) suture passers "handing off" the suture from the posterior to the anterior Penetrator.

- Then, insert an empty Penetrator through the anterior portal to pierce the anterior cuff tissue.

- The posterior Penetrator then "hands off" the suture to the anterior Penetrator (Fig. 17V-2).

- Pull the anterior Penetrator out the anterior portal, thereby completing one margin convergence pass.

- Repeat this process, as necessary, working laterally.

- Once an appropriate number of margin convergence sutures are placed, sequentially tie them, beginning with the most medial suture and then working laterally.

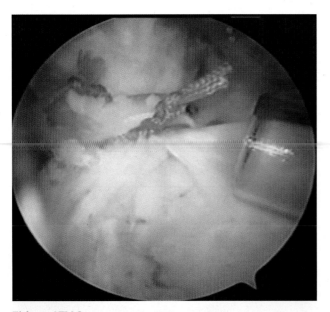

Figure 17V-3 Lateral view demonstrates that once all margin convergence sutures are tied, the lateral margin of the rotator cuff tendon is pulled over the prepared bone bed.

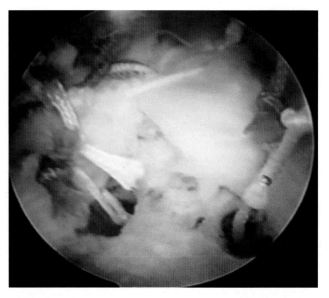

Figure 17V-4 Lateral view demonstrates that once the lateral cuff margin is secured to the bone anchors, a complete tendon-to-bone repair has been achieved.

- At the end of this process, the lateral margin of cuff is generally lying tension-free over the prepared bone footprint (Fig. 17V-3).

- Then, place suture anchors in the bone bed and pass simple sutures through the lateral cuff margin.

- Once margin convergence has been completed, a complete tendon to bone repair can be achieved in what initially seemed like an irreparable tear (Fig. 17V-4).

TIPS AND TRICKS

- The "hand-off" technique is one technique of margin convergence. Another technique we often use involves passing sutures through the anterior leaf with a Viper (Arthrex) suture passer from the posterior portal. Once the suture has been placed through the anterior leaf, an empty Penetrator pierces the posterior leaf and grasps the articular sided limb of each suture and sequentially pulls it out the posterior portal.

17W

Double-Row Margin Convergence to Bone

- Margin convergence techniques are particularly effective with U-shaped tears. These tears exhibit more mobility in the anterior to posterior direction than the medial to lateral direction.

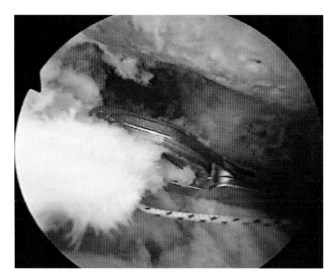

Figure 17W-1 Lateral view of a left shoulder demonstrates a Viper (Arthrex, Inc.; Naples, FL) suture passer placing a free FiberWire (Arthrex) through the anterior leaf of the rotator cuff tear.

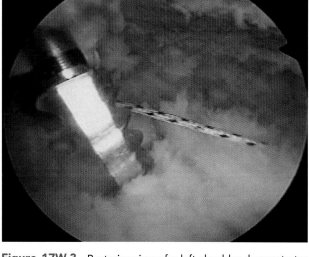

Figure 17W-3 Posterior view of a left shoulder demonstrates placement of a 5.5-mm BioCorkscrew-FT (Arthrex, Inc.; Naples, FL) suture anchor at the articular margin of the cuff footprint.

- One technique used to place margin convergence sutures is to pass a free FiberWire (Arthrex, Inc.; Naples, FL) through the anterior leaf using a Viper (Arthrex) suture passer (Fig. 17W-1). While viewing laterally, introduce the Viper through the posterior portal and grasp the anterior leaf. Then, pass the suture through this leaf and pull it back out the posterior portal.

- Next, insert a Penetrator (Arthrex) device through the posterior portal and to pierce the posterior leaf. Then, with the Penetrator, grasp the articular sided limb of the previously passed FiberWire (Arthrex) suture (Fig. 17W-2).

- Then place a 5.5-mm BioCorkscrew-FT (Arthrex) suture anchor at the articular margin of the footprint as a medial anchor point (Fig. 17W-3). Pass one limb of each color suture through the anterior leaf and the other limb of each color suture through the posterior leaf. For the anterior leaf, we use the Viper or Scorpion (Arthrex) suture passer (Fig. 17W-4). For the posterior leaf, we use the Penetrator from the posterior portal.

- Place another anchor at the lateral "drop off" of the footprint and pass the sutures in a similar fashion as the medial anchor sutures (Fig. 17W-5).

- Then, individually tie the sutures from medially to laterally using the Sixth Finger (Arthrex) knot pusher to optimize loop and knot security.

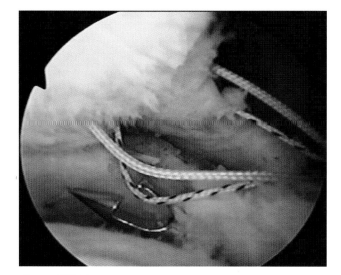

Figure 17W-2 Lateral view demonstrating a Penetrator (Arthrex, Inc.; Naples, FL) suture passer piercing the posterior leaf of the rotator cuff to grasp the articular limb of the FiberWire (Arthrex) suture.

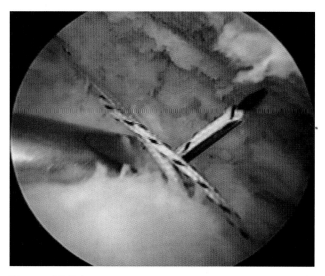

Figure 17W-4 The Scorpion (Arthrex, Inc.; Naples, FL) suture passing device is used to pass one limb of suture through the anterior leaf of the cuff in an antegrade direction.

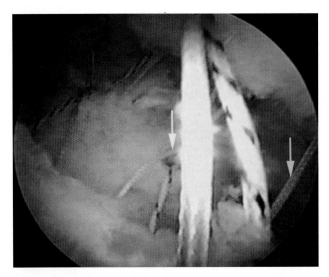

Figure 17W-5 Posterior view of the left shoulder after placement of all margin convergence sutures (*green arrow*), medial margin to bone sutures (*yellow arrow*), and lateral margin to bone sutures (*red arrow*).

● The final construct demonstrates a complete repair of a massive U-shaped tear with complete restoration of the greater tuberosity footprint (Fig. 17W-6).

TIPS AND TRICKS

● Multiple methods can be used to pass margin convergence sutures. The Viper plus Penetrator method outlined above has been effective and is most often used by us as our preferred technique.

17X

Two Anchor Transtendon PASTA Repair via the Double-Pulley Technique

● Glenohumeral arthroscopy demonstrates a significant partial articular surface tendon avulsion (PASTA). The anterior to posterior dimension is sufficiently large to accept two medial anchors (Fig. 17X-1).

● Next, reposition the scope to the subacromial space and perform a complete subacromial bursectomy. At the same time, thoroughly examine the bursal surface of the cuff to be sure the cuff tear is solely intra-articular. If any bursal component to the tear exists, complete the tear and perform a standard double row rotator cuff repair.

● Again reposition the scope to the glenohumeral space and prepare the footprint with a combination of electrocautery, shaver, and an arthroscopic burr (Fig. 17X-2).

● Next, insert an 18-gauge spinal needle off the lateral aspect of the *acromial process* (acromion) and into the joint to assess the appropriate deadman's angle (Fig. 17X-3). The arm may need to be adducted to gain a better angle.

● Position both anchors just off the articular margin. Place one anchor just posterior to the biceps tendon and the other anchor at the posterior aspect of the PASTA lesion (Fig. 17X-4).

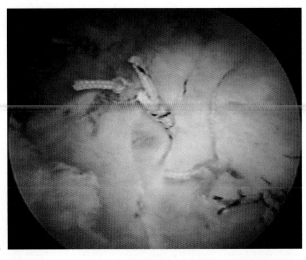

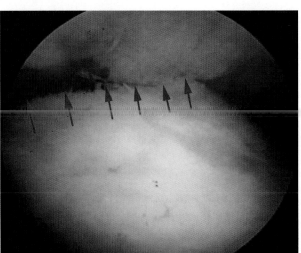

Figure 17W-6 **A:** Posterior subacromial view after the complete rotator cuff repair demonstrates complete closure of the cuff tear. **B:** The arthroscope is repositioned intra-articularly and the footprint is examined from inside. Restoration of the footprint along the articular margin (*red arrows*) is confirmed.

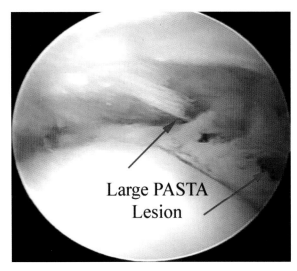

Figure 17X-1 Posterior glenohumeral view of a right shoulder demonstrates a large partial articular sided tendon avulsion (PASTA) lesion (*red arrows*).

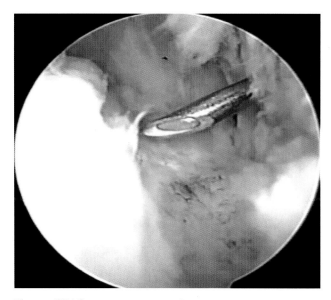

Figure 17X-3 An 18-gauge needle is used to assess the appropriate insertion angle for the anchors.

- Then, position the arthroscope into the subacromial space. Pull one suture strand from the anterior anchor and one same color suture strand from the posterior anchor through the lateral cannula and tie them extracorporeally (Fig. 17X-5).

- Then, pull the corresponding free suture strands and advance the knot into the subacromial space and on top of the cuff. Then, pull out the other two suture strands of the same color from the lateral cannula and tie them. Because the sutures can no longer slide, a static knot is essential.

- Repeat the process with the other color sutures. At the conclusion of the procedure, a bridge of tissue is compressed against the bone bed (Fig. 17X-6). This reconstitutes the footprint very well (Fig. 17X-7).

TIPS AND TRICKS

- The subacromial bursectomy is essential before placement of any anchors. If this space is not cleared, the shaver can easily capture and cut one or more of the sutures from the anchors.

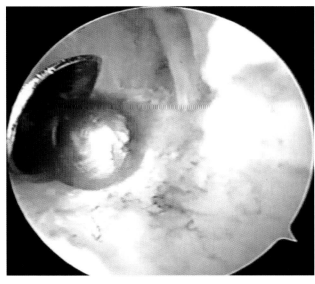

Figure 17X-2 The tear footprint is prepared with a burr to a bleeding bone surface without decorticating the bone.

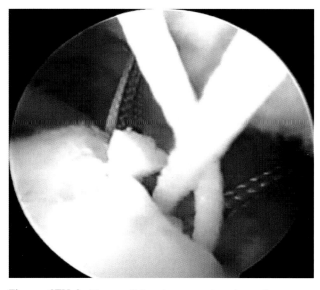

Figure 17X-4 Two medial anchors are placed, one just posterior to the biceps tendon and the second at the posterior aspect of the rotator cuff tear.

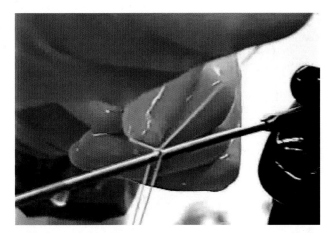

Figure 17X-5 One suture from the anterior anchor and one same color suture from the posterior anchor are pulled out the lateral cannula and tied over a metal post with six throws.

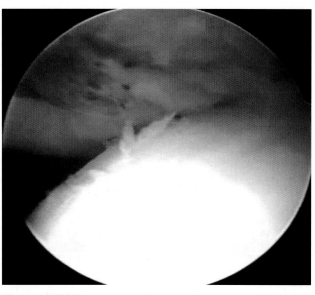

Figure 17X-7 Intra-articular view demonstrates excellent reconstruction of the footprint.

- If the anchor insertion angle is too steep, an assistant should adduct the arm against the patient's body to obtain a better angle of approach.

- It is IMPERATIVE to remember when tying the second pair of sutures that they do not slide any longer. A static knot is essential. This is easily performed with the Sixth Finger (Arthrex, Inc.; Naples, FL) knot pusher. The added benefit of this device is that it allows for tissue compression while the knot is being tied.

17Y

Anterior Interval Slide in Continuity

- An anterior interval slide in continuity is typically performed in conjunction with a massive anterosuperior rotator cuff tear, which includes a subscapularis tendon tear in addition to a supraspinatus and infraspinatus tear.

- First, place a traction suture in the comma tissue and apply lateral traction, which reveals the junction of the

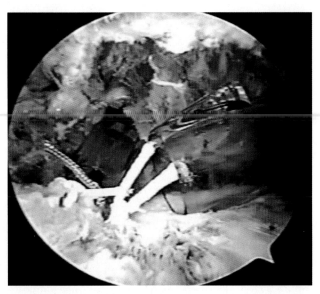

Figure 17X-6 At the conclusion of the procedure, a bridge of cuff tissue is compressed against the bone bed.

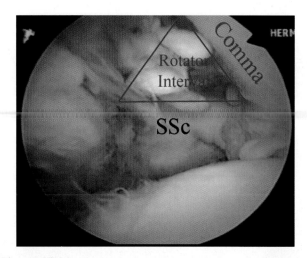

Figure 17Y-1 Posterior glenohumeral view of a right shoulder. A traction suture is placed in the comma tissue and lateral traction reveals the confluence of the subscapularis tendon (*SSc*) with the comma tissue. Also apparent is the intervening rotator interval tissue.

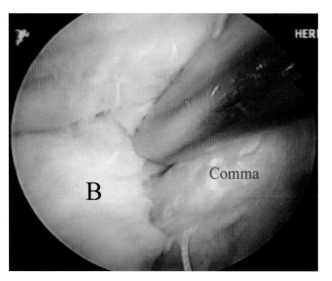

Figure 17Y-2 Posterior glenohumeral viewing portal with a 70° arthroscope demonstrates the proper line of resection during the anterior interval slide in continuity. The excision proceeds from just anterior to the root of the biceps tendon *(B)* medially to the base of the coracoid. (Note: In the photo the biceps has been tenotomized, so the biceps root is just a stump of tendon.)

subscapularis tendon, the comma, and the rotator interval tissue (Fig. 17Y-1).

● Then, excise the rotator interval tissue with a combination of the arthroscopic shaver and OPES (Arthrex, Inc.; Naples, FL) electrocautery.

● Next, excise the tissue just anterior to the supraspinatus tendon with arthroscopic scissor, shaver, and electrocautery while preserving the comma tissue. This process removes the coracohumeral ligament tissue.

● Be aware of an important landmark, the root of the biceps tendon, to use as a guide (Fig. 17Y-2). While excising the coracohumeral ligament tissue, aim the excision devices over the root of the biceps and continue the excision until reaching the base of the coracoid.

● Once soft tissue excision has been completed, the entire base of the coracoid can be visualized (Fig. 17Y-3), signifying that a complete anterior interval slide in continuity has been performed.

TIPS AND TRICKS

● When a complete subscapularis tendon release is performed, an anterior interval slide in continuity, essentially, is also performed.

● Typically, we prefer the anterior interval slide in continuity rather than the anterior interval slide procedure because it preserves the comma tissue, which is often incorporated into the rotator cuff repair.

17Z
Anterior Interval Slide

● In the face of a massive rotator cuff tear, place traction sutures in the supraspinatus and infraspinatus tendons (Fig. 17Z-1). Lateral traction on these sutures will reveal the extent of the cuff tear mobility.

● If the cuff is contracted and somewhat immobile, use a cuff grasper to try to determine where points of contraction exist. If the supraspinatus tendon lacks mobility,

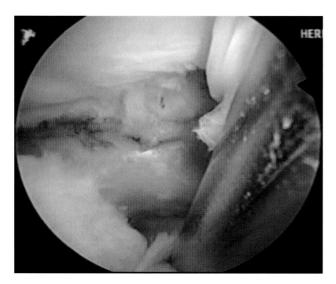

Figure 17Y-3 After completion of the anterior interval slide in continuity, the entire base and arch of the coracoid can be visualized. The entire coracohumeral ligament and any adhesions between the anterior supraspinatus tendon and coracoid have now been removed.

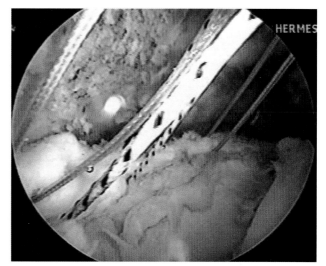

Figure 17Z-1 Posterior view of the right shoulder with a massive rotator cuff tear. Two traction sutures are placed in the supraspinatus tendon and two traction sutures are placed in the infraspinatus tendon.

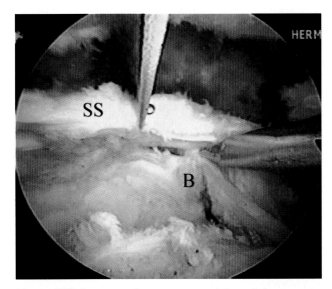

Figure 17Z-2 A 70° arthroscope inserted through the posterior portal gives a perspective very similar to a 30° arthroscope in the lateral portal. The arthroscopic scissor is inserted through the lateral portal and positioned directly over the stump of the biceps root (*B*) at the anterior aspect of the supraspinatus (*SS*).

often substantial scarring is seen of the anterior supraspinatus tendon against the base of the coracoid.

● Position arthroscopic scissor at the anterior aspect of the supraspinatus tendon directly over the origin of the long head of the biceps tendon (Fig. 17Z-2). This is where the comma tissue joins the supraspinatus tendon. The comma tissue is then cut.

● Cut just anterior to the supraspinatus tendon tissue, aiming over the biceps. The base of the coracoid is just anteromedial to the biceps root.

● Cut all tissue reaching the base of the coracoid.

● Next, insert a 15° arthroscopic elevator through the lateral portal. While pulling on the traction sutures, push the elevator underneath the supraspinatus tendon to break up any adhesions underneath it.

● Once the anterior interval slide is completed, apply lateral traction to the supraspinatus tendon sutures to determine the amount of increased excursion obtained (Fig. 17Z-3). Usually, an anterior interval slide gives ~1 to 2 cm of increased excursion to the supraspinatus tendon.

TIPS AND TRICKS

● The difference between the anterior interval slide and the anterior interval slide in continuity is the comma tissue. In the anterior interval slide, all the tissue anterior to the supraspinatus tendon is cut. This includes the lateral attachment of the comma tissue with the anterior edge of the supraspinatus tendon. In the anterior interval slide in continuity, the comma attachment with the anterior supraspinatus tendon is left intact. This comma tissue is often incorporated into the rotator cuff repair. Whenever possible, we attempt to perform an anterior interval slide in continuity to take full advantage of this comma tissue.

● Although we free up the tissue underneath the supraspinatus tendon with an arthroscopic elevator, this typically adds very little to the overall release. For some reason, the adhesions underneath the supraspinatus (if any) are not nearly as constricting as the adhesions at the anterior and posterior aspects of the tendon.

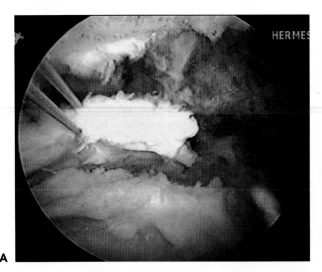
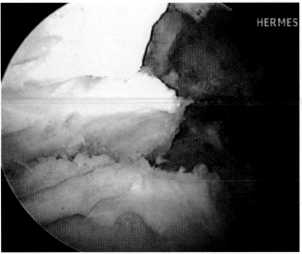

Figure 17Z-3 **A:** After the anterior interval slide is completed, the entire anterior aspect of the supraspinatus tendon is free. **B:** Lateral traction is applied to supraspinatus tendon demonstrating significantly increased lateral excursion.

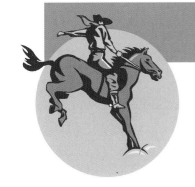

18

Biceps

18A

Arthroscopic-Assisted Biceps Tenodesis for Retracted Biceps Tendon Tear: The Cobra Procedure

● Perform intra-articular arthroscopy to confirm complete rupture of the long head of biceps tendon.

● In cases of a retained intra-articular biceps stump, arthroscopically débride it.

● Palpate the retracted proximal biceps tendon in the upper arm, then make a short 4-cm diagonal incision over it and extract the tendon. Assess the tendon for adequate length and tissue quality.

● Place a Krakow whipstitch, with three or four interlocking throws on each side of the biceps tendon (Fig. 18A-1). Trim the bulbous end of the tendon to ~5 mm from the entry point of the whipstitch. The BioTenodesis (Arthrex, Inc.; Naples, FL) driver will later be used to push the end of the tendon to the bottom of a prepared bone socket after threading the whipstitch ends through the tip of the driver.

● Palpate the lower bicipital groove with a finger passed through the incision in the arm. The bicipital groove will be located deep to the pectoralis major, just medial to that muscle's insertion into the humerus. While palpating the distal bicipital groove, pass a switching stick through the distal incision so that it

passes medial to the palpating finger and runs proximally through and then past the bicipital groove to tent the skin just anterolateral to the anterolateral corner of the *acromial process* (acromion). Adduct the arm while torquing the tip of the switching stick in a lateral direction to direct it to the proper exit point for an anterolateral subacromial portal. Now, the switching stick exits both proximally and distally, and defines a safe channel within the arm and shoulder for passage of the biceps tendon.

● Insert the arthroscope's sheath over the proximal end of the switching stick (at the shoulder), then place a 7-mm clear cannula over the distal end of the switching stick (in the upper arm). Advance the sheath and cannula toward each other until the cannula telescopes over the smaller-diameter scope sheath (Fig. 18A-2). Then, remove the switching stick. This leaves a safe tunnel composed of the telescoped sheath and cannula, which will prevent inadvertent neurovascular injury when passing sharp instruments through this tunnel.

● Pass a long suture passer or a Beath pin from proximal to distal through the enclosed cylindrical tunnel formed by the telescoped sheath and cannula. Then, remove the distal clear cannula.

● Thread the two ends of the whipstitch into the suture passer or Beath pin (Fig. 18A-3).

● Withdraw the suture passer or Beath pin through the proximal portal puncture, pulling the biceps tendon through the bicipital groove and into the subacromial space.

● Close the distal incision.

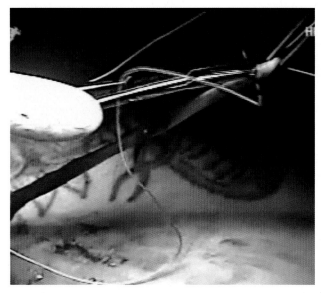

Figure 18A-1   A Krakow interlocking whipstitch is placed in the end of the retrieved long head of biceps tendon.

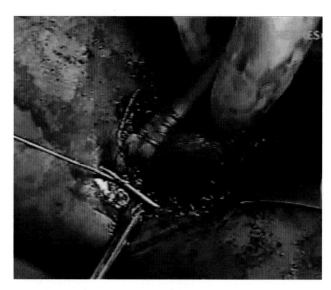

Figure 18A-3   The whipstitch suture limbs are threaded into the suture passer where it exits the distal incision.

- Now that the biceps tendon has been retrieved into the subacromial space, proceed with a standard arthroscopic biceps tenodesis using a BioTenodesis (Arthrex) screw for fixation.

- Use the BioTenodesis inserter to "size" the biceps tendon before passing it proximally in order to choose the proper diameter BioTenodesis screw (usually 7 or 8 mm diameter).

- Drill a bone socket to a depth of 25 mm at the proximal aspect of the bicipital groove. In cases of an associated supraspinatus tendon tear, make the bone socket at the anterolateral aspect of the greater tuberosity, so that the sutures from the BioTenodesis construct can be used as part of the lateral row repair for the rotator cuff.

- Thread the BioTenodesis driver with the whipstitch suture ends, and use it to push the biceps tendon into the bone socket.

- Insert the BioTenodesis screw alongside the biceps tendon to achieve interference fixation (Fig. 18A-4).

- In cases of an associated rotator cuff tear, repair it, incorporating the sutures from the BioTenodesis construct into the lateral row of the cuff repair.

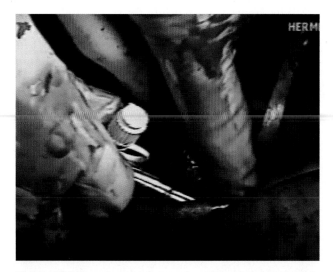

Figure 18A-2   A 7-mm clear cannula is inserted over the switching stick at the distal incision so that it telescopes over the arthroscope sheath, which has been placed over the switching stick through the proximal skin puncture.

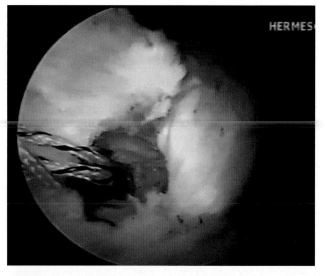

Figure 18A-4   Completed biceps tenodesis with interference fixation by a BioTenodesis (Arthrex, Inc.; Naples, FL) screw. The suture ends are incorporated into the lateral row of the rotator cuff repair.

TRICKS AND TIPS

- The key to safely passing the tendon proximally through the bicipital groove is to create a safe cylindrical tunnel (telescoping sheath and cannula) through which the sharp passing instrument (long suture retriever or Beath pin) can be passed without risk of neurovascular injury.

- To create a safe cylindrical tunnel, the switching stick must be safely passed deep to the pectoralis major. This maneuver is facilitated by torquing the tip of the switching stick in a lateral direction so that it "hugs" the lateral insertion of the pectoralis major as it is pushed proximally. Adduction of the shoulder will make this manipulation easier.

- After the BioTenodesis screw has been inserted, the suture ends from the whipstitch (which exit through the center of the cannulated BioTenodesis screw) can be used in the rotator cuff repair. It is important to recognize that these two suture limbs will not slide, so a static knot-tying technique must be used.

18B

Biceps Tenodesis without Supraspinatus Tendon Tear

- Using a spinal needle for localization, create an anterosuperolateral portal through the bicipital roof, directly over the top of the biceps tendon at its exit point at the top of the bicipital groove.

- Prepare a bleeding bone bed just proximal to the top of the bicipital groove, using a power shaver and ring curette (Fig. 18B-1).

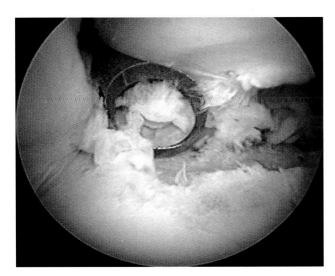

Figure 18B-1 Left shoulder, posterior viewing portal. A ring curette is used to create a bleeding bone bed.

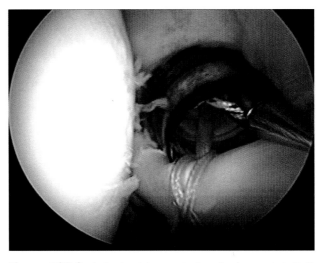

Figure 18B-2 Left shoulder, posterior viewing portal. Half-racking sutures have been placed in the biceps tendon. Because the tension in the suture loop is perpendicular to the direction of the tendon fibers, the fibers create a strong strangulation effect to prevent suture cut-out through the tendon.

- Insert two half-racking sutures into the biceps tendon to maintain a grip on the tendon after it is tenotomized (Fig. 18B-2).

- Use an electrocautery wand to perform a biceps tenotomy.

- Exteriorize the biceps tendon through the anterosuperolateral portal and place a Krakow whipstitch along both sides of the tendon (Fig. 18B-3).

- Size the tendon using the sizing holes in the thumb plate of the BioTenodesis (Arthrex, Inc., Naples, FL) screwdriver. For most patients, tendon size will be 8 mm (men) or 7 mm (women).

- Place a guide pin in the prepared bone bed.

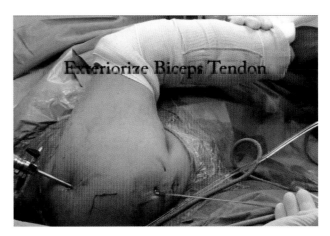

Figure 18B-3 Flexion of the elbow and shoulder by an assistant will add tendon length during exteriorization of the tendon for placement of the whipstitch.

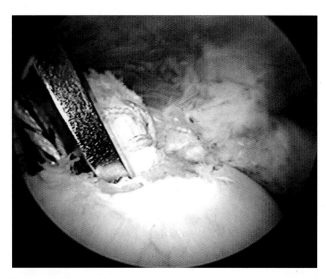

Figure 18B-4 The biceps tendon is inserted into the bone socket by pushing the end of the tendon with the tip of the BioTenodesis (Arthrex, Inc.; Naples, FL) inserter, through which the whipstitch sutures have been passed.

- Use a cannulated headed reamer from the BioTenodesis set to create a bone socket the same diameter as the "sized" tendon and 25-mm deep.

- Clear the mouth of the bone socket of soft tissue and bone debris with a power shaver.

- Insert the biceps tendon by loading its whipstitch through the cannulated tip of the BioTenodesis driver, then use the tip of the driver to push the tendon end to the bottom of the bone socket (Fig. 18B-4).

- Advance the BioTenodesis screw by turning the screwdriver while holding the thumbplate on the driver so

that the thumbplate will not rotate (Fig. 18B-5). This manipulation advances the screw by the reverse threaded sleeve above the screw, while the tip of the driver holds the end of the tendon stationary at the bottom of the bone socket.

- Use the sutures from the BioTenodesis screw construct to repair the upper subscapularis tendon if it is torn (Fig. 18B-6).

TRICKS AND TIPS

- A ring curette is useful in preparing the bone bed at the proposed site for the biceps tenodesis.

- The half-racking sutures in the biceps create a "strangulation hold" on the tendon so that the sutures will not cut through the tendon (which would allow it to retract distally) as it is prepared for tenodesis.

- In some patients, especially those who are very muscular or very obese, exteriorization of the tendon through the anterosuperolateral portal can be difficult, because the tendon does not have sufficient length and excursion to pull through the skin for a sufficient distance for the placement of the whipstitch. If this situation is encountered, additional working length to the tendon can be obtained by flexion of the elbow in combination with forward flexion of the shoulder (Fig. 18B-3).

- We prefer to use BioTenodesis screws that are ≤8 mm in diameter. Before placing the Krakow whipstitch, we "size" the tendon in the thumbplate sizing holes. If it is >8 mm in diameter, we trim the tendon lengthwise for a distance of 25-mm (a little longer than the length of the

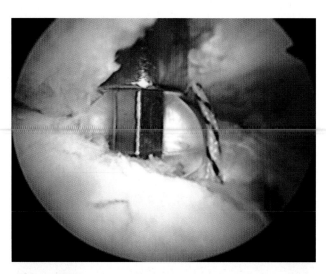

Figure 18B-5 Turning the BioTenodesis (Arthrex, Inc.; Naples, FL) screwdriver while holding its thumbplate will advance the reverse-threaded sleeve on the shaft of the inserter. In this figure, the sleeve can be seen advancing the BioTenodesis screw down the shaft of the inserter.

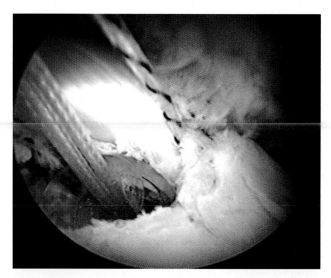

Figure 18B-6 Final construct, showing interference fixation of the biceps tendon against the biodegradable screw within the bone socket. The suture from the biceps tendonesis may be used to repair the upper subcapularis tendon if it is torn.

BioTenodesis screw, which is 23-mm) before placing the whipstitch, so that its final diameter will be ≤8 mm.

- We begin and end the whipstitch on the superior aspect of the tendon, 5-mm from its end, so that the tendon can be pushed to the bottom of the bone socket with the tip of the BioTenodesis driver (Fig. 18B-4).

- In drilling the bone socket, we advance the headed reamer the last 10-mm by turning the drill-chuck by hand so as to not "wander" in bone and create an oversized bone socket. Also, we remove the headed reamer by hand twisting.

- We load the whipstitch ends directly through the driver and keep tension on the suture ends at the back of the driver handle while pushing the tendon into the prepared bone socket. This technique will maintain the biceps tendon at the tip of the driver, allowing easy manipulation.

- If the sutures from the BioTenodesis construct are incorporated into a subscapularis tendon repair, remember that these sutures will not slide and that a nonsliding static knot must be tied.

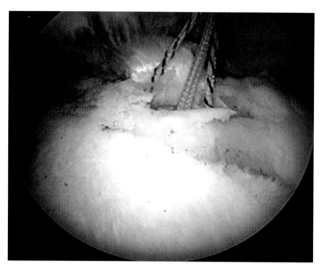

Figure 18C-1 The BioTenodesis (Arthrex, Inc.; Naples, FL) screw construct has achieved a biceps tenodesis posterolateral to the bicipital groove, where its sutures can be incorporated into the lateral row of the rotator cuff repair.

that the BioTenodesis (Arthrex, Inc.; Naples, FL) construct is located at the anterolateral aspect of the greater tuberosity (Fig. 18C-1). Then, incorporate the sutures from the BioTenodesis construct into the lateral row repair of the rotator cuff.

18C

Biceps Tenodesis with Torn Supraspinatus Tendon

- The steps are the same as in the previously described procedure in Chapter 18B, *Biceps Tenodesis without Supraspinatus Tendon Tear*, with two exceptions:

  1. It is not necessary to place a separate incision through the bicipital roof because all of the arthroscopic work can be performed through the defect in the supraspinatus tendon.
  2. Place the bone socket for tenodesis just posterior or posterolateral to the top of the bicipital groove, so

TRICKS AND TIPS

- The BioTenodesis construct will have two suture pairs that can be incorporated into the lateral row repair of the rotator cuff. Use of these suture pairs eliminates the need for an additional anterolateral suture anchor for rotator cuff repair.

- If a double-row rotator cuff repair is to be done following biceps tenodesis, consider using the smaller diameter 3.7-mm BioCorkscrew (Arthrex) suture anchors for the medial row to preserve more native footprint for maximal tendon-to-bone contact.

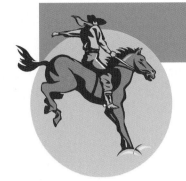

19

Tricks and Tips

Arthroscopic Knot-Tying Using the Sixth Finger Knot Pusher

- The Sixth Finger (Arthrex, Inc.; Naples, FL) knot pusher is a double diameter knot pusher. Its wire loop through the inner cannula allows suture material to be passed through the center of the device (Fig. 19A-1).

- During knot-tying, two limbs of suture—the *post* limb and the *loop* limb (or wrapping limb)—are available. Thread the limb that you have chosen to be the post limb through the inner metal cannula (Fig. 19A-2).

- Next, throw a half-hitch around the metal cannula. The half-hitch can be overhand or underhand, whichever is more easily performed. Loop this half-hitch around the inner metal cannula and push the half-hitch down the shaft of the metal cannula with the outer plastic cannulated tube (Fig. 19A-3).

- Once the first half-hitch is thrown, the metal cylinder can assist in manipulating the soft tissue over to the bone bed (Fig. 19A-4).

- The greatest characteristic of the Sixth Finger knot pusher is that it allows the surgeon to maintain a tight loop while performing subsequent throws. After the first

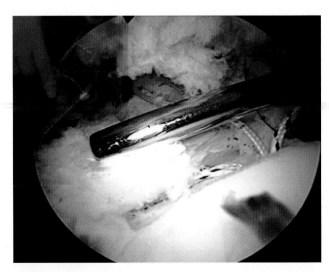

Figure 19A-1 A FiberWire (Arthrex, Inc.; Naples, FL) suture strand is threaded through the wire loop that goes through the inner metal cannula of the Sixth Finger (Arthrex) knot pusher.

Figure 19A-2 The desired post limb should be threaded through the inner metal cannula. In this example, the post limb is the limb coming from the cuff (subscapularis) tissue.

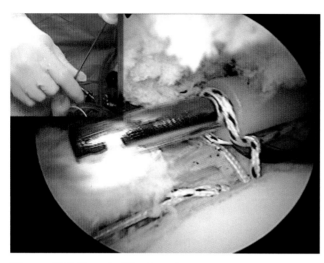

Figure 19A-3 A half-hitch is thrown and pushed down the metal cylinder with the outer plastic tube.

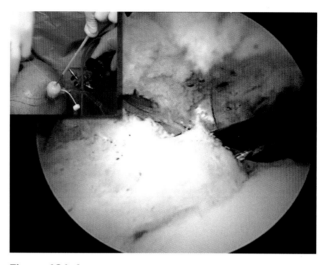

Figure 19A-4 Once one half-hitch is thrown, the metal cylinder can be used to manipulate the soft tissue over the bone bed. In this case, the surgeon pulls the subscapularis laterally over the lesser tuberosity bone bed.

half-hitch is thrown, hold tension on the post suture limb while pushing down on the plastic disc at the back of the knot pusher. This maintains excellent loop security while subsequent half-hitches are thrown.

- As subsequent half-hitches are thrown, it is important to pay attention to each loop as it slides down the metal cylinder to assure that any twists are removed before sliding the hitch down completely. Twists can be removed by turning the plastic tube and metal cylinder in the opposite direction of the twist (Fig. 19A-5).

- Create a "base knot" by throwing three half-hitches in the same direction. Once these three half-hitches are tightened, sufficient internal friction has been developed to prevent knot slippage (and subsequent loss of loop security). The next three throws serve to "lock" the knot.

- Throw the fourth half-hitch in the *same* direction as the previous three. Once the loop is pushed down to within 1 to 2 cm of the base knot, the metal cylinder is backed off (Fig. 19A-6). Tension is then released from this suture strand and applied to the free strand (the previous loop strand). The surgeon will both see and feel the knot "flip." The previous post is now the loop; the previous loop is now on tension and has been transformed into the "new" post (Fig. 19A-7).

- Now, use the metal cylinder to pull the loop down the post and past the knot. Position the cylinder past the knot and apply tension to both suture strands. This technique of "past pointing" provides optimal knot security (Fig. 19A-8).

- Throw the fifth half-hitch in the *same* direction as all the previous throws. Reapply tension to the suture strand in

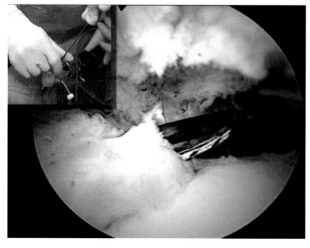
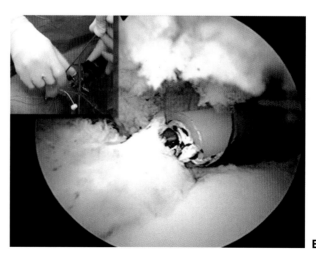

Figure 19A-5 **A:** A one-quarter twist is noted in the clockwise direction around the metal cylinder. **B:** By twisting the outer plastic tube and metal cylinder in the counterclockwise direction, the twist is removed before securing the half-hitch down.

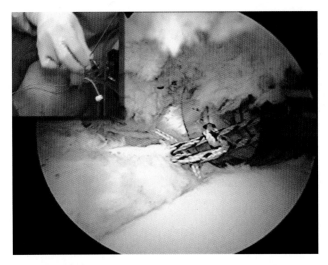

Figure 19A-6   The metal cylinder is pulled back. The suture strand going through the metal cylinder is still under tension; therefore, this strand is still considered the post. The tension will be released from this strand and applied to the other strand to "switch posts."

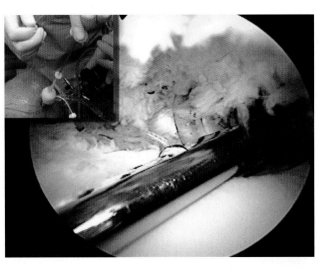

Figure 19A-8   The metal cylinder is passed beyond the knot and tension is applied to both suture strands. This technique of "past pointing" secures the half-hitch and provides optimal knot security.

the metal cylinder and use the outer plastic tube to push the loop down this cylinder. Secure the half-hitch on top of the knot by past pointing. This fifth throw is *not* flipped.

● Throw the sixth and final half-hitch in the *same* direction as all previous throws. Once the half-hitch is positioned ~1 to 2 cm from the knot, the metal cylinder is backed off and the knot is flipped, as described previously. Secure the half-hitch by past pointing.

● Use the open-ended FiberWire (Arthrex) suture cutter to cut the suture strands 3 or 4 mm from the knot (Fig. 19A-9).

TIPS AND TRICKS

● It is always preferable to tie knots onto soft tissue rather than bone. When choosing which suture limb to load into the metal cylinder of the Sixth Finger knot pusher, it is important to pull the sutures so that the soft tissue strand can be loaded, rather than the strand emanating directly from the anchor.

● Once the first half-hitch is thrown, the tissue can be manipulated with the end of the metal cylinder. This allows the tissue to be pulled or pushed into the appropriate position over the bone bed.

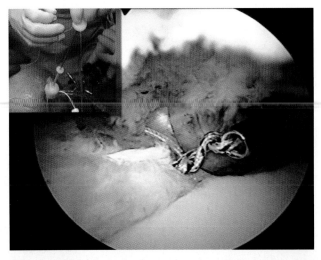

Figure 19A-7   Tension has now been applied to the suture strand not traversing the metal cylinder. The cylinder strand is now looped around the free strand and is now considered the loop strand. The metal cylinder is used to push the loop down the post.

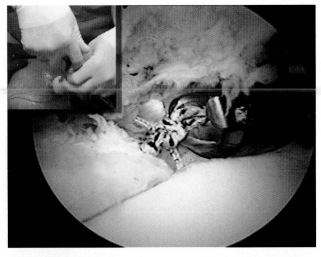

Figure 19A-9   The open ended 4.2-mm FiberWire (Arthrex, Inc.; Naples, FL) suture cutter is used to cut the free strands 3 or 4 cm from the knot.

- When choosing which portal from which to tie, it is optimal if the metal cylinder of the Sixth Finger knot pusher can compress the tissue directly over the anchor. Therefore, an angle more perpendicular to the tissue and less parallel to the tissue is usually best.

- Past pointing should be used on *every* throw. On the first throw, this will optimize loop security and on subsequent throws this will optimize knot security.

- When pushing the loop down the metal cylinder, it is critical to remove any twists before securing the throw. This is done by twisting the metal cylinder and plastic tube in the direction opposite the twist. If this is a full twist, then "pre-untwist" the next throw by rotating the free suture strand once around the knot pusher before throwing the next half-hitch.

- Whether a static knot or a sliding knot is chosen, the literature is clear that every knot should be "locked" with three reversing half-hitches on alternating post (RHAP) throws. This is essential to prevent the knot from failing by slippage. In the six-throw surgeon's knot, the post is flipped, or reversed, on the fourth and the sixth throws.

19B

Anchor Removal from Glenoid Using OATS Harvester

- A broken metal screw-in anchor that is "sitting proud" above the articular surface will rapidly cause articular cartilage damage. The difficulty in removing such a broken anchor results from a variety of reasons:

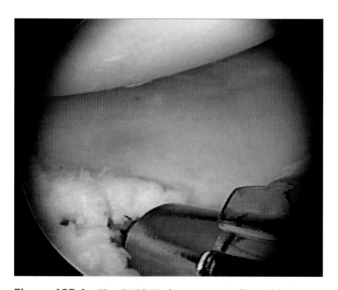

Figure 19B-1 The OATS (Arthrex, Inc.; Naples, FL) harvester tube is placed over the end of the broken anchor, in line with its long axis.

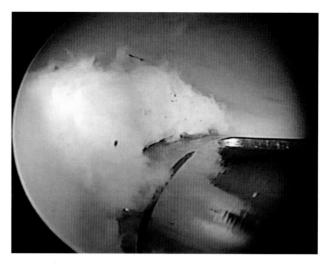

Figure 19B-2 The OATS (Arthrex, Inc.; Naples, FL) harvester tube is impacted to a depth of 12 to 15 mm around the anchor.

1. It cannot be driven in by impaction because its screw threads prevent this.
2. It cannot be screwed further in because its hex head for insertion is broken off.
3. It cannot be unscrewed because it is impossible to grasp its broken trailing end.

- The best way to remove such an anchor is with the 6-mm OATS (Osteochondral Autogenous Transfer System) (Arthrex, Inc.; Naples, FL) harvester tube.

- Insert the OATS harvester tube directly over the exposed end of the broken anchor, in line with the long axis of the anchor (Fig. 19B-1).

- After the harvester tube is impacted to a depth of 12 to 15 mm around the anchor (Fig. 19B-2), rotate the harvester tube counterclockwise while removing the screw-in

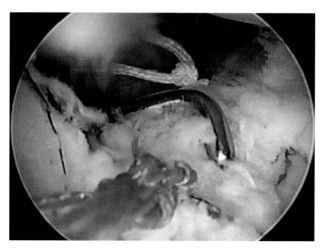

Figure 19B-3 The labrum has been repaired above and below the bone cylinder, which has been reinserted as its own graft.

anchor and its surrounding cylinder of bone. This counterclockwise rotation assures that the screw will be unscrewed in case some of the threads still extend beyond the cylinder of bone that is within the OATS harvester tube. The top of the screw can be observed through the "windows" in the tube as the harvester is withdrawn, to ensure that the screw is backing out along with the bone plug. The same technique should be used for removing a push-in type of anchor.

- If the anchor can be unscrewed from the bone, the cylinder of bone can be reinserted into the bone socket to serve as its own graft. Otherwise, the bone socket should be grafted with allograft bone chips by a compaction grafting technique (see Chapter 19E).

- Repair the Bankart lesion with anchors above and below the bone graft (Fig. 19B-3).

TRICKS AND TIPS

- This entire procedure is a series of tricks and tips on how to get out of a difficult situation gracefully, and they are all incorporated into the above surgical protocol.

19C

Anchor Removal from Greater Tuberosity Using OATS Harvester

- In revision of failed rotator cuff repairs, metal anchors from the original surgery may need to be removed if they are "sitting proud" above the bone surface.

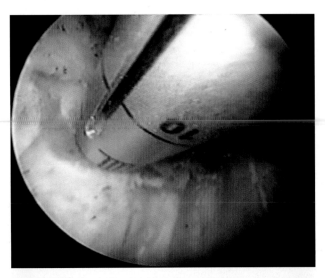

Figure 19C-1 Right shoulder, posterior subacromial viewing portal. The OATS (Arthrex, Inc.; Naples, FL) harvester surrounds the visible proximal portion of the anchor and is in the same axial alignment as the anchor.

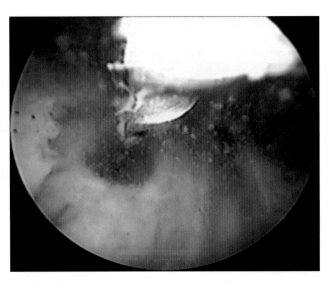

Figure 19C-2 By turning the OATS (Arthrex, Inc.; Naples, FL) harvester in a counterclockwise direction, the anchor is removed from the bone. The tip of the anchor can be seen extending past the OATS harvester.

- If an extractor or inserter for that anchor is not available, it can be removed by coring over the anchor with a 6-mm OATS (Osteochondral Autogenous Transfer System) (Arthrex, Inc.; Naples, FL) harvester tube (Fig. 19C-1). It should be impacted 15-mm around the anchor, then turned counterclockwise to remove the anchor with the surrounding core of bone (Fig. 19C-2).

- Bone graft the defect with allograft bone chips compacted into the bone socket using the disposable OATS system and the appropriate bone tamp (Fig. 19C-3) (see Chapter 19E).

TRICKS AND TIPS

- After the OATS harvester tube has been driven 15-mm into the bone, it is important to turn it counterclockwise during removal. This will assure that the anchor will come out with the bone plug, even if threads extend beyond the captured cylinder of bone (see Fig. 19C-2).

19D

Arthroscopic Suprascapular Nerve Release at the Suprascapular Notch

- Débride the fibrofatty tissues from the scapular spine so that the spine is clearly delineated (Fig. 19D-1). Because the transverse scapular ligament has a rather medial location, visualization will be best if the arthroscope

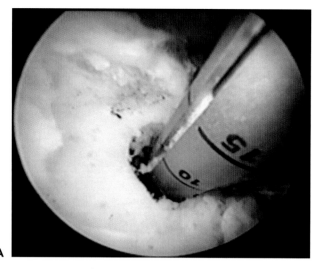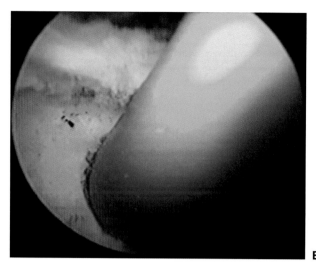

Figure 19C-3 **A:** The OATS (Arthrex, Inc.; Naples, FL) harvester is loaded with allograft bone chips and these are placed in the bone defect. **B:** The accompanying impactor is then used to compact the bone graft securely.

"hugs" the scapular spine medially and if a 70° arthroscope is used to "look around the corner."

● Expose the distal clavicle and remove the fibrofatty soft tissues from the posterior undersurface of the distal clavicle (Fig. 19D-2).

● By carrying the dissection of the posterior clavicle medially, the posterior aspect of the coracoclavicular (CC) ligament complex comes into view (Fig. 19D-3).

● Follow the posterior aspect of the CC ligament inferiorly to its insertion point at the base of the coracoid. At that point, three ligamentous structures will be seen radiating outward:

1. The trapezoid ligament portion of the CC ligament

2. The conoid portion of the CC ligament
3. The transverse scapular ligament (Fig. 19D-4).

● Clear off the posterosuperior aspect of the transverse scapular ligament with an elevator, but do not shave the fibrofatty tissue around this ligament, because this could inadvertently damage the suprascapular nerve.

● Establish an accessory posterior portal over the lateral suprascapular fossa by spinal needle localization. The angle of approach should allow direct insertion of arthroscopic scissor toward the transverse scapular ligament.

● Identify the suprascapular nerve (as it exits beneath the transverse scapular ligament) by gently pulling on the fibrofatty tissue below the ligament with a suture

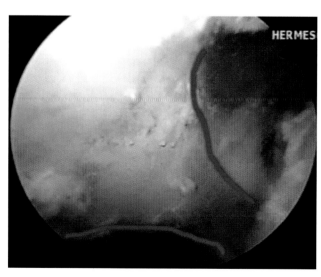

Figure 19D-1 Right shoulder, posterior viewing portal, 70° arthroscope. The scapular spine has been exposed.

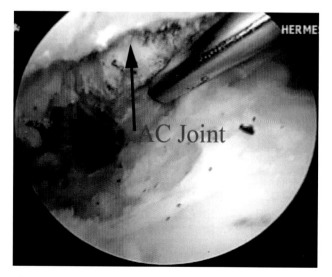

Figure 19D-2 Right shoulder, posterior viewing portal, 70° arthroscope. Here, the soft tissues are to be removed from the posterior undersurface of the distal clavicle just medial to the AC (acromioclavicular joint).

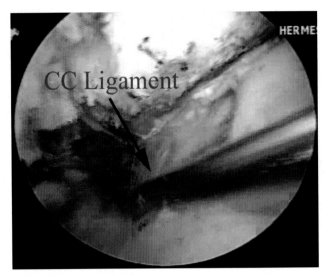

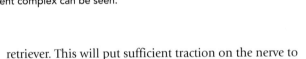

Figure 19D-3 Right shoulder, posterior viewing portal, 70° arthroscope. The posterior aspect of the coracoclavicular (CC) ligament complex can be seen.

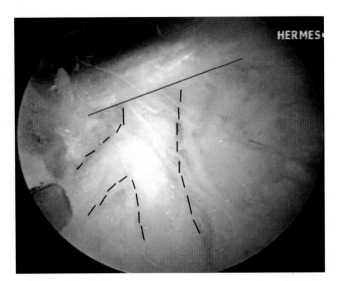

Figure 19D-5 Right shoulder, posterior viewing portal, 70° arthroscope. A suture retriever gently pulling on the fibrofatty tissue reveals the outline of the suprascapular nerve. (Dotted lines indicate the outline of the nerve.)

retriever. This will put sufficient traction on the nerve to reveal its outline (Fig. 19D-5).

- Using an arthroscopic scissor brought in through the accessory supraspinatus fossa portal, divide the transverse scapular ligament (Fig. 19D-6). Lift the tips of the scissor upward while cutting to avoid injury to the nerve.

TRICKS AND TIPS

- This procedure is most easily done in a patient with atrophy of the supraspinatus muscle, which is typical

in the cases where a suprascapular nerve lesion truly exists. If no atrophy is noted, the supraspinatus muscle belly will likely obscure visualization of the transverse scapular ligament. In that case, question the diagnosis of suprascapular nerve compression must be questioned.

- A 70° arthroscope through a posterior portal gives the best view.

- Do not excise fat inferior to the transverse scapular ligament because of the risk of damaging the suprascapular nerve.

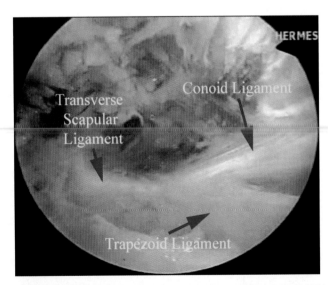

Figure 19D-4 Right shoulder, posterior viewing portal, 70° arthroscope. The triradiate ligament array from the base of the *processus coracoideus scapulae* (coracoid) can be seen: trapezoid ligament, conoid ligament, and transverse scapular ligament.

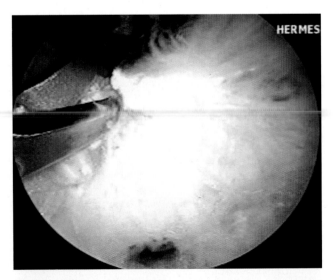

Figure 19D-6 Right shoulder, posterior viewing portal, 70° arthroscope. An arthroscopic scissor divides the transverse scapular ligament, thereby decompressing the suprascapular nerve.

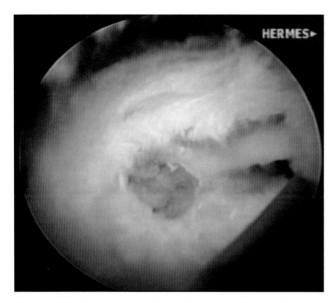

Figure 19E-1 This relatively small rotator cuff tear will require an anchor in the middle of the exposed bone bed on the greater tuberosity. The problem is that the area where the anchor must be placed is almost completely occupied by a degenerative bone cyst.

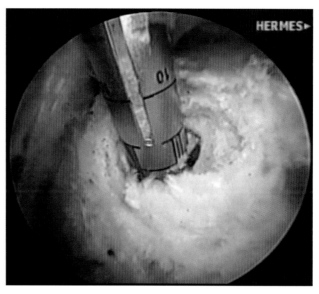

Figure 19E-3 The OATS (Arthrex, Inc.; Naples, FL) harvester cylinder, which has been packed with allograft bone, is placed at the mouth of the cyst to deliver bone to the cyst cavity.

19E

Compaction Bone Grafting Using OATS Harvester

- Compaction bone grafting using the OATS (Osteochondral Autogeneous Transfer System) (Arthrex, Inc.; Naples, FL) harvester is useful in the case of a rotator cuff tear where an anchor needs to be placed at a point on the greater tuberosity where there is a degenerative bone cyst (Fig. 19E-1).

- Thoroughly remove the cyst (Fig. 19E-2).

- Pack an appropriate-size disposable OATS harvester cylinder with allograft bone chips. Place the OATS harvester against the mouth of the cyst and advance the plunger in the cylinder with the screw-in mechanism at the top of the handle (Fig. 19E-3). This delivers the bone into the cyst.

- Use an impactor from the OATS set to compact the bone into the bottom of the cyst cavity (Fig. 19E-4).

- Repack the OATS harvester cylinder with bone and repeat the steps outlined above as many times as necessary to

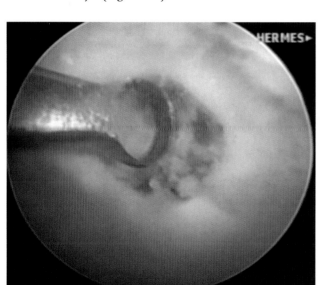

Figure 19E-2 Curettes are used to clear soft tissue from the cyst cavity.

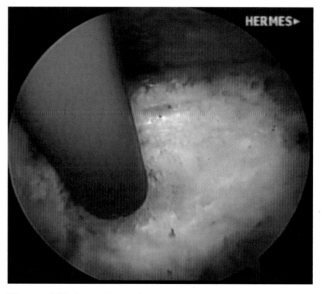

Figure 19E-4 A blue cylindrical impactor is used to further compact the allograft bone.

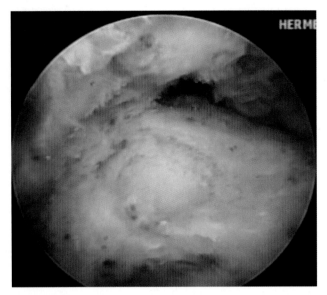

Figure 19E-5 This arthroscopic view shows that the cyst has been densely packed with bone all the way to the mouth of the cyst.

obtain dense bone packing of the cyst cavity, all the way to the mouth of the cyst (Fig. 19E-5).

● The goal is to create bone density within the cyst cavity that is sufficient to securely hold a suture anchor. We insert a BioCorkscrew or BioCorkscrew-FT (Arthrex) anchor without tapping (Fig. 19E-6), and then perform a standard rotator cuff repair.

TRICKS AND TIPS

● Compaction is achieved in two ways:

1. The screw-in mechanism that advances the plunger on the OATS harvester cylinder provides an efficient compaction mechanism;
2. The solid OATS impactor further compacts the bone by manual blows with a mallet.

● Do not tap a channel for a suture anchor. In fact, it is best simply to make a small superficial "starter hole" in the bone with a punch. In this way, anchor insertion produces even more bone graft compaction.

19F
Exposing the Scapular Spine

● Perform a subacromial bursectomy, excising the fibrofatty tissue medially until the posterior acromioclavicular (AC) joint is well visualized.

● Follow the medial margin of the *acromonial process* (acromion) as it arches posteromedially from the posterior AC joint. Continue débriding the fibrofatty tissue around this bone arch, which is the scapular spine (Fig. 19F-1).

TRICKS AND TIPS

● The lower portion of the scapular spine, with its characteristic lateral keel-like ridge, gives it the same appearance as the keel of a boat (Fig. 19F-2).

● The scapular spine is a useful landmark in the repair of massive retracted cuff tears because it defines the border between supraspinatus and infraspinatus muscle bellies.

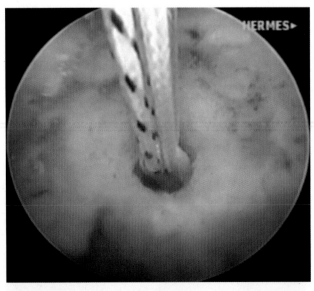

Figure 19E-6 A BioCorkscrew (Arthrex, Inc.; Naples, FL) anchor placed within the grafted cyst will provide secure fixation of the rotator cuff to bone.

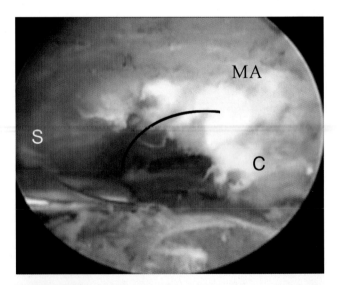

Figure 19F-1 Right shoulder, lateral viewing portal. Scapular spine (*solid black line*) arches downward in a posteromedial direction from the medial acromion (*MA*). C, distal clavicle; S, scapular spine.

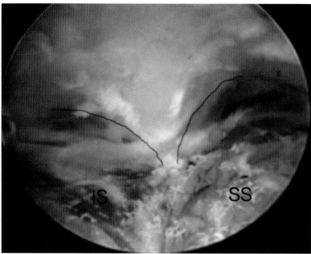

Figure 19F-2 Right shoulder, lateral viewing portal. This arthroscopic image demonstrates the keel shape of the scapular spine. SS, supraspinatus muscle; IS, infraspinatus muscle.

19G

Salvaging a Loose Anchor by the "Buddy Anchor" Technique

- The "buddy anchor" technique is used to salvage a loose anchor in which the eyelet migrates above the surface of the bone when tugging on the anchor's sutures to test its security in bone ("tug test") (Fig. 19G-1).

- Push the original anchor to the desired depth with a bone punch so that its eyelet is below the surface of the bone.

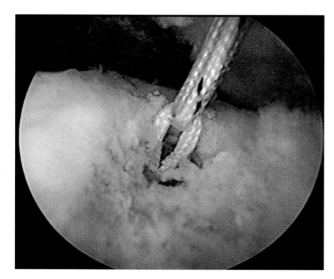

Figure 19G-1 Loose BioCorkscrew (Arthrex, Inc.; Naples, FL) anchor that has pulled back so that its eyelet is located in a "proud" position above the bone.

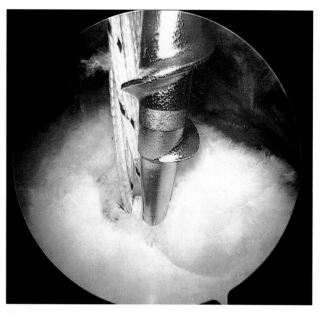

Figure 19G-2 Creating an undersized notch adjacent to the original bone socket.

- Notch the cortex directly adjacent to the original bone socket, using a BioCorkscrew (Arthrex, Inc.; Naples, FL) bone punch (Fig. 19G-2).

- In notching the cortex, drive the punch only halfway in, creating an undersized hole for insertion of a second anchor, which will wedge the first anchor tightly in place by means of an interference fit.

- Insert the second anchor adjacent to the first anchor while maintaining sufficient tension in the sutures of the first

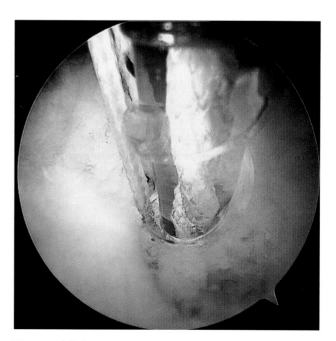

Figure 19G-3 Inserting the second anchor to create an interference fit against the first anchor.

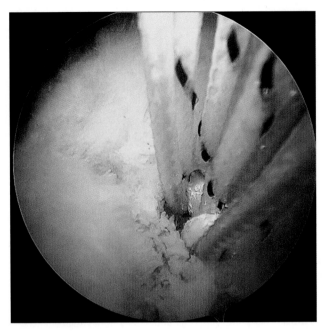

Figure 19G-4   Final construct of the two anchors in the "Buddy Anchor" Technique.

anchor to avoid driving the first anchor deep into bone ahead of the second anchor (Figs. 19G-3 and 19G-4).

TRICKS AND TIPS

- The concept of the final construct is interference fixation of an anchor against an anchor.

- The notch should be undersized to create a tight fit when the second anchor is placed.

- It is important to maintain tension on sutures of the original anchor as the second anchor is inserted.

19H

The "Suture Weave" Technique of Reloading an Anchor

- The suture weave technique is useful if one suture has become unloaded from the anchor eyelet, but one suture remains in place in the eyelet.

- Using a Graft Preparation Needle (Arthrex), pass a "free suture" of a different color through one limb of the suture that is still within the eyelet (suture through a suture) (Fig. 19H-1).

- Pull the other limb of the intact suture so that it, in turn, pulls the new suture through the eyelet of the anchor to reload the anchor (Fig. 19H-2).

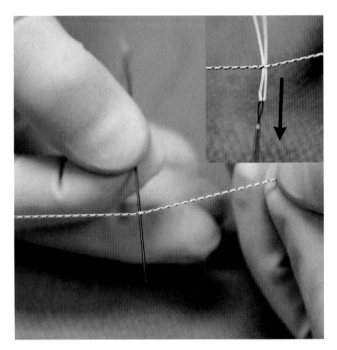

Figure 19H-1   Suture-through-a-suture is achieved with a straight, thin needle (e.g., Graft Preparation Needle; Arthrex, Inc.; Naples, FL).

- Disengage the two interwoven sutures.

TRICKS AND TIPS

- This particular technique is most reliably done with an anchor that has a flexible eyelet.

- One suture must remain in the anchor for this technique to be done.

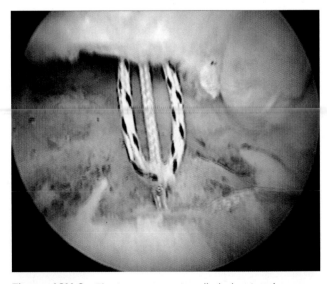

Figure 19H-2   The intact suture is pulled, drawing the suture-through-a-suture construct into the shoulder and through the eyelet of the anchor.

191

Pull the Right One: How to Ensure That You Don't Unload a Suture Anchor

- When pulling a suture through soft tissue (the superior labrum in this case) in a retrograde fashion, a loop will protrude from the portal where the suture was passed (Fig. 19I-1).

- Position the arthroscope such that the anchor eyelet is visible.

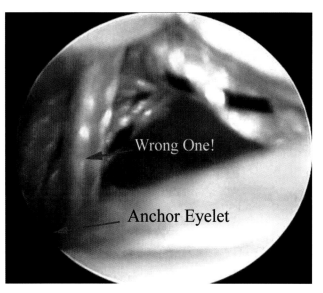

Figure 19I-2 While watching the anchor eyelet, if the suture strand traversing this eyelet slides, the *wrong* suture is being pulled.

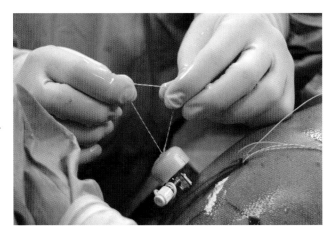

Figure 19I-1 When a BirdBeak (Arthrex, Inc.; Naples, FL) suture passer is used to pull a suture retrograde through soft tissue, a loop of suture protrudes from the cannula.

- Next, pull (or have an assistant pull) on one strand of suture while visualizing the anchor eyelet. If the suture strand traversing the eyelet slides when this strand is pulled, the wrong strand is being pulled (Fig. 19I-2).

- While pulling on the other strand and visualizing the eyelet, make sure that there is no motion of the suture through the eyelet, which ensures that the anchor is not going to be unloaded.

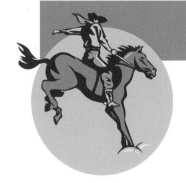

20

Assorted Conditions

Calcific Tendinitis

- The intra-articular view of calcific tendinitis shows intense synovitis and abnormal capsulotendinous tissue underlying calcific deposit.

- The subacromial view of calcific tendinitis often shows a dense subacromial bursa, which must be débrided.

- Locate the calcific deposit with an 18-gauge needle placed percutaneously into the subacromial space (Fig. 20A-1).

- Débride abnormal tendon (i.e., tendon that is infiltrated with calcium among its fibers) (Fig. 20A-2).

- Repair the residual defect based on the mobility of the remaining cuff margin in accordance with standard principles of cuff tear pattern recognition and repair (Fig. 20A-3).

TRICKS AND TIPS

- Locate the calcific deposit with an 18-gauge spinal needle.

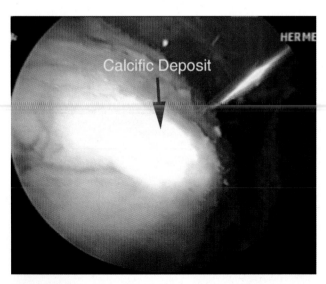

Figure 20A-1 Right shoulder, posterior viewing portal. An 18-gauge spinal needle is used to locate the calcific deposit.

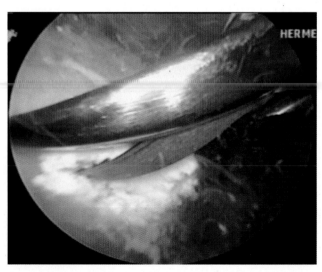

Figure 20A-2 Tendon infiltrated with calcium is débrided.

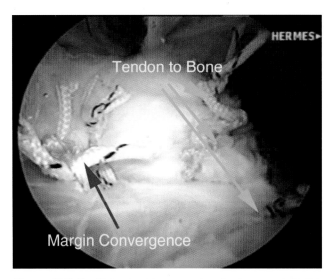

Figure 20A-3   Right shoulder, posterior viewing portal. Cuff is repaired according to standard principles (*red arrow* indicates margin-convergence-to-bone sutures; *green arrows* indicate simple tendon-to-bone sutures).

- Débride the portion of the tendon that is infiltrated with calcium.
- Repair the healthy tendon based on its tear pattern.

20B
Minicapsular Plication in the Overhead Athlete

- An easy drive-through sign can result from a superior labrum anterior and posterior (SLAP) lesion or instability.

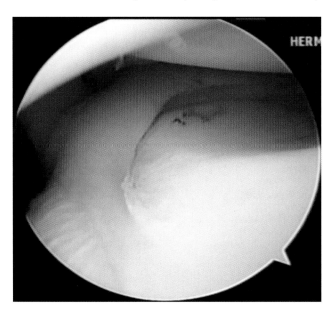

Figure 20B-1   Right shoulder, posterior viewing portal. The peel-back test is positive, suggesting the presence of a superior labrum anterior and posterior (SLAP) lesion.

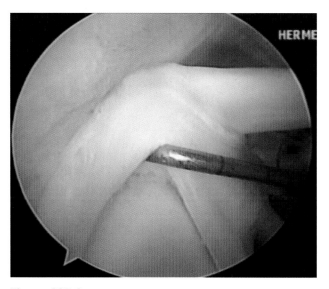

Figure 20B-2   Right shoulder, posterior viewing portal. A displaceable biceps root confirms a superior labrum anterior and posterior (SLAP) lesion.

- A positive peel-back test (Fig. 20B-1) and a displaceable biceps root (Fig. 20B-2) indicate that this patient has a SLAP lesion.
- Perform a SLAP repair in the usual manner (Fig. 20B-3).
- Perform the drive-through test after SLAP lesion repair. In most cases, the SLAP repair will convert the drive-through test from positive to negative. If the drive-through test is still positive after SLAP repair, however, consider anterior minicapsular plication. A second indication for anterior minicapsular plication is external rotation of >130° with the shoulder in 90° abduction.

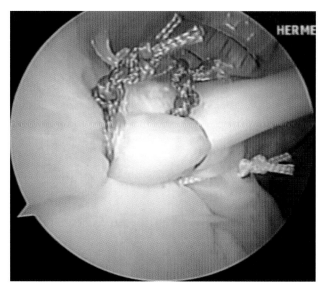

Figure 20B-3   Right shoulder, posterior viewing portal. A superior labrum anterior and posterior (SLAP) repair has been completed.

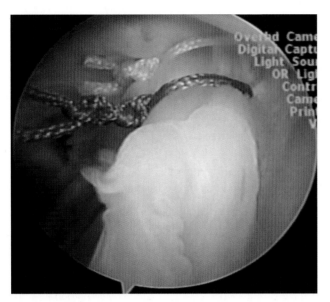

Figure 20B-4   Right shoulder, anterosuperior viewing portal. An anterior minicapsular plication has been completed. Two sutures have been placed to plicate the middle glenohumeral ligament to the anterior band of the inferior glenohumeral ligament.

● Perform minicapsular plication by placing two sutures to plicate the middle glenohumeral ligament to the anterior band of the inferior glenohumeral ligament (Fig. 20B-4).

TRICKS AND TIPS

● The three potential components in surgical treatment of the disabled throwing shoulder are as follows:

1. SLAP repair.
2. Posteroinferior capsular release (if glenohumeral internal rotation deficit [GIRD] >25° in a patient who is a stretch nonresponder).
3. Anterior minicapsular plication (if external rotation is >130° with the shoulder abducted 90°, or the drive-through test is still positive after SLAP repair).

● Any individual thrower may require one or more of these treatment components, depending on clinical and arthroscopic findings.

20C

Stretching and Strengthening Exercises: Patient Education Video

● This video segment demonstrates the exercises we show our patients for postoperative stretching and strengthening.

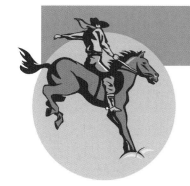

The Future

21

21A

BioForkLok Bankart Repair

- A new knotless technology, the BioForkLok (Arthrex, Inc.; Naples, FL) Bankart repair, uses FiberChain (Arthrex), a flexible suture-chain with identical links, and a forked push-in anchor to achieve a secure repair without knots. The video clip on the DVD should be viewed for a description of this new technology.

21B

FiberChain Plus Swivel-Lok Double-Row Rotator Cuff Repair

- The FiberChain plus Swivel-Lok system is new knotless technology that uses FiberChain (Arthrex, Inc.; Naples, FL), a flexible suture-chain with identical links, and a screw-in anchor with a snap-on forked swivel, to achieve a solid double-row rotator cuff repair without knots. The video clip on the DVD should be viewed for a description of this new technology.

Index

Page numbers followed by t indicate table. Page numbers in *italics* indicate figure.

A

Acromioplasty, arthroscopic, 239–240, *240*, *241*
Adhesive capsulitis, capsular release for, *245*, 245–246, *246*
ALPSA (anterior labral periosteal sleeve avulsion), 54–55, *57*
Anchor insertion (*See also* Suture anchors)
  deadman system for, 38–39, *40*
  in poor bone, 178–180, *180*, *181*
  in subscapularis tendon repair, 125–126, *130*
Angle of approach, 7–32
  arthroscope angles, 7–8
    0 degrees, 7
    30 degrees, 7, *8*, *10*
    70 degrees, 7–8, *9*, *10*
  instrumentation, 19–32
  portals, 8–18
    glenohumeral, 9–12, *11*
    subacromial, 13, *14*, 15–16
Anterior and posterior interval slide, 115, *115*, *116*
Anterior glenohumeral portal, *11*, 12, *12*
Anterior interval slide, 111, 114, *114*, *287*, 287–288, *288*
  in continuity, *286*, 286–287, *287*
  coracoid identification for, 150–151, 153, *153*, *154*
Anterior labral lesions, 53–55, *55*, *56*, *57*
Anterior labral periosteal sleeve avulsion (ALPSA), 54–55, *57*
Anterior release, of subscapularis tendon, 123–124, *129*
Anterior subacromial portal, *14*, 15, *16*
Anterior supraspinatus tears, angle of approach, 8, *10*
Anterosuperolateral glenohumeral portal, *11*, 12, *14*
Arthrex
  Bio-Tenodesis Screw System, *131*, *132*, 133, 183
  BioCorkscrew, 36–37, *37*, 178–180, *180*, *181*, 182
  BioTenodesis inserter, 290, *290*
  BirdBeak, 21, *22*, 23
  Needle Punch, *29*, 30
  OATS harvesting tube, 181–182, *182*, *183*, 185–186, *297*, 297–298, *298*, *301*, 301–302, *302*
  Penetrator suture passer, *22*, 23, 176, *176*
  Scorpion, 24, *26–28*, 28, 30–31
  Sidewinder, *22*, 23
  Surgeon's Sixth Finger, 43, *46*, *47*, *185*, *186*, 188–189, *294–296*, 294–297
  Suture Lasso, 31, *31*, *32*, 178, *179*, 187
  Viper, 23–26, *23–24*, 30
Arthroscope angles, 7–8
  0 degrees, 7
  30 degrees, 7, *8*, *10*
  70 degrees, 7–8, *9*, *10*
Arthroscopic capsular release, for glenohumeral internal rotation deficit (GIRD), 59–60, *63*, *64*
Arthroscopic knots (*See* Knots)
Articular surface tears, *93*
  rotator cuff, 91–94, *93*
    measuring tendon involvement, 94, *95*

B

Banana Lasso, *30*, 31
Bankart lesion, *58*
  inverted pear configuration and, 160, *160*
  repair of bony, 227, *228–230*, 229–230
Bankart repair
  arthroscopic, tricks and tips, 217–220, *218–220*
  BioForkLok, 309
  capsular laxity and, 72–73, *75*
  posterior, with SLAP repair, *226*, 226–227, *227*
Bear Hug test, for subscapularis tendon tear, *118*, 118–119
Bernoulli effect, *4*, 4–6, *5*
Biceps root, in superior labrum anterior and posterior (SLAP) lesions, 66, *72*
Biceps tendon repair, 129–141 (*See also* Biceps tenodesis)
  Bio-Tenodesis Screw System for, *131*, *132*, 133
  rationale for, 129, 133
  in subscapularis tendon repair, 119–120, *120*, *121*
Biceps tendon tears, 79–81, *80–83*
  evaluation of, 79–80, *80*, *81*, *82*, 102, *105*
    dislocation, 80, *83*
    stability, 80, *82*
    subluxation, 80, *83*
Biceps tenodesis, 120, 133–141
  biceps tenotomy in preparation for, 119–120, *120*, *121*
  Bio-Tenodesis Screw System for, *131*, *132*, 133
  Cobra procedure, 138, *140*, 140–141, *141*
  technique
    with intact rotator cuff, 138, *139*
    for rupture of long head of biceps tendon, 138, *140*, 140–141, *141*
    for ruptured biceps tendon, 289–290, *290*
    with supraspinatus tear, 293, *293*
    with torn rotator cuff, *133–138*, 135–136, 138
    without supraspinatus tear, *291*, 291–293, *292*
Biceps tenotomy, 119–120, *120*, *121*
Bio-Tenodesis Screw System, *131*, *132*, 133, 183
Bio-Tenodesis Screwdriver, *131*, 133, 183
BioCorkscrew, 36–37, *37*, 178–180, *180*, *181*, 182
BioForkLok Bankart repair, 309
BioTenodesis inserter, 290, *290*
BirdBeak suture-passer, 21, *22*, 23
Bleeding during surgery
  minimizing, 3–4
  turbulence control, *4*, 4–6, *5*
  visualization and, 3
Bone bed
  preparation for compaction bone graft, 181
  preparation for subscapularis tendon repair, 124–125, *130*
Bone cyst, compaction bone graft for, 180–184, *182*
Bone deficiency, 156–168
  glenoid
    inverted pear configuration, 77–79, *78*, *79*, 158, 160 161, *161 163*
    measurement of, 78, *79*
    normal anatomy, 158, *160*
  Hill-Sachs lesions, 76, *77*
    diagnosis of, 76, *77*
    engaging, 76, 157–158, *158*
    modified Latarjet procedure for, 158, *160*
    nonengaging, 76, 157, *159*
    surgical options, 158, *159*, *160*
  instability and, 75
  significance of, 156
Bone graft
  compaction, for bone cyst, 180–184, *182*, *301*, 301–302, *302*
  coracoid, 166, 167, *167*

Bone tunnels, *vs.* suture anchors, 33, *34*
Bristow procedure, 161
Bubble sign, in rotator cuff interstitial tears, 96, *96, 97, 270, 270–271, 271*
Buddy anchor technique, for salvaging loose anchor, *303,* 303–304, *304*
Bursal leaders, 147–148, *148*
Bursal surface tears, rotator cuff, *93*
 measuring tendon involvement, 95, *95, 96*
Bursectomy, 170, *170, 171*

C

Calcific tendinitis
 postoperative rehabilitation, 206
 repair, *306,* 306–307, *307*
Cannula use
 knot tying and, *184–187,* 187–189
 with portals, 18–19, *21*
 sizes of, 19, *21*
Capsular laxity
 Bankart repair and, 72–73, *75*
 rotator interval and, 72–73, *75,* 75–76, *76*
Capsular release
 for adhesive capsulitis, *245,* 245–246, *246*
 for postoperative stiffness, *246,* 246–247, *247*
Capsulitis, adhesive, capsular release for, *245,* 245–246, *246*
Capsulotomy
 in modified Latarjet procedure, *165, 166,* 167
 selective posteroinferior, for glenohumeral internal rotation deficit (GIRD), 59–60, *63, 64*
Cavitas glenoidalis (*See* Glenoid bone)
Closed-chain scapular control exercise, *207,* 210
Cobra procedure, biceps tenodesis, 138, *140,* 140–141, *141,* 289–290, *290*
Comma sign, in subscapularis tendon tears, 106, *107, 108,* 122–123, *125–128,* 266, *266*
Compaction bone graft, for bone cyst, 180–184, *182, 301,* 301–302, *302*
Coracohumeral interval, 103–105, *105*
Coracoid
 identification of
  for anterior interval slide, 150–151, *153, 153, 154*
  for subscapularis tendon repair, 120–121, *122, 123*
 Roller-Wringer phenomenon, 274, *274*
Coracoid graft, in modified Latarjet procedure, *166, 167,* 167
Coracoid osteotomy, in modified Latarjet procedure, *164,* 166
Coracoplasty
 with nonretracted subscapularis tendon, 250, *250*
 in subscapularis tendon repair, 121, *123,* 267, *267*
Crescent-shaped rotator cuff tears, 88, *88*
 massive contracted adhered, 110–111, *111, 113*
 repair of, *196, 197,* 269–270, *270*

D

Dead arm syndrome, 57–58
Deadman system, for anchor insertion, 38–39, *40*
Dilator knot, *184,* 187
Distal clavicle
 arthroscopic excision, 7–8, *10, 241,* 241–242, *242*
 coplaning of, *242,* 242–243, *243*
Distal locking sliding knots, 43, *50*
Double-diameter knot pusher, 43, *46, 47*
Double interval slide, 114–115, *115,* 279–280, *279–281*
 modified, 257–261, *257–260*
Double-row rotator cuff repair, 98–99, *99,* 252–254, *253, 254*
 double-pulley technique, *251,* 251–252, *252*
Drive-through sign, in superior labrum anterior and posterior (SLAP) lesions, 67

E

Exercises, postoperative
 closed-chain scapular control, *207,* 210
 four-pack, 20, *205, 206*
 low row, *209,* 210
 open-chain scapular strengthening, *208,* 210
 pectoralis minor stretches, *209,* 210
 sleeper stretch, *206,* 209–210

F

Fatty degeneration, of subscapularis tendon, 127
FiberChain/Swivel-Lok double row rotator cuff repair, 309
5 O'clock portal, *11, 12, 13,* 17–18
Footprint reconstruction, rotator cuff repair, 97–99, *98*
Force couples
 in rotator cuff repair, 86, *88*
 in rotator cuff tears, 81–82, *83, 84, 84*
Four-pack exercise, 20, *205, 206*

G

Glenohumeral internal rotation deficit (GIRD), 58–60
 arthroscopic capsular release for, 59–60, *63, 64*
 stretching program for, 58–59, *62*
 superior labrum anterior and posterior (SLAP) lesions and, 58–60
Glenohumeral joint, force couples, 81–82, *83, 84, 84*
Glenohumeral ligaments
 humeral avulsion of the, 71–72, *74, 75*
 reverse humeral avulsion of the, 72, *74*
Glenohumeral portals, 9–12, *11*
 5 O'clock, *11, 12, 13,* 17–18
 anterior, *11, 12, 12*
 anterosuperolateral, *11, 12, 14*
 Port of Wilmington, *11, 12, 14,* 17–18, *20*
 posterior, 9–11, *11*
 posterolateral, *11, 12, 14*

Glenoid bone
 inverted pear configuration, 77–79, *78, 79,* 158, 160–161, *161–163*
 measurement of, 78, *79*
 normal anatomy, 158, *160*
Glenoid bone bare spot, 78, 78t
Glenoid labrum
 anatomy and variants, 53, *54, 55*
 anterior labral lesions, 53–55, *55, 56, 57*
 posterior labral lesions, 55, *58*
 superior labral tears, 56 [*See also* Superior labrum anterior and posterior (SLAP) lesions]
 triple labral lesions, 69, 71, *74*
Greater tuberosity
 anchor removal from, 298, *298*
 treatment for malunion, 275–277, *276, 277*

H

Half-hitches, 41–43
 double-diameter knot pusher, 43, *46, 47*
 over-under, 41, *45*
 reversing, 43, *49,* 188, 189–190
 three RHAP, 42, *46, 48, 51, 52*
 tying stacked, 42–43, *46, 47, 48*
 under-over, 41, *45*
 variations of, 41, *45*
Hill-Sachs lesions
 diagnosis of, 76, *77,* 222, *223*
 engaging, 76, 157–158, *158,* 222–223, *223*
 modified Latarjet procedure, 158, *160*
 nonengaging, 76, 157, *159*
 surgical options, 158, *159, 160*
Humeral avulsion of the glenohumeral ligaments (HAGL), 71–72, *74, 75*
 arthroscopic repair of, 234–235, *235*
 reverse, 72, *74*
 repair of, *230,* 230–231, *231*
Humerus, hyper-external rotation of, in superior labrum anterior and posterior (SLAP) lesions, 63–64, *67*
Hyper-external rotation of humerus, in superior labrum anterior and posterior (SLAP) lesions, 63–64, *67*

I

Infraspinatus tendon tears, combined with subscapularis and supraspinatus tendon tear, 141–145, *142–145*
Instability
 bone deficiency and, 75
 multidirectional, 72
 unidirectional, 72–73
Instability repair, postoperative rehabilitation following
 anterior, 208–209
 posterior, 209
Instrumentation, 19–32
 antegrade suture passage, 23–24, 30–31
 BirdBeak, 21, *22, 23*
 Needle Punch, *29,* 30
 Penetrator, *22, 23*
 retrograde suture passage, 20–21, *22*

Scorpion, 24, *26–28*, 28, *30–31*
shuttling, *31*, 31–32, *32*
suture-passing, 20–24, *30–31*
Viper, *23–26*, 23–24, *30*
Interstitial tear, rotator cuff, *93*
identifying tear location, 96, *96*, *97*,
270, 270–271, *271*
Interval slide
anterior, 111, 114, *114*, *287*, 287–288,
288
in continuity, *286*, 286–287, *287*
coracoid identification for, 150–151,
153, *153*, *154*
anterior and posterior, 115, *115*, *116*
in continuity, *142–145*, 143–145
coracohumeral ligament release, 144,
144
rotator interval resection and release,
144, 144–145
double, 114–115, *115*, 279–280,
279–281
modified, *257–260*, 257–261
posterior, exposing scapular spine for,
153–155, *154*, *155*
Intra-articular depth gauge, 94, *94*
Inverted pear configuration, 77–79, *78*,
79, 158, 160–161, *161–163*
Bankart lesion and, 160, *160*
glenoid bone deficiency and, 77–79,
78, *79*
modified Latarjet procedure for (*See*
Modified Latarjet procedure)

J
Jobe relocation test, modified, for supe-
rior labrum anterior and posterior
(SLAP) lesions, 65, *70*

K
Knot proper, 40, *41*
Knot pusher, 52, *52*
double-diameter, 43, *46*, *47*
Knot security
defined, 40
factors in, 40, *41*, *42*
optimizing, 43, 48, 52
Knot tying
in cannula, *184–187*, 187–189
with Surgeon's Sixth Finger, 43, *46*, *47*,
185, *186*, 188–189, *294–297*,
294–297
suture type and, 37–38, *39*
"tying as you go," 171–172, *173*
visualization of, 170, *171*
Knotless lateral row fixation, rotator cuff
repair, *274*, 274–275, *275*
Knots, 39–43, *44–52*, 48, 52
choosing, 43, 48, 52
classification of, 40–41
dilator knot, *184*, 187
Duncan loop, 41, 43, *44*
half-hitches, 41–43 (*See also* Half-
hitches)
knot proper, 40, *41*
loop, 40, *41*
loop security, 40, *42*, 43, 48, 52
Nicky's knot, 41, 43, *44*

nonsliding, 40–41, *43*
overview, 39–43, *44–52*, 48, 52
past pointing, 40, *42*
post limb, 39–40, *41*
Revo, 41, *43*
Roeder knot, 41, 43, *44*
sliding, 41, 43, *44*
SMC knot, 41, *44*
surgeon's, 41, *44*
suture material and, 37–38, *39*
Tennessee slider, 41, 43, *44*
Weston knot, 41, *44*
wrapping limb, 40, *41*

L
L-shaped rotator cuff tears, 88, *90*, *91*
assessment, 254, *254*, *255*
repair of, 200, *200*
reverse, 88
reverse repair, *255*, 255–257, *256*, 269,
269
Labral lesions
anterior, 53–55, *55*, *56*, *57*
posterior, 55, *58*
repair, 192
triple, 69, 71, *74*, 192
repair of, *232–234*, 232–234
Labral repair, 192
Latarjet procedure
arthroscopic, tricks and tips, 220
modified, 161, 164–168
approach, 167
capsulotomy, *165*, *166*, 167
coracoid bone graft placement, *166*,
167, 167
coracoid osteotomy, *164*, 166
for Hill-Sachs lesions, 158, *160*
postoperative procedures, 168
preoperative imaging, 164
subscapularis tendon management,
165, 167
upper scapularis repair, 167, *168*
open, tricks and tips, *223*, 223–226,
226
Lateral subacromial portal, 13, *14*, 15, *16*
Lift-off test, for subscapularis tendon tear,
117, *117*
Ligaments, of glenoid labrum, 53, *54*
Loop security, 40, *42*
optimizing, 43, 48, 52
Low row exercise, *209*, 210

M
Margin convergence
double row, *277*, 277–278, *278*,
282–284, *283*, *284*
in reverse L-shaped tear, *255*, 255–257,
256
in rotator cuff repair, 89–91
routine technique, *281*, 281–282, *282*
in small U-shaped tear, *277*, 277–278,
278
strain reduction following, 89–91
Mason Allen stitch, modified, 34–35
Massive contracted adhered rotator cuff
tears, 89, 110–145
biceps tendon repair, 129–141

combined subscapularis, supraspinatus,
and infraspinatus tendon tears,
141–145, *142–145*
crescent-shaped, 110–111, *111*, *113*
longitudinal, 110, *111*, *112*
repair, 111, 114–115, *114–116*
anterior and posterior interval slide,
115, *115*, *116*
anterior interval slide, 111, 114, *114*
assessment of, 111, *114*
double interval slide, 114–115, *115*,
257–260, 257–261
immobile, 200, *201*, 202
partial, 202, *202*
tendon-to-bone fixation, 115, *116*
subscapularis tendon tears, 117–129
Middle locking sliding knots, 43, *50*
Minicapsular plication, *307*, 307–308, *308*
Mobility assessment, in rotator cuff tear,
193–202, *194–202*
anterior to posterior, 197, *197–200*, 200
medial to lateral, 193, *195*, 197
minimal mobility, 200, *201*, 202, *202*
step-wise progression, 193, *194*
Modified Jobe relocation test, for superior
labrum anterior and posterior
(SLAP) lesions, 65, *70*
Modified Latarjet procedure, 161,
164–168
approach, 167
capsulotomy, *165*, *166*, 167
coracoid bone graft placement, *166*,
167, 167
coracoid osteotomy, *164*, 166
for Hill-Sachs lesions, 158, *160*
postoperative procedures, 168
preoperative imaging, 164
subscapularis tendon management,
165, 167
upper scapularis repair, 167, *168*
Modified Mason Allen stitch, 34–35
Modified Neviaser subacromial portal, *14*,
15–16, *17*, 17–18
Multidirectional instability, 72
arthroscopic treatment of, 220,
221–222, 222
Mumford procedure
angle of approach, 7–8, *10*

N
Napoleon test, for subscapularis tendon
tear, 117–118, *118*
Needle Punch suture-passer, *29*, 30
Neviaser subacromial portal
modified, *14*, 15–16, *17*, 17–18

O
OATS harvesting tube
for anchor removal, *183*, 185–186, *297*,
297–298, *298*
for compaction bone graft, 181–182,
182, *301*, 301–302, *302*
O'Brien test, for superior labrum anterior
and posterior (SLAP) lesions, 65,
69
Open-chain scapular strengthening exercise, *208*, 210

Operating room set-up, 215, *216*
Os acromiale excision, *243*, 243–244
Osteochondral autograft transfer system (OATS) (*See* OATS harvesting tube)
Over-under half-hitch, 41, *45*

P
Panalok RC anchor, 37, *37*
Past pointing, 40, *42*
PASTA lesion, converting to full-thickness tear, 249, *249*
PASTA repair, 261–262, *261–263*
   double-pulley technique, 284–286, *285, 286*
Pathology
   anterior labral lesions, 53–55, *55, 56, 57*
   biceps tendon disorders, 79–81, *80–83*
   bone deficiency (*See* Bone deficiency)
   humeral avulsion of the glenohumeral ligaments (HAGL), 71–72, *74, 75*
   posterior labral lesions, 55, *58*
   rotator cuff tears, 81–82, *84*, 86–99
   rotator interval and capsular laxity, 72–73, 75, *75–76, 76*
   subscapularis tendon, 99–106
   superior labral tears, 56 [*See also* Superior labrum anterior and posterior (SLAP) lesions]
   triple labral lesions, 69, 71, *74*
Pear configuration, inverted, 77–79, *78, 79*, 158, 160–161, *161–163*
   Bankart lesion and, 160, *160*
   glenoid bone deficiency and, 77–79, *78, 79*
Pectoralis minor stretches, *209*, 210
Peel-back mechanism, of superior labrum anterior and posterior (SLAP) lesions, 64–65, *68*
Peel-back test, in superior labrum anterior and posterior (SLAP) lesions, 66–67, *73*
Penetrator suture-passer, *22, 23*, 176, *176*
Port of Wilmington portal, *11, 12, 14*, 17–18, *20*
Portal placement, for subscapularis tendon repair, 119, *119, 120*
Portals
   cannula use, 18–19, *21*
   creating, 17–18, *19, 20*
   glenohumeral, 9–12, *11*
     5 O'clock, *11, 12, 13*
     anterior, *11, 12, 12*
     anterosuperolateral, *11, 12, 14*
     Port of Wilmington, *11, 12, 14*
     posterior, 9–11, *11*
     posterolateral, *11, 12, 14*
   spinal needle use with, 171, *172*
   subacromial, 13, *14*, 15–16
     anterior, *14, 15, 16*
     lateral, 13, *14, 15, 16*
     modified Neviaser, *14*, 15–16, *17*
     posterior, 13, *14, 15*
     subclavian, *14*, 16–17, *18*
   visualization and, 170–171
Post limb, 39–40, *41*
Posterior glenohumeral portal, 9–11, *11*

Posterior instability repair, postoperative rehabilitation following, 209
Posterior interval slide, exposing scapular spine for, 153–155, *154, 155*
Posterior labral lesions, 55, *58*
Posterior release, of subscapularis tendon, 124, *129*
Posterior subacromial portal, 13, *14, 15*
Posteroinferior capsule contracture, in superior labrum anterior and posterior (SLAP) lesions, 60–61, 63, *64, 65, 66*
Posterolateral glenohumeral portal, *11, 12, 14*
Postoperative rehabilitation
   for calcific tendinitis, 206
   exercises
     closed-chain scapular control, *207*, 210
     four-pack, 20, *205*, 206
     low row, *209*, 210
     open-chain scapular strengthening, *208*, 210
     pectoralis minor stretches, *209*, 210
     sleeper stretch, *206*, 209–210
   following anterior instability repair, 208–209
   following modified Latarjet procedure, 168
   following posterior instability repair, 209
   following rotator cuff repair, 203–208, *204, 205*
   following SLAP repair, *206–209, 209–211, 210t, 211t*
   following subscapularis tendon repair, 128–129
   for throwing athlete, 210, *210t, 211t*
Postoperative stiffness, capsular release for, *246*, 246–247, *247*
Proximal humeral migration, 128
Proximal sliding knots, 43, *50*
Pull-out strength, of suture anchor, 35

R
Retrieving sutures, 174–177, *175, 176*
Retrograde suture passage, 20–21
Reverse humeral avulsion of the glenohumeral ligaments, 72, *74*
   repair of, *230*, 230–231, *231*
Reverse L-shaped rotator cuff tears, 88
   assessment of, *254, 254, 255*
   repair of, *255*, 255–257, *256*, 269, *269*
Reversing half-hitches, 43, *49, 188*, 189–190
RHAP half-hitch, three, *42, 46, 48, 51, 52*
Rim rents, 91–92
Roller-wringer phenomenon, in subcoracoid impingement, 100, *100, 101*, 274, *274*
Rotator cable, 84, *85, 86*
Rotator cuff, 81–82, *84*, 86–99
   adhesed, 148–150, *149–153*
   force couples in, 81–82, *83*, 84, *84*
   suspension bridge model of, 84, *85*, 86, *86, 87*
Rotator cuff repair, 249–288
   anterior and posterior interval slide, 115, *115, 116*

anterior interval slide, 111, 114, *114*, 286–288, *286–288*
   bursal sided, 265, *265–266, 266*
   converting PASTA lesion to full-thickness tear, 249, *249*
   coracoplasty, 250, *250*
   crescent-shaped, *196*, 197, 269–270, *270*
   double interval slide, 114–115, *115, 257–260, 257–261, 279–280, 279–281*
   double row, 98–99, *99*, 252–254, *253, 254*
     double-pulley technique, *251*, 251–252, *252*
     FiberChain/Swivel-Lok, 309
   footprint reconstruction, 97–99, *98*
   goals of, 86, 88
   interstitial, *268*, 268–269, *269*
   knotless lateral row fixation, *274*, 274–275, *275*
   L-shaped, 200, *200*
   with labral repair, 192
   margin convergence in, 89–91, *255*, 255–257, *256*
   massive contracted adhered, 111, 114–115, *114–116*
     anterior and posterior interval slide, 115, *115, 116*
     anterior interval slide, 111, 114, *114*, 286, 286–288, *288*
     assessment of, 111, *114*
     double interval slide, 114–115, *115, 257–260, 257–261*
     immobile, 200, *201*, 202
     partial, 202, *202*
     tendon-to-bone fixation, 115, *116*
   mobility assessment in, 193–202, *194–202*
     anterior to posterior, 197, *197–200*, 200
     medial to lateral, 193, *195*, 197
     minimal mobility, 200, *201*, 202, *202*
     step-wise progression, 193, *194*
   order of steps, 191–192
   PASTA repair, 261–262, *261–263*
     double-pulley technique, 284–286, *285, 286*
   postoperative stiffness, *246*, 246–247, *247*
   rationale for, 97
   reverse L shaped, *255*, 255–257, *256*, 269, *269*
   shoestring technique, *274*, 274–275, *275*
   soft tissue debridement, 170, *170, 171*
   subscapularis tear
     complete, 266, 266–268, *267*
     partial, 263–265, *263–265*
   triple double technique, 271–273, *271–273*
   U-shaped, 197, *198*, 277, 277–278, *278*
Rotator cuff tears (*See also* Massive contracted adhered rotator cuff tears)
   articular surface tears, 91–94, *93*
   bursal surface tear, *93*
   crescent-shaped, 88, *88*

determining margins of, 147–148, *148*
interstitial tear, *93*
  identifying tear location, 96, *96, 97, 270, 270–271, 271*
  L-shaped, 88, *90, 91*
  massive contracted adhered, 89
  measuring tear thickness, 92–94, *94*
  measuring tendon involvement
    articular surface tears, 94, *95*
    bursal surface tears, 95, *95, 96*
  partial thickness, 91–99
  reverse L-shaped, 88, 200, *200*
  strain in, 90
  U-shaped, 88, *89*
Rotator interval
  capsular laxity and, 72–73, *75,* 75–76, *76*
  closure of, 76, *76*
Row exercise, low, *209,* 210

S

Scapular spine, exposing, 153–155, *154, 155, 302, 302, 303*
Scorpion suture-passer, 24, *26–28, 28, 30–31*
Shoestring technique, rotator cuff repair, *274, 274–275, 275*
Shuttle sutures, *184, 187*
Shuttling instrumentation, *31, 31–32, 32*
Sidewinder suture-passer, *22, 23*
Sixth Finger knot pusher, 43, *46, 47, 185, 186, 188–189, 294–296, 294–297*
SLAP lesions [*See* Superior labrum anterior and posterior (SLAP) lesions]
SLAP repair
  with Bankart lesion, *226, 226–227, 227*
  postoperative rehabilitation, 206, *206–209,* 209–211, 210t, 211t
  rationale for, 67–69
  tricks and tips, 236–238, *237, 238*
Sleeper stretch, *206,* 209–210
Sliding knots, 41, 43, *44, 50*
  distal locking, 43, *50*
  locking, 43, *52, 52*
  middle locking, 43, *50*
  proximal, 43, *50*
  research on, 48, *50, 51*
  unlocking, 43
Speed test, for superior labrum anterior and posterior (SLAP) lesions, 65, *69*
Spinal needle, use with portals, 171, *172*
Stiffness
  capsular release for adhesive capsulitis, *245, 245–246, 246*
  manipulation under anesthesia for, *247,* 247–248, *248*
  postoperative, capsular release for, *246,* 246–247, *247*
Strain, in rotator cuff tears, 90
Stretch
  pectoralis minor, *209,* 210
  sleeper, *206,* 209–210
Subacromial portals, 13, *14,* 15–16
  anterior, *14, 15, 16*
  lateral, 13, *14, 15, 16*
  modified Neviaser, *14,* 15–16, *17, 17–18*

posterior, 13, *14, 15*
subclavian, *14,* 16–18, *18*
Subacromial procedures
  acromioplasty, arthroscopic, 239–240, *240, 241*
  distal clavicle
    arthroscopic excision, *241,* 241–242, *242*
    coplaning of, *242,* 242–243, *243*
    os acromiale excision, *243,* 243–244
Subclavian subacromial portal, *14,* 16–18, *18*
Subcoracoid impingement, 99–101, *100–103,* 143, *143*
  diagnosis of, 101, *102, 103*
  roller-wringer effect, 100, *100, 101,* 274, *274*
  tensile undersurface fiber failure lesions of subscapularis tendon, 100–101, *101*
Subcoracoid space
  creating anterior, for subscapularis tendon repair, 122, *124*
  defined, 103
  evaluation of, 102–106, *105*
Subcoracoid stenosis, defined, 104
Sublabral sulcus, superior labrum anterior and posterior (SLAP) lesions, 66, *71*
Subscapularis tendon
  anatomy and function, 99
  evaluation of, 80, *83*
  fatty degeneration of, 127
  finding, 122–123, *125–128*
  non-repairable, 127
  tensile undersurface fiber failure lesions of, 100–101, *101*
  three-sided release for retracted, 123–124, *128, 129, 267, 267*
Subscapularis tendon repair, 117–129
  anchor insertion, 125–126, *130*
  assessment, *117,* 117–119, *118*
    Bear Hug test, *118,* 118–119
    lift-off test, 117, *117*
    Napoleon test, 117–118, *118*
  biceps tendon repair, 119–120, *120, 121*
  bone bed preparation, 124–125, *130*
  complete, *266,* 266–268, *267*
  coracoid identification, 120–121, *122, 123*
  coracoplasty, 121, *123*
  creating anterior subcoracoid space, 122, *124*
  finding subscapularis, 122–123, *125–128*
  partial, 263–265, *263–265*
  portal placement, 119, *119, 120*
  postoperative protocol, 128–129
  preoperative planning, *117,* 117–119, *118*
  proximal humeral migration, 128
  safety of approach, 117
  subscapularis mobilization, 123–124, *128, 129*
    anterior release, 123–124, *129*
    posterior release, 124, *129*
    superior release, 124, *129*
  suture passage, 126–127, *131*

Subscapularis tendon tears, 99–106, 117
  arthroscopic evaluation, 101–106, *104*
    biceps tendon evaluation, 102, *105*
    subcoracoid space evaluation, 102–106, *105*
  combined with infraspinatus and supraspinatus tendon tear, 141–145, *142–145*
  etiology, 99–101, *100–103*
  identification of margin, 106, *107, 108*
  roller-wringer phenomenon, 274, *274*
Superior labral tears, 56 [*See also* Superior labrum anterior and posterior (SLAP) lesions]
Superior labrum anterior and posterior (SLAP) lesions, 56–69
  bone deficiency and, 164
  classification of, 56, *59, 60*
  dead arm syndrome, 57–58
  diagnosis, 65–67, *69, 70*
    biceps root, 66, *72*
    drive-through sign, 67
    modified Jobe relocation test, 65, *70*
    O'Brien test, 65, *69*
    peel-back test, 66–67, *73*
    Speed test, 65, *69*
    sublabral sulcus, 66, *71*
    superior sulcus, 66, *71*
  hyper-external rotation of humerus, 63–64, *67*
  patient population, 56–58, *61*
  peel-back mechanism of, 64–65, *68*
  postoperative rehabilitation, 206, *206–209,* 209–211, 210t, 211t
  surgery for
    with Bankart lesion, *226, 226–227, 227*
    rationale, 67–69
    tricks and tips, 236–238, *237, 238*
  throwing athlete and, 58–65
  type I, 56, *59, 60*
  type II, 56, *59, 60,* 65, 66
    glenohumeral internal rotation deficit (GIRD), 58–60
    posteroinferior capsule contracture, 60–61, *63, 64, 65, 66*
  type III, 56, *59, 60*
  type IV, 56, *59, 60*
Superior release, of subscapularis tendon, 124, *129*
Superior sulcus, in superior labrum anterior and posterior (SLAP) lesions, 66, *71*
Suprascapular nerve release, 298–300, *299, 300*
Supraspinatus tendon tears
  biceps tenodesis with, *293, 293*
  combined with subscapularis and infraspinatus tendon tear, 141–145, *142–145*
Surgeon's Sixth Finger, 43, *46, 47, 185, 186, 188–189, 294–296, 294–297*
Suspension bridge model, of rotator cuff, 84, *85,* 86, *86, 87*
Suture abrasion
  effect of suture anchor design on, 35–36, *36, 37*
  effect of suture type on, 37, *38*

Suture anchors
  anchor insertion
    deadman system for, 38–39, *40*
    in poor bone, 178–180, *180, 181*
    in subscapularis tendon repair,
      125–126, *130*
  BioCorkscrew, 36–37, *37*
  biodegradable, 36–37, *37*
  characteristics of different, 35–36, *36, 37*
  cyclic loading, 33–34, *34*
  fixation points, 35, *35*
  knot tying (*See also* Knots)
    in cannula, 184–187, 187–189
    with Surgeon's Sixth Finger, 43, *46,*
      47, 185, 186, 188–189
    suture type and, 37–38, *39*
    visualization of, 170, *171*
  minimizing suture cut out, 34–35
  modified Mason Allen stitch, 34–35
  Panalok RC anchor, 37, *37*
  preventing anchor unloading, 174–177,
    175, 305, *305*
  pull-out strength, 35
  reloading, 177–178, *179, 180,* 304, *304*
  removal, *183,* 184–186
    from glenoid, *297,* 297–298
    from greater tuberosity, 298, *298*
    salvaging loose, *303,* 303–304, *304*
  suture abrasion, 35–36, *36, 37*
  suture loop eyelet, 37
  suture material for, 37–38
  vs. bone tunnels, 33, *34*
Suture cut out, minimizing, 34–35
Suture Lasso, 31, *31, 32,* 178, *179,* 187
Suture loop eyelet, 37
Suture management, 172–177
  finding matching sutures, 177
  lost sutures, 177, *178*
  organization, *173,* 173–174, *174*

  preventing anchor unloading, 174–177,
    175
  retrieving sutures, 174–177, *175, 176*
  untangling sutures, 177, *177*
Suture material
  resorbable, 37, *38*
  types for suture anchors, 37, *38*
Suture passage, 174, *174*
  instrumentation for, 20–24, 30–31
    BirdBeak, 21, *22, 23*
    Needle Punch, *29,* 30
    Penetrator, *22, 23*
    retrograde suture passage, 20–21, *22*
    Scorpion, 24, *26–28,* 28, 30–31
    Sidewinder, *22, 23*
    Viper, 23–24, *23–26,* 30
  in subscapularis tendon repair,
    126–127, *131*
  "tying as you go," 171–172, *173*
Suture weave, for reloading anchors, 304,
  304

T

Tendinopathy, of biceps tendon, 79, *81, 82*
Tendinitis, calcific
  postoperative rehabilitation, 206
  repair, *306,* 306–307, *307*
Tensile undersurface fiber failure lesions
  of subscapularis tendon, 100–101,
  101
Three RHAP half-hitch, 42, *46,* 48, *51, 52*
Three-sided release, for retracted subscapularis tendon, 123–124, *128,*
  129
Throwing athlete
  glenohumeral internal rotation deficit
    (GIRD), 58–60
  hyper-external rotation of humerus,
    63–64, *67*

  postoperative throwing program, 210,
    210t, 211t
  rationale for surgery, 67–69
  superior labrum anterior and posterior
    (SLAP) lesions, 58–65
Throwing program, postoperative, 210,
  210t, 211t
Traction shuttle technique, *184,* 187
Triple double technique rotator cuff
  repair, 271–273, *271–273*
Triple labral lesions, 69, 71, *74,* 192
  repair of, 232–234, *232–234*
Tuberoplasty, 275–277, *276, 277*
Tuberosity, greater
  anchor removal from, 298, *298*
  treatment for malunion, 275–277, *276,*
  277
Turbulence control, 4, *4–6, 5*
  Bernoulli effect and, *4,* 4–5
  controlling, *5,* 5–6

U

U-shaped rotator cuff tear, 88, *89*
  margin convergence in, *277,* 277–278,
  278
  repair, 197, *198*
Under-over half-hitch, 41, *45*
Unidirectional instability, 72–73

V

Viper suture-passer, 23–24, *23–26,* 30
Visualization, 3–6
  bleeding and, 3–4
  portal use and, 170–171
  suture tying and, 169–170
  turbulence control and, *4,* 4–6, *5*

W

Wrapping limb, 40, *41*